INTRODUCTION TO

Nursing Research

Incorporating Evidence-Based Practice

SECOND EDITION

Edited by:

Carol Boswell, EdD, RN, CNE, ANEF

*Professor and Co-Director of the Center of
Excellence in Evidence-Based Practice
Texas Tech University Health Sciences Center
Anita Thigpen Perry School of Nursing
Odessa, Texas*

Sharon Cannon, EdD, RN, ANEF

*Regional Dean and Professor
Texas Tech University Health Sciences Center
Anita Thigpen Perry School of Nursing
Odessa, Texas*

JONES AND BARTLETT PUBLISHERS
Sudbury, Massachusetts
BOSTON   TORONTO   LONDON   SINGAPORE

World Headquarters

Jones and Bartlett Publishers
40 Tall Pine Drive
Sudbury, MA 01776
978-443-5000
info@jbpub.com
www.jbpub.com

Jones and Bartlett Publishers
Canada
6339 Ormindale Way
Mississauga, Ontario L5V 1J2
Canada

Jones and Bartlett Publishers
International
Barb House, Barb Mews
London W6 7PA
United Kingdom

Jones and Bartlett's books and products are available through most bookstores and online booksellers. To contact Jones and Bartlett Publishers directly, call 800-832-0034, fax 978-443-8000, or visit our website www.jbpub.com.

Substantial discounts on bulk quantities of Jones and Bartlett's publications are available to corporations, professional associations, and other qualified organizations. For details and specific discount information, contact the special sales department at Jones and Bartlett via the above contact information or send an email to specialsales@jbpub.com.

The authors, editor, and publisher have made every effort to provide accurate information. However, they are not responsible for errors, omissions, or for any outcomes related to the use of the contents of this book and take no responsibility for the use of the products and procedures described. Treatments and side effects described in this book may not be applicable to all people; likewise, some people may require a dose or experience a side effect that is not described herein. Drugs and medical devices are discussed that may have limited availability controlled by the Food and Drug Administration (FDA) for use only in a research study or clinical trial. Research, clinical practice, and government regulations often change the accepted standard in this field. When consideration is being given to use of any drug in the clinical setting, the health care provider or reader is responsible for determining FDA status of the drug, reading the package insert, and reviewing prescribing information for the most up-to-date recommendations on dose, precautions, and contraindications, and determining the appropriate usage for the product. This is especially important in the case of drugs that are new or seldom used.

Production Credits
Publisher: Kevin Sullivan
Acquisitions Editor: Emily Ekle
Acquisitions Editor: Amy Sibley
Associate Editor: Patricia Donnelly
Editorial Assistant: Rachel Shuster
Associate Production Editor: Katie Spiegel
Marketing Manager: Rebecca Wasley
V.P., Manufacturing and Inventory Control: Therese Connell
Composition: Toppan Best-set Premedia Limited
Cover Design: Scott Moden
Cover Image: © Matej Pavlansky/ShutterStock, Inc.
Printing and Binding: Malloy, Inc.
Cover Printing: Malloy, Inc.

Library of Congress Cataloging-in-Publication Data
Introduction to nursing research : incorporating evidence-based practice / [edited by] Carol Boswell and Sharon Cannon. — 2nd ed.
      p. ; cm.
   Includes bibliographical references and index.
   ISBN 978-0-7637-7615-2
   1. Nursing—Research—Methodology.   2. Evidence-based nursing.   I. Boswell, Carol.   II. Cannon, Sharon, 1940-
   [DNLM: 1. Nursing Research—methods.   2. Evidence—Based Nursing.   WY 20.5 I6196 2010]
   RT81.5.I5844 2010
   610.72—dc22
                                              2009024377

6048
Printed in the United States of America
13   12   11   10   10   9   8   7   6   5   4   3

Contents

Acknowledgments

We would like to express our appreciation to our wonderful network of colleagues who so readily accepted the task of rewriting selected chapters. The value of this book stems from the expertise provided by the contributing authors, to whom we are profoundly indebted.

We again would like to thank the first edition reviewers for their careful and methodical examination of the chapters. These reviewers supplied real-life examples in clinical settings and assisted us in focusing each chapter's content. From their comments we were able to maintain the scholarly level of the book. Specific to this second edition, we are grateful for the comments and suggestions provided by the numerous users of the textbook. The insight provided by the end-users has been valuable in helping us keep the original purpose of this text intact.

Also with this second edition, we continue our grateful recognition of Mary E. Nunnally. Using her strong editorial perspective, she assured consistency in changes to all chapters and proved to be an invaluable resource.

Dr. Carol Boswell and Dr. Sharon Cannon

Every once in a while, our lives are enhanced by very special people. One such person is my friend and colleague, Dr. Carol Boswell. Not only is she a kindred spirit, she is also one of my "balcony" people.

Along with Carol, my family has played a significant part in the shaping of my life. So, I wish to say a special thank you to Carol; my parents G.E. and Laurine Cannon (who are always with me in spirit); my children and their spouses, Joe and Lynn Tischner, and Ryan and Desi Ganey; my grandchildren, Kelly Tischner, Andrew Ganey, Shelby Ganey, and Shannon Ganey; and my brother and sister-in-law, Gene and Cathi Cannon.

Dr. Sharon Cannon

As people carefully consider different paths within the journey of life, we must focus our attention on the roads that we select to travel. Dr. Sharon Cannon, my incredible colleague and friend, has dared me to embrace visionary pathways on my journey to professionalism. I also recognize the love, encouragement, and steadfastness of my husband, Marc E. Boswell; he permits me to soar with the eagles while still maintaining my check on reality. Finally, my heart cherishes the love and support provided by my family: my parents, Dwight and Wanda Miller; my children, Michael and Casey Boswell, Jeremy Boswell, and Stephanie Boswell; and my grandchildren, Matthew Boswell, Kobe Boswell, Kayia Howard, and Caleb Boswell. Without the support and confidence of my family and friends, I would not be able to challenge the madness of the world while holding onto the reality of what is important for a person's humanity.

Dr. Carol Boswell

Contributors

Kathaleen C. Bloom, PhD, ARNP, CNM
Associate Professor
University of North Florida
College of Health
School of Nursing
Jacksonville, Florida

James Eldridge, PhD
Associate Professor
University of Texas of the Permian Basin
Odessa, Texas

Dorothy Greene Jackson, PhD, RN, FNP
Assistant Professor
Texas Tech University Health Sciences Center
School of Nursing
Odessa, Texas

JoAnn Long, PhD, RN
Associate Professor and Chairman
Lubbock Christian University
Department of Nursing
Lubbock, Texas

Margaret Robinson, MSN, RN
Senior Vice President, Patient Care Services
Midland Memorial Hospital
Midland, Texas

Jane Sumner, PhD, RN
Associate Professor of Nursing
Louisiana State University Health Sciences Center
School of Nursing
New Orleans, Louisiana

Donna Scott Tilley, PhD, RN, CNE
Associate Professor
Texas Women's University
College of Nursing
Denton, Texas

Lucy B. Trice, PhD, ARNP, BC
Associate Dean
University of North Florida
College of Health
School of Nursing
Jacksonville, Florida

Chapter 1

Connection Between Research and Evidence-Based Practice

Sharon Cannon and Carol Boswell

Chapter Objectives

At the conclusion of this chapter, the learner will be able to

1. Identify the need for research to validate evidence-based practice
2. Define evidence-based practice
3. Discuss obstacles to evidence-based research
4. Examine the nurse's role in evidence-based practice
5. State how evidence-based practice affects nursing practice

Key Terms

➤ Evidence-based practice (EBP)

➤ Obstacle

➤ PICOT

➤ Research process

➤ Research utilization

Introduction

Regardless of the specific healthcare setting a nurse may select for practicing the art and science of nursing care, the overarching principle for the practice is the provision of quality nursing care to all clients without consideration of social, financial, cultural, ethnic heritage, or other individual characteristics. As the nurse initiates contact with the client, the client should be confident that the care provided by that nurse is based on the most current, up-to-date health information available. Having established the currency of the health information to be utilized, the nurse and client must also agree that individualized application of this information is necessary. Thus the need for evidence-based practice (EBP) is confirmed by our expectations related to nursing care.

The nurse who receives the assignment to care for an elderly woman, a young child, or a critically ill husband must come to the nursing practice arena with more than the latest information. The information must be tested and confirmed. To see how this works, let's consider the idea of asthma information, although any disease process could be utilized for this purpose.

Within nursing practice, certain health information concerning the management of asthma is accepted. The initial question that should be asked by a nurse would be: Is this disease management information corroborated by research results? The answer to this question is frequently a negative response. The informational basis for each aspect of the nursing care to be provided should be analyzed to determine its source. Does the information come from general usage, or is it based on information that has been established through research endeavors to be accurate? Having determined the basis for the care to be provided, the nurse must then determine the application of the information based on the individuality of the client situation. The application of the information for each client situation would depend on the specifics of the client's needs, the client's expectations concerning health, and many other aspects requiring modification of the confirmed research application. The foundation of nursing care delivery must be research-tested and research-confirmed knowledge, tempered by an awareness of the unique characteristics of the client and the situation. Although the healthcare field defines "client" and "patient" differently, for purposes of this text these terms are used interchangeably.

Pravikoff, Tanner, and Pierce (2005) describe the process of EBP as including assessing and delineating a problem through verbalization of an identifiable question, pursuing and evaluating the available facts, implementing a practice intervention as a result of the evidence, and evaluating the entire process for effectiveness. Initially EBP requires the identification of the practice problem, followed by the utilization of tested research results to improve the care provided for the clients. According to Ciliska, Cullum, and Marks (2001), the three fundamental appraisal questions are identical whether the clinical question concerns treatment, diagnosis, prognosis, or causation:

- Are the outcomes of the study compelling?
- Which outcomes were identified?
- Will the outcomes aid in the management of the patient's care?

It was this need to incorporate proven practices into the provision of health care that fostered the expectations and development of EBP in the current healthcare arena. Bucknall (2007) notes that cognitive approaches, intuition, and analysis of information play key roles in how research is acknowledged, evaluated, and incorporated into the clinical decision-making process that impacts patient outcomes. Clinical decisions are frequently not corroborated by unambiguous, persuasive evidence. Nurses are asked to make real-world decisions with limited information in a fast-paced environment. Time is valuable to the nurse at the bedside, so any course of action has to be both practical and rational (Cannon & Boswell, In press). This responsibility to make knowledgeable, well-supported decisions based on sound facts emphasizes the need to become effective and efficient at evidence-based practice and research utilization.

Providing a Line of Reasoning for EBP and Evidence-Based Research

Health care is a complex system addressing multiple health-related aspects in an attempt to accomplish the anticipated outcome for the client. Throughout the healthcare arena, nursing care is provided to individuals in need of assistance related to their health status. This attention requires nurses to identify a core foundation of information that reflects quality care. Thus, the need for EBP to be developed around a research-centered foundation was envisioned.

Porter-O'Grady (2006) suggested that the management of EBP requires the use of unique clinical applications based on accessible, up-to-date research. In the quest for quality nursing care, the nurse must use both reliable clinical knowledge and high-quality clinical information. This process of establishing a core foundation of knowledge has been called many things over the years, such as *best practices, evidence-based practice,* and *quality of care*. No matter what the practice is called, the basis for the care to be provided must be grounded in research. According to Melnyk and Fineout-Overholt (2005), "When healthcare providers know how to find, critically appraise, and use the best evidence, and when patients are confident that their health-care providers are using evidence-based care, optimal outcomes are achieved for all" (p. 3). It is this assurance that the care being pro-vided is confirmed from a tested research foundation that inspires patient confidence in nurses' commitment to quality health care. Nurses should not rely on unsubstantiated treatment plans, but rather must endeavor to critically analyze aspects of the care to be provided to ensure that quality, tested practices are utilized in the provision of nursing care for each individual.

? Think Outside the Box

Make a list of the tasks that are routinely done by nurses during a typical clinical day. Carefully consider what evidence you have used as the foundation for these tasks. Are the skills for the tasks based on research, personal preferences, clinical guidelines, or traditions?

The practicing nurse has to value the idea of the EBP process to facilitate its complete incorporation and implementation. Nurses must understand the value of integrating research results with personal experiences and client values when determining the treatment plan that best addresses a situation's identified challenges. According to the Oncology Nursing Society (2005), even though a healthcare provider may utilize the optimal evidence available, each encounter with an individual continues to be unique. The treatments and outcomes will change based on the uniqueness of the client's values, preferences, interests, and/or diagnoses. According to Fonteyn (2005), "A bonus of nurses' involvement in EBP activities is their improved ability to think critically and their increased understanding of and comfort with research, all of which seems to perpetuate their interest and success in subsequent EBP pursuits" (p. 439). Nurses are taught, encouraged, and expected to think critically. This process of critical thinking corresponds to the use of EBP on clinical units and in primary care settings. Critical thinking embraces the need for health care to be based on a foundation of proven researched data and to include the client's perspective. The use of unconfirmed reports, hearsay, and unfounded information, combined with a lack of client input, does not fit with the provision of sound, quality nursing care at this point in time.

Fineout-Overholt and Melnyk (2005) state that "Ongoing onsite and off-site learning opportunities for all providers to hone EBP skills in asking searchable, answerable questions, finding the best available evidence, efficiently appraising research reports, and determining relevance and applicability of evidence [are] essential to cultivating an evidence-based culture" (p. 28). A key element within the effective provision of EBP is the nurse's expertise. Each nurse brings serviceable knowledge to the practice arena. During the process of providing nursing care to a group of individuals, nurses build an underpinning of knowledge on which they draw when delivering future care. This underpinning knowledge base intensifies and expands with each client encounter that the nurse has. Thus it is not stagnant but rather increases throughout an individual's nursing career.

Jolley (2002) articulated the expectation that practicing nurses should "be able to access, produce, and use different sorts of evidence, including research, to determine best clinical practices" (p. 2 of 12). Even when nurses do not want to be actively involved in an actual research project, they must understand the method for accessing published information and assessing it for applicability. Rolston-Blenman (2009) supports this idea by stating that management has "to recognize the hard truth that every system is perfectly designed to achieve exactly the results it gets" (p. 20). We all know that individuals rise to the level to which we expect them to rise: If we set low expectations, that is all they will meet. If we establish challenging expectations, they will strive to attain them. At times, a knowledge base is unconsciously incorporated, because the nurse seems to manage the nursing care without directly acknowledging the underlying foundation. This process grows as the nurse gains experience and expertise.

Research is a methodical examination that uses regimented techniques to resolve questions or decipher dilemmas. The conclusions resulting from this focused chain of examination provide a base upon which to build a practice of care that is centered on tested solutions. According to Omery and Williams (1999), "Research, as a scientific process, with its inherent ability to explain and predict, enhances a practice discipline's ability to anticipate and guide interactions" (p. 1 of 13). This anticipation and guidance are related to a discipline's ability to incorporate into practice the sound evidence derived from valid research endeavors. Although EBP goes beyond research results, the foundation for the practice is the grounded knowledge that comes from the research process. This underpinning allows for the safe and effective provision of quality health care. According to Melnyk and Fineout-Overholt (2005), "The gap between the publishing of research evidence and its translation into practice to improve patient care is a cause for concern in healthcare organizations and federal agencies" (p. 4). Moving the use of researched evidence into the actual patient care setting requires that nurses become increasingly familiar and comfortable with the process of critiquing and applying the evidence to the practice arena.

Each of these aspects—thought process, client preferences, research, and nursing expertise—is included in the EBP definition

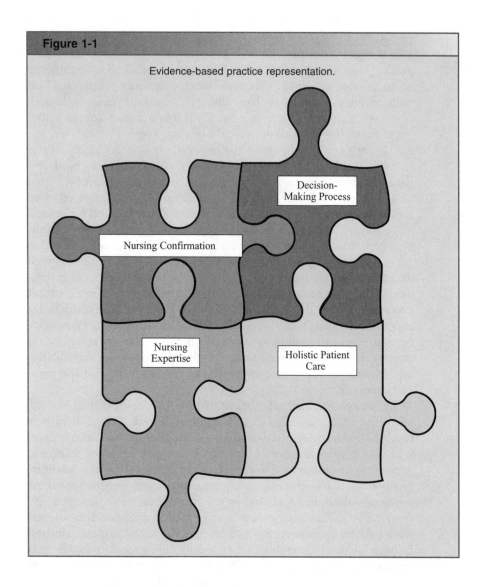

Figure 1-1

Evidence-based practice representation.

used in this textbook (**Figure 1-1**). Although all of these aspects are required, the actual situation directs the weighting of the aspects, because each situation is unique. Melnyk (2004) acknowledges that a consistent, hard-and-fast weighting of the different pieces—research, patient values, and clinician's expertise—included in EBP is not possible, because the decision-making process is contingent on the situation. In this textbook, EBP is defined as a process of using confirmed evidence (research and quality improvement), decision making, and nursing expertise to guide the delivery of holistic patient care by nurses. Holistic nursing care encompasses the clinical expertise of the nurse, patient preferences, cultural aspects, psychosocial facets, and biological components. The research process and scientific data generated serve as the foundation on which the decision-making process for nursing care is based.

Assessing the Need for Research in the Practice Arena

According to Davies (2002), "The transfer of research evidence into practice is a complex process and changing provider behavior is a challenge, even when the relative advantages are strong" (p. 558). The nurse is paramount to the success of the EBP process. Each nurse, whether in the acute care, home health, community health, or other healthcare setting, regularly identifies nursing aspects of care. Those aspects of care may seem to (1) appropriately address the care needs of the client, (2) not fit the current accepted provision of care, or (3) be better addressed via some other method of care. Most nurses have at some point in their practice identified a situation that needs to be reevaluated. Within the day-to-day provision of nursing care, the question arises about why we perform a procedure a certain way when something else seems to work better. It could also be a question of how the care can be better provided to meet the client's needs and expectations. The healthcare community is also encouraging this line of questioning in an effort to identify the best methods for the provision of care. The expectation behind EBP is that everyone will become involved in the identification, examination, and implementation of research-founded health care that can result in the provision of effective, validated client care. Nurses must accept the responsibility of being active in providing quality care to their clients. To do so effectively, they must base the provision of care on results that support the care being administered in a wide variety of healthcare settings.

Cronenwett (2002) has stated that "Evidence for practice mounts slowly over time, as scientists discover first what works in controlled environments and second what works in daily clinical practice" (p. 3 of 19). The application of research results in the everyday provision of nursing care takes both time and energy by each and every nurse to ensure that the quality of care is appropriate. All nurses have the responsibility of ensuring that the care they provide to their clients is based on sound nursing knowledge, not just "the way we have always done it." Cronenwett (2002) has further identified the need to challenge clinical community partners to become increasingly involved upfront in the recognition of the problem and the development of the intervention, which includes new research opportunities. Practicing nurses must become actively engaged at multiple levels of the different phases of the research endeavor. At each phase, the nurse's clinical expertise should be readily valued as the process moves forward to establish the evidence for use in the clinical setting.

According to the Agency for Healthcare Research and Quality (AHRQ, 2000), outcomes research is a growing expectation within health care. The provision of quality health practices requires that individuals "seek to understand the end results of particular health care practices and interventions" (AHRQ, 2000, para. 1). Outcomes research is viewed as a mechanism for determining both which quality care is possible and how to get to that point of quality care for the patient. The linkage of outcomes experienced with the care expected empowers research to cultivate improved channels for monitoring and improving the quality of care provided within the healthcare arena. Translational research is an endeavor that seeks to move the evidence that has been collected by effective research projects into the actual provision of health care. Nurses at the bedside must become champions for the inclusion of timely, documented, substantiated results into the active provision of health care to benefit clients confronted with the health issues.

Titler, Everett, and Adams (2007) discuss the notion of implementation science as "the investigation of methods, interventions, and variables that influence adoption of evidence-based healthcare practices by individuals and organizations to improve clinical and operational decision making and including testing the effectiveness of interventions to promote and sustain use of evidence-based healthcare practices" (p. S53). It is through the use of concepts such as implementation science that research utilization, evidence-based practice, and research are coming together for the improvement of healthcare delivery. As nurses learn to appreciate the importance of investigating the different routines, interventions, and obstacles within the provision of quality care, innovative and tested systems of healthcare delivery and skills will become increasingly available and accepted. According to Malloch and Porter-O'Grady (2006), "The goal of a research course is to introduce nursing students to the basics of the scientific approach of research in the belief that they will be able to use the information produced to provide guidance to their nursing practice upon graduation" (p. 75). The idea behind clarifying the process of research is to enable practicing nurses to utilize the scientific thought process to validate and augment the nursing care provided to clients. The entire process of critiquing research articles and conducting research projects is designed to strengthen the nursing professional's critical thinking abilities, thereby allowing for the delivery of the most holistic care possible in the work environment. Malloch and Porter-O'Grady (2006) note that the critical skill required for effective EBP is the ability of nursing professionals to analytically examine research results and evidence to determine the optimal data to use in the provision of holistic health care on a day-to-day basis. Without this foundation, which enables them to methodically examine the evidence, nurses are left to vacillate among varying interpretations of healthcare information.

? Think Outside the Box

Look at the different definitions for evidence-based practice. How do you see patient preferences meshing with research utilization?

Exploring EBP in Light of Research

Definitions of EBP

Many different definitions of EBP exist, and each definition tends to add another dimension to the concept of EBP. Each different dimension should be carefully and thoroughly considered as EBP is implemented to ensure that actual nursing practice is comprehensive. Within each definition, however, certain aspects are consistently identified. The consistent and unique aspects can be visualized as shown in **Table 1-1**.

Melnyk and Fineout-Overholt (2005) conceptualize EBP as a method that allows healthcare providers to deliver the maximum quality of care when addressing the multifaceted requests of their patients and families. In another article by Melnyk (2003), EBP is defined as "a problem solving approach to clinical decision making that incorporates a search for the best and latest evidence, clinical expertise and assessment, and patient preference and values within a context of caring" (p. 149). Both of these definitions reflect the use of problem solving with clinical involvement and patient contribution.

Rutledge and Grant (2002) define EBP as "care that integrates best scientific evidence with clinical expertise, knowledge of pathophysiology, knowledge of psychosocial issues, and decision making preferences of patients" (p. 1). This definition incorporates the ideas of pathophysiology and psychosocial components into the mix for consideration.

According to Porter-O'Grady (2006), "Evidence-based practice is simply the integration of the best possible research to evidence with clinical expertise and with patient needs. Patient needs in this case refer specifically to the expectations, concerns, and requirements that patients bring to their clinical experience" (p. 1). This definition tends to further emphasize the importance of the patient within the entire process.

Table 1-1 Comparison of Qualities Included in Evidence-Based Practice Definitions

Author (Year)	Quality of Care	Multifaceted	Decision-Making Process	Clinical Focus	Foundation of Practice	Client Involvement	Other Aspects
Johns Hopkins Nursing (2007)			X	X		X	
Melnyk & Fineout-Overholt (2005)	X	X					
Melnyk (2003)			X	X	Evidence, expertise, assessment	X	
Rutledge & Grant (2002)			X	X	Evidence, expertise, pathophysiology, psychosocial		
Porter-O'Grady (2006)				X	Evidence, expertise	X	
Burns & Grove (2009)	X				Research	X	Cost
Magee (2005)			X		Evidence	X	
Pravikoff, Tanner, & Pierce (2005)			X	X	Evidence	X	
Omery & Williams (1999)			X		Expertise		
DiCenso, Cullum, & Ciliska (1998)			X	X	Evidence, proficiency	X	Assets

Burns and Grove (2009) define EBP as "conscientious integration of best research evidence with clinical expertise and patient values and needs in the delivery of quality, cost-effective health care" (p. 699). Consequently, these authors integrate the idea of cost-effectiveness as an additional consideration when determining the appropriate EBP components.

Magee (2005) defines evidence-based medicine as "the conscientious, explicit, and judicious use of current best evidence in making decisions about the care of individual patients" (p. 73). The entire focus of this definition is evidence-based medicine. It is directed toward physician care, not nursing care.

Another definition submitted by Pravikoff et al. (2005) for EBP is "a systematic approach to problem solving for health care providers, including RNs, characterized by the use of the best evidence currently available for clinical decision-making in order to provide the most consistent and best possible care to patients" (p. 40). For their part, Omery and Williams (1999) define EBP as "a scientific process [that], with its inherent ability to explain and predict, enhances a practice discipline's ability to anticipate and guide interventions" (p. 1 of 13). Both of these definitions consolidate the idea of systematic processing with the idea of anticipatory consideration when providing nursing care.

DiCenso, Cullum, and Ciliska (1998) offer a model for evidence-based decision making that integrates research evidence, clinical proficiency, patient choices, and accessible assets. Within this model, each element is weighted differently based on the particular client circumstances. The evidence desired for an EBP process can be accessed via sources as diverse as bibliographical databases and a quality improvement department located within a healthcare agency. The evidence used within this process can include research, integrative reviews, practice guidelines, quality improvement data, clinical experience, expert opinion, collegial relationships, pathophysiology, common sense, community standards, published materials, and case studies. According to Ferguson and Day (2005), the forms of evidence, in descending order of credibility, include these:

1. Randomized, controlled trials
2. Single randomized, controlled trials
3. Controlled trials without randomization
4. Quasi-experimental studies
5. Nonexperimental studies
6. Descriptive studies
7. Expert consensus
8. Quality improvement data
9. Program evaluation data

While each of these forms of evidence is necessary and functional, the credibility of the evidence must be considered carefully when determining a plan of action. Each provides information to use in a decision-making process, and the support for the information (evidence) is better in those with research than in those based on opinion.

Each of the proposed definitions supports the definition identified for this text, in which EBP is viewed as a process of using confirmed evidence (research and quality improvement), decision making, and nursing expertise to guide the delivery of holistic patient care. The four consistent aspects found within all of these definitions are (1) a decision-making process, (2) a clinical focus, (3) nursing expertise, and (4) client involvement (see Figure 1-1).

As evidence-based practice has evolved within the field of health care, the idea of what constitutes appropriate evidence has also matured (**Figure 1-2**). While research results constitute the strongest category of evidence, other evidence—such as quality improvement results, policy/procedure confirmation, and protocol guideline confirmation—is nevertheless beneficial to the provision of safe and effective health care. Within the realm of EBP, each component of the

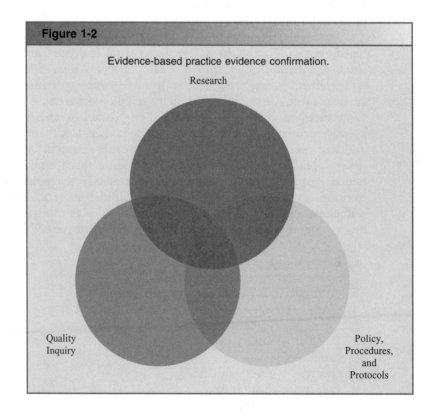

Figure 1-2

Evidence-based practice evidence confirmation.

Research

Quality Inquiry

Policy, Procedures, and Protocols

evidence must be carefully assessed in terms of the strength and applicability of the information to the unique client setting. Each agency and nurse must critically consider the results and evidence available concerning an identified healthcare problem. As the results and evidence are thoroughly examined for practicality and efficiency, nursing care practices can be modified to manage the various aspects of care.

Posing Forceful Clinical Questions

Melnyk and Fineout-Overholt (2005) have declared that "The importance of asking the 'right' question cannot be overemphasized" (p. 27). The clarification of the question focuses the search for valid evidence so that it speaks to the issue under examination. According to DiCenso, Guyatt, and Ciliska (2005), "The searchable question requires focus to avoid complicating and time consuming searches that retrieve irrelevant materials" (p. 23). As the issue under examination is carefully considered to determine the principal focus for the investigation, two components need to be considered. First, the initial attention should be directed to answering the "what, where, when, why, and how" aspects of the issue. Second, the scrutiny should then turn to the outcome of interest, which reflects the nursing diagnosis and/or research project.

Melnyk and Fineout-Overholt (2005) describe the two types of initial questions as background questions and foreground questions. Background questions address the core knowledge within the healthcare field. This type of information provides a strong foundation of knowledge related to biological, psychological, and sociological facets of care that can be located in any textbook. Obtaining answers to these questions does not require access to research databases, because the information is preparatory to the provision of basic holistic care. In contrast, foreground questions address the "scientific evidence about diagnosing, treating, or assisting patients with understanding their prognosis" (Melnyk & Fineout-Overholt, 2005, p. 28). At this point in the process of EBP, the search for answers to the identified question focuses on the combination of core knowledge and scientific evidence.

? Think Outside the Box

Within every organization, obstacles to incorporating changes such as evidence-based practice are present. Look at your institution. Which obstacles do you see? What can you do to confront and overcome these obstacles?

The use of the acronym PICOT is helpful in focusing the development of the foreground questions (**Table 1-2**). The PICOT acronym has the following meaning (Melnyk & Fineout-Overholt, 2005):

P   Patient population of interest
I   Intervention of interest
C   Comparison of interest
O   Outcome of interest
T   Time

In considering the population aspect within the question, time is needed to determine specific information about the persona of the

Table 1-2

<table>
<tr><td colspan="1" align="center">Examples of Searchable Questions for Research in EBP</td></tr>
<tr><td align="center">Example 1: Labor and Delivery</td></tr>
<tr><td>You are a staff nurse in a rural hospital that performs 120 to 150 vaginal deliveries each year. Within the past 6 months, the institution has hired a certified registered nurse anesthetist (CRNA) to help with anesthesia for the facility. The CRNA and physicians have decided to begin offering epidural anesthesia for routine vaginal deliveries. You offer to seek out studies that address the use of epidural anesthesia in the labor and delivery process.
Preliminary Question: Is epidural anesthesia appropriate for all laboring patients?
Clarification of Question: This question identifies the population and time as all laboring patients and the intervention as the use of epidural anesthesia. It fails to document any comparison with other anesthesia methods or the outcome that the hospital is interested in achieving. Here is the PICOT analysis:
   Population: All laboring patients
   Intervention: Use of epidural anesthesia
   Comparison: Versus other anesthesia methods
   Outcome: Reduction in labor complications
   Time: Individuals in labor
Revised Searchable Question: For all laboring patients, will the administration of epidural anesthesia be more effective in reducing labor complications than other forms of anesthesia administered during the labor process?</td></tr>
<tr><td align="center">Example 2: Routine Checkup</td></tr>
<tr><td>A 50-year-old man comes to the clinic for his yearly physical examination. His blood pressure is recorded as 158/90 mm Hg. He complains of frequent headaches during stressful periods. The patient has been fired from his place of employment. When you confer about the findings with him, he asks you about the potential of having a heart attack or stroke. Because these areas are regular potential complications identified within the clinic population, you elect to search for the best evidence to use for discussion with the clinic population.
Preliminary Question: Which type of patient information needs to be included in the teaching related to hypertension and cardiovascular accidents?
Clarification of Question: The limitations of this question include the failure to stipulate the population and to supply adequate particulars about the situation. Here is the PICOT analysis:
   Population: Ambulatory clients between the ages of 30 and 60 years
   Intervention: Development of cardiovascular symptoms such as hypertension and headaches
   Comparison: Ambulatory clients without cardiovascular symptoms
   Outcome: Development of cardiovascular complications
   Time: Within the initial year following diagnosis
Revised Searchable Question: Within the initial year following diagnosis, are ambulatory clients between the ages of 30 and 60 years who have developed cardiovascular symptoms at an increased risk for developing cardiovascular complications, such as stroke and acute myocardial infarction, compared with ambulatory clients who do not exhibit cardiovascular symptoms?</td></tr>
</table>

Table 1-2

Examples of Searchable Questions for Research in EBP *(Continued)*

Example 3: Pediatrics

You work for the pediatric unit at the local hospital. The same children keep getting readmitted for earaches, injuries, and respiratory diseases. You have been assigned to prepare and deliver parenting classes for adolescent parents who have had their child admitted to the hospital. As you are thinking about the classes to be prepared, you question whether the adolescent parents are at greater risk and if they need different information than the general community of parents. You want to provide the most recent and best practices for child rearing.

Preliminary Question: Which type of information must be included in a parenting class for adolescent parents?

Clarification of Question: Although the population has been somewhat specified, additional clarification is needed. Other limitations within the preliminary question are the lack of clarification about the interventions, comparisons, outcomes, and time component of the PICOT. Here is the PICOT analysis:

Population: Parents who have had children admitted to the hospital for reoccurring health problems
Intervention: Parenting classes
Comparison: Age of parents affects the information needed in the classes
Outcome: Reduction in the number of admissions for reoccurring health problems
Time: Within a 6-month period

Revised Searchable Question: Does the age of the parents (adolescent versus non-adolescent) influence the number of child admissions for reoccurring health problems within a 6-month period for parents who attend a parenting class program?

Example 4: Cancer-Related Illness

A 75-year-old woman who had been admitted to the hospital for cervical cancer treatment asks to talk with you about general cancer-related issues. She has three children between the ages of 40 and 55 years. She is worried about their potential for developing cancer and wants to know what she should tell them about getting routine checkups. She does tell you that her father died of colon cancer at the age of 71 years.

Preliminary Question: Which type of routine screening examinations should be performed for children who have a family history of cancer?

Clarification of Question: Within this question, the population is briefly delineated. The question does not clearly denote the intervention, the outcome, or the time aspects of a PICOT question. Here is the PICOT analysis:

Population: Individuals with a family history of cancer
Intervention: Scheduling of routine cancer screening examinations
Comparison: No comparison used in this example
Outcome: Early diagnosis of cancer
Time: Routine cancer screening examinations

Revised Searchable Question: For individuals with a family history of cancer, what effect does the timing of routine cancer screening examinations have on the early diagnosis of cancer compared with those individuals who do not have an identified family history of cancer?

group under investigation. This description could relate to age, gender, diagnosis, or ethnicity. The process needs to be specific enough to provide direction, while not restricting the search too much. According to Dawes et al. (2005), "There is a balance to be struck between getting evidence about exactly your group of patients and getting all the evidence about all groups of patients" (p. 13). Care must be given to providing enough specificity to ensure that the search addresses the appropriate population while not excluding relevant information.

The depiction of the intervention for the question is another key aspect that necessitates careful thought and attention. This facet is the clear determination of the topic under consideration. It does not have to be an action step (and, therefore, an activity), but rather is the key topic for clarification. This aspect of the query should seek to potentially include "any exposure, treatment, patient perception, diagnostic test, or prognostic factor" (Melnyk & Fineout-Overholt, 2005, p. 29). Clarification of this aspect within the questioning process reduces the potential for having to backtrack later when the results are not as clearly delineated as anticipated.

The third aspect of the question formation—the comparison of interest—is an optional facet within the questioning process. Within this component, the comparison of different treatment options would be analyzed. In many situations, alternative treatment decisions may not be available. The lack of supplementary preferences does not restrict the development of EBP guidelines.

The fourth aspect for consideration in foreground questions is the outcome of interest. According to Dawes et al. (2005), it is very important to carefully consider this aspect to determine exactly the outcome that is expected.

The final aspect on which to reflect is time. Timing for the outcome of interest is a principal characteristic to prudently contemplate. While time is not included in all PICOT questions, it is valuable for inclusion on those questions that can be directly affected by the passage of time. Time is, therefore, not always seen in PICOT questions.

Having presented these considerations for preparing the question(s) for concentrating the evidence-based search, it must be acknowledged that too specific a question can also be a major problem. According to Gennaro, Hodnett, and Kearney (2001), "A one-size-fits-all technical procedural protocol will not help" (p. 236). There is no single way to ask a searchable question. The PICOT format fosters clarification of the heart of the area for investigation. The overarching motivation must be the narrowing of the investigation to allow for the effective determination of evidence to strengthen the delivery of holistic nursing care for the client population.

As our thoughts move to the research process, the use of different types of questions for various research types must be clarified. Questions focusing on how many or how much are frequently answered through the use of quantitative studies. According to DiCenso et al. (2005), a quantitative question involves three components—population, intervention/exposure, and outcomes. Questions that are directed toward discovering how people feel or experience a specific state of affairs or environments are answered through the use of qualitative research designs. Qualitative questions are worded to

include only two parts—population and situat
2005). These questions focus on characteristics t
tion for composing EBP questions and analyzir
confirm EBP practices.

Research Utilization

In the past, much lip service has been given to the need for nurses
to apply research to practice. More recently, with the emergence and
acceptance of EBP, the literature regarding research utilization in the
clinical arena has proliferated. The need for improved patient outcomes, decreased healthcare costs, greater patient safety, and higher
patient satisfaction are driving forces for the use of scientific data in
the decision-making process of nursing care provision (**Table 1-3**).

As a result of the promotion of using research as a basic component in nursing practice, one might ask, "Is nursing research being
applied to nursing practice?" Surprisingly, the answer is both "yes"
and "no." Logic seems to dictate that if EBP can improve patient

---

Table 1-3

Suggested Resources to Support the Retrieval and Appraisal of Evidence

Agency for Healthcare Research and Quality (www.ahrq.gov)
Cochrane Database of Systematic Reviews (www.update-software.com/publications/cochrane)
Institute of Medicine of the National Academies (holds the documents produced by the IOM related to patient safety; www.iom.edu)
Joanna Briggs Institute (www.joannabriggs.edu.au)
The Joint Commission (http://jointcommission.org)
Medscape (integrated information and educational tools; www.medscape.com/nurseshome)
Morrisey, L. J., & DeBourgh, G. A. (2001). Finding evidence: Refining literature searching skills for the advance practice nurse. *AACN Clinical Issues, 12*(4), 560–577.
National Comprehensive Cancer Network (www.nccn.org)
National Guidelines Clearinghouse (www.guideline.gov)
National Library of Medicine Web site, which allows free searches of MEDLINE through PubMed (www.ncbi.nlm.nih.gov/entrez/query.fcgi)
Oncology Nursing Society (ONS)—EBP Online Resource Center "Evidence Search" section (http://onsopcontent.ons.org/toolkits/evidence/ProcessModel/references.shtml)
Registered Nurses' Association of Ontario (RNAO), Best Practice Guidelines (www.rnao.org/Page.asp?PageID = 861&SiteNodeID = 133)
Sarah Cole Hirsh Institute (http://fpb.case.edu/Centers/Hirsh)
School of Health and Related Research (ScHARR), University of Sheffield—Netting the Evidence (www.shef.ac.uk/scharr/ir/netting)
Schulmeister, L., & Vrabel, M. (2000). Searching for information for presentations and publications. *Clinical Nurse Specialists, 16*(2), 79–84.
Sigma Theta Tau Virginia Henderson Library. (www.nursinglibrary.org/portal/main.aspx)
Studentbmj.com: International Medical Student's Journal (http://studentbmj.com/back_issues/0902/education/313.html)
University of Alberta—Evidence Based Medicine Tool Kit (www.ebm.med.ualberta.ca/ebm.html)
University of North Carolina at Chapel Hill Health Sciences Library (www.hsl.unc.edu/services/tutorials/ebn/index.htm)

Note: Access verified February 17, 2009.

care, EBP should be implemented. Some healthcare organizations are beginning to incorporate EBP in their institutions. Unfortunately, obstacles for the use of EBP often focus primarily on research utilization.

Obstacles to Using Research

Much of the literature discusses barriers to using research for the guidance of practice. *Webster's II New College Dictionary* (1999) defines a barrier as "something that hinders or restricts; a boundary; limit" (p. 91). A barrier seems to imply a structure that impedes success. Perhaps another word better defines the utilization of research to nursing practice—*obstacle*. An obstacle is "one that opposes, stands in the way of or diverts passage or progress" (*Webster's II New College Dictionary*, 1999, p. 755). An obstacle can be overcome. As a result, the term "obstacle" will be used instead of "barrier" when discussing reasons for not employing research utilization in evidence-based nursing care.

The nurse strives to identify ways to overcome each impediment in the path to success; thus it becomes a challenge to overcome the hindrance and be successful. The use of theories can be viewed as a barrier within the application of research, for example. The complexity of theories and functionality of using theories within the field of research can be perceived as a challenge by the nurse providing care at the bedside. An in-depth discussion of theories is beyond the scope of this textbook, although a general dialogue about the use of theories within the research process will be provided in several chapters. Nurses at the bedside do need to understand the connection between theory, research, and practice.

? Think Outside the Box

Discuss the role of clinical expertise in evidence-based practice.

While it may seem simple to apply research to practice, it is actually a complex problem. Three major categories of obstacles deter nurses from readily incorporating research into their practice—education, beliefs/attitudes, and support/resources.

Education

Educational preparation ranks high on the list of obstacles. Omery and Williams (1999) suggest that the more education a nurse has, the greater the chance the nurse will use research in providing patient care.

Keeping in mind that the majority of nurses (57%) practicing in the United States are prepared at the associate degree (ADN) or diploma level, most ADN programs do not include research in their curricula (Estabrooks, 1998). If, as Estabrooks suggests, nurses practice as they were taught, then few nurses today have knowledge about research. You will frequently hear, "That's the way I was taught." When you consider that the average age of nurses is 47, the fallacy of that line of thinking becomes apparent: Such a nurse may have been taught 20 to 25 years ago. Research may appear to be too "mystical" and have no relevance to nurses educated during that time period.

Another aspect of educational preparation that influences a nurse's use of research is the way in which research is taught. Even though baccalaureate and graduate programs include research courses in their curriculum, many graduates continue to resist engaging in or exploring research. Learning research can be likened to learning a foreign language. Carroll et al. (1997) state, "Researchers often present their findings in technical language that is difficult to understand" (p. 3 of 10). Research seems to be presented as if only an academician at a state-of-the-art university can conduct research. The idea that research is practical and beneficial, if linked to clinical practice, appears to be poorly explained to novice nurses. No wonder nurses do not understand research, much less want to use it in their practice. Without adequate motivation to use all aspects of an educational program, nurses are unwilling to translate research to practice.

Beliefs/Attitudes

A major portion of the literature attributes the lack of research use to beliefs and attitudes regarding research. Several authors (Carroll et al., 1997; Cronenwett, 2002; Jolley, 2002; Omery & Williams, 1999; Pravikoff et al., 2005) suggest that negative attitudes about research use represent obstacles for incorporating EBP into nursing care. This is true of both healthcare organizations and individual nurses. If organizations perceive that research has a lack of value for their operations (Jolley, 2002), then little support will exist for EBP within the organization. If nurses feel intimidated (Yoder, 2005) or lack confidence in their ability to use research (Cronenwett, 2002), then nurses will not actively incorporate research into their practice.

Support/Resources

The third major category of obstacles to the incorporation of EBP is support and resource availability. Too often, administrators list "cost" as a reason for limiting or hindering the use of EBP. When a nursing shortage exists, staffing becomes a major issue. Allowing staff adequate time to do the requisite reading to update their clinical or EBP knowledge or to attend continuing nursing education offerings is not always possible in such circumstances.

Another problem relates to the lack of access to or availability of research materials. Many organizations do not have a library, librarian, or personnel familiar with accessing current research findings. Nurses who lack computer skills may not know how to conduct online searches. For this reason, without the assistance of a library, librarian, or information technology personnel, nurses may not seek out EBP data. Both new and older generations of nurses have little, if any, expertise in using search engines. Even when a nurse has the requisite knowledge and skill to be able to conduct EBP database searches, state and federal policies may prevent the searches from being conducted within the healthcare organization. For example, privacy issues relating to HIPAA guidelines inhibit access to the Web from agency computer systems.

No wonder EBP has a steep learning curve, as practitioners struggle to overcome these obstacles. Lack of nursing educational preparation, lack of value assigned to research by whole organizations and individuals nurses, and lack of support/resources must be critically examined, and solutions must be found to these problems must be found, if nursing is to promote widespread use of EBP. According to Vratny and Shriver (2007), "Leadership, enthusiasm, mentorship, clinical inquiry, and reflective practice are what really make evidence-based practice grow, thrive, and come to light" (p. 166).

In the future, as agencies support nurses in recognizing the extent of improvement possible in clinical care and patient outcomes through the use of EBP, nurses will seize the opportunity to move nursing care forward and seek empowerment as part of their professional growth. Of course, expecting all organizations and every nurse to conduct research is unrealistic. Nevertheless, use of research in EBP provides the opportunity for research utilization by all.

Responsibility for Using Research

At this point, you may be asking yourself, "Given the formidable obstacles to research, why do research at all?" Few would argue with the premise that having evidence to improve patient outcomes is desirable. As Brockopp and Hastings-Tolsma (2003) say, "Professional nurses have the responsibility to participate in the promotion of evidence-based practice. Such expectations are both societal and professional" (p. 459). A better-informed consumer will inevitably demand higher-quality care. Thus, given their greater accessibility to healthcare information, today's healthcare consumers expect nurses to use the most current data available to provide quality care. To do so, nurses must continuously explore new evidence and incorporate that evidence into nursing practice. Carroll et al. (1997) have suggested, "The possession of a body of knowledge from research is the hallmark of a profession" (p. 2 of 10). Fain (2009) recommends that nurses take an active role in developing a body of knowledge. As a relatively new profession, nursing has the responsibility to provide scientific data and to use that data to achieve optimal outcomes. EBP uses the best clinical data available in making decisions about nursing care. Thus the profession demands that nurses not only be responsible for the use of research, but also participate in research to add to the body of nursing knowledge through EBP.

According to Kitson (2007), "Health administrations across the world are looking to understand how best to improve the quality, effectiveness, and safety of the healthcare they deliver" (p. S1). Two key movements in health care have led to this quest for excellence: quality/safety initiatives and the evidence-based practice innovation. By striving to acquire a foundation of knowledge while holding fast to honesty, integrity, and respect for the wide variety of perspectives and experiences within the healthcare delivery system, nursing can establish a firm base on which to build the practice of health care for each individual patient encountered.

Overcoming obstacles to the use of research in practice can improve patient outcomes, decrease costs, and increase the body of knowledge for the nursing profession as a whole. Nursing practice generates research questions, and vice versa. Practice and research as evidence confirmation are inseparable pieces of the puzzle of EBP, as depicted in Figure 1-1. Posing questions about nursing care frequently generates scientific data, which in turn often generate further questions to be explored.

The Importance of Generating Evidence

Discovering Significant Evidence

As stated earlier, to practice nursing based on "how we are taught" assumes that there is no further need to produce evidence. That dangerous assumption was investigated as early as 1975, when Ketefian's study revealed that nurses did not use research for making decisions about nursing care (Polit & Beck, 2008).

Lack of innovation and failure to develop a rationale for nursing care will result in a decrease in respect for nursing as a profession. Currently, consumers of health care list nurses/nursing as one of the most respected roles in today's society. Consequently, generating and using scientific evidence can only improve the image of nursing and provide better outcomes from the ensuing nursing care.

Another force underlying the need for generating evidence and incorporation into practice is the increasing cost of health care. Healthcare costs are spiraling upward at an uncontrollable rate that demands nurses perform their work in the most cost-effective way. As Bucknall (2007) notes, "Without an assessment of the extent to which the facts are relevant and contribute to a particular conclusion, they remain simply facts rather than evidence" (p. S61). Each and every fact must be carefully gauged to ensure that the cost of delivering the care remains within an acceptable level while still leading to high-quality, high-safety health care. In fact, the nursing profession cannot afford to ignore innovative approaches in nursing care that will reduce costs while simultaneously improving outcomes.

Impact on Practice

The potential impact of using research in evidence-based nursing practice is enormous. No longer can nurses rely on "how I was taught" or a "gut feeling." Research provides tangible scientific data to promote optimal patient outcomes. The nurse at the bedside must be an integral participant in the development of EBP. Nurses are the individuals who observe what works and what does not work in the real world of health care. The expertise that this hands-on practice brings to the research process is of paramount importance to the effective development of a body of nursing knowledge.

Patients interact with nurses and, as surveys indicate, trust them with their care. As a result, nursing practice that incorporates research also increases patient satisfaction. In turn, assisting a patient to recover health brings satisfaction to the nurse and helps keep the cost of health care at an acceptable level.

Within the current healthcare environment, nurses are expected to embrace continuous performance improvement (CPI) processes such as Six Sigma and the Plan–Do–Study–Act (PDSA) cycle. These continuous improvement processes are being driven by the Institute of Medicine (IOM)'s *Health Profession Education: A Bridge to Quality* (2003) document, which identified five core areas of concern: providing patient-centered care, working in interdisciplinary teams, employing evidence-based practice, applying quality improvement, and utilizing informatics. According to Finkelman and Kenner (2007), "The report [IOM] recommends (1) adopting transformational leadership and evidence-based management, (2) maximizing the capability of the workforce, and (3) creating and sustaining cultures of safety" (p. 8). As a result, nurses are confronted with the challenges of transforming care at the bedside (TCAB); situation, background, assessment, recommendation (SBAR) communication strategies; electronic medical records (EMR); and other healthcare trends. Change is imperative for each of us working within the healthcare field. It is our responsibility to become knowledgeable about the evidence that is available as we select mechanisms to address these core areas identified by the IOM report and The Joint Commission.

Nurses must step up to the plate and ask targeted, concise questions about the nursing care that is being provided. According to Rolston-Blenman (2009), "Successfully embracing a culture of change and innovation requires enlisting nurses to champion the objectives and empowering them to design the tools they need for success on the frontline" (p. 25). Settling for the status quo is no longer acceptable. Instead, nurses must take the lead in querying the healthcare delivery venue as to the appropriateness and safety of the care being provided. According to Yoder (2008), "By deploying the broadest range of solutions possible, organizations can significantly improve communication among providers, decrease care delays, and enable clinicians to spend more time with patients, all of which can lead to improved outcomes" (p. 26). Evidence-based nursing practice requires that each nurse develop this "inquiring mind" posture to ensure that the resulting patient outcomes are of high quality, safe, and appropriate in the current healthcare arena.

Nursing is truly both an art and a science. EBP not only provides elements of each aspect, but also contributes to the profession's overall development. As a result, EBP improves everyday practice by providing empirical data to guide nursing interventions.

Summary Points

1. A core body of nursing knowledge is derived from the process in which research is incorporated into practice; this process has been called best practice, quality of care, and evidence-based practice.
2. A working definition of evidence-based practice (EBP) is that EBP is a process of utilizing confirmed evidence (research and quality improvement), decision making, and nursing expertise to guide the delivery of holistic patient care.
3. The PICOT acronym provides a mechanism for posing forceful, clinical questions to generate scientific questions.
4. Obstacles for research utilization can be categorized into three areas: education, beliefs/attitudes, and support/resources.
5. Generating evidence adds to the core of nursing knowledge, which promotes nursing as a profession.
6. The combination of nursing practice and research is essential to developing EBP.
7. Safe, effective patient care is not a luxury, but rather a necessity.

RED FLAGS

Within the documentation of a research project, certain decisions concerning the planning and implementation of the process must be supported by rationales. In EBP, randomized controlled trials are viewed as the most powerful evidence. As a result, some research aspects are viewed as stronger designs (quantitative, experimental, and randomized sampling) than other facets of the process. In this text, the designation of a *red flag* will reflect features of the research project that are less stringent than others. These areas are not strictly forbidden within research, but rather are concerns that need to be taken into account. Within the documentation, these aspects should be supported by rationales reflecting the thought process for utilization of those pieces.

When a nurse is appraising an article for inclusion in an EBP situation, the presence of red flags should be seen as an opportunity to assess the justification for the decisions made by the research team. If the research team has provided an adequate justification for its research decisions, a study characterized by multiple red flags can still be a strong study. The documentation of the research report by a researcher is a process of validation and justification of the various judgments made during the planning process. The researcher has the responsibility to document the reasoning for the decisions incorporated into the study such as ethics, sampling, design, and data collection.

Red flags are areas within the documentation of the study that may raise concerns. These areas are not items that should never be done, but rather are items that should be supported by sound, clear rationales as to why the researcher used the research components.

Multiple Choice Questions

1. One of the primary foundations for evidence-based nursing practice is
    A. Medical knowledge.
    B. Research results.
    C. Everyday health care.
    D. Textbook information.

2. Within the process of providing evidence-based nursing care, which types of research results are incorporated to ascertain the plan of treatment?
    A. Personal experiences and medical knowledge
    B. Client values and medical knowledge
    C. Personal experiences and client values
    D. Medical knowledge and identified challenges

3. As a novice nurse on a medical–surgical hospital unit, you do want to get involved in a research study that is being proposed for your unit. Because your hospital is involved with evidence-based nursing practice, which aspects of EBP are essential for you to have?
    A. Sound bedside nursing skills
    B. Basic knowledge of your unit
    C. Method for accessing published information
    D. Fundamental safety knowledge

4. Which of the EBP components carries the greatest weight in determining the management of the clinical situation?
    A. Thought process
    B. Client preferences
    C. Research
    D. The situation

5. Evidence comes in many forms. Examples of the data that could best be utilized for EBP are
    A. Quality improvement data and integrated reviews.
    B. Integrated reviews and non-peer-reviewed journal articles.
    C. Collegial relationships and lay journals.
    D. Heresy data and practice guidelines.

6. When developing a question to drive the compilation of evidence for a specific practice situation, the five components that can be used to focus the investigation are
    A. Patient, situation, intervention, comparison, and practice.
    B. Situation, intervention, comparison, outcome, and time.
    C. Patient, intervention, comparison, outcome, and time.
    D. Patient, situation, intervention, outcome, and data.

7. A nurse working in a cancer follow-up setting has been asked to consider the development of a transition program to help young people adjust to the adult program. The initial question suggested for use in focusing the identification of evidence is "What is it like to have care transferred from a pediatric center to an adult clinic?" Which aspects of this question need to be strengthened to make it more searchable?

   A. Population and outcome
   B. Population and intervention
   C. Intervention and outcome
   D. Comparison and outcome

8. Research utilization has often been

   A. Neglected in the literature.
   B. Denied by publishers.
   C. Reported in the literature.
   D. Spurned by EBP.

9. Obstacles to using nursing research in practice include lack of

   A. Education, beliefs/attitudes, and support/resources.
   B. Faculty, knowledge, and cost.
   C. Time, beliefs/attitudes, and consumers.
   D. Outcomes, values, and motivation.

10. As a nurse on a medical–surgical hospital unit, you begin to question the amount of time your hospital policy requires for taking a patient's oral temperature. Your hospital uses an EBP approach to nursing care. Which hospital resources would you expect to be able to connect with to assist with the accessing of a computer?

    A. Ward clerk or CNA
    B. Doctor or lawyer
    C. Charge nurse or supervisor
    D. Librarian or library

11. You are a BSN-prepared nurse who wants to initiate a research project on your unit. To get the other nurses to participate, you would

    A. Ask the doctors what they think.
    B. Check the educational level of other nurses on the unit.
    C. Ignore your desire to learn more at this time.
    D. Give a presentation to your peers on the benefits of research.

12. In the past, nurses were often taught that while research might be a good thing to do, only faculty could do research because

    A. Faculty members are the only ones prepared to do research.
    B. Most nurses have not been taught research.
    C. Most nurses don't need to use research.
    D. Faculty members know what's best for nursing.

13. Many nurses don't understand research because

    A.   Research isn't necessary for their practice.

    B.   Most nurses are too old.

    C.   Research is like a foreign language.

    D.   Patients don't expect them to use research.

14. Research is often not valued because

    A.   It costs too much.

    B.   Administration wants it.

    C.   Search engines are easy to access.

    D.   Staffing is not an obstacle.

15. Nurses have a responsibility to use research because

    A.   Doctors order it done.

    B.   Administrators don't have time for research.

    C.   Research is nice to know.

    D.   Research is the "hallmark of a profession."

Discussion Questions

1. You are a public health nurse working in an outpatient hospice facility. You are responsible for clients and their families in a six-county area. During the course of a week, you have from six to ten clients or their families who experience stressful situations related to the disease process. These families and their loved ones experience anguish and guilt as they confront and deal with the terminal nature of the healthcare situation. You have been asked to explore the following question: How do others in this type of situation deal with the numerous stressful challenges? Which type of searchable question could you develop to drive the data search related to this request?

2. As a BSN staff nurse, you are excited that your hospital wants you to participate in an evidence-based project. You have been chosen to chair a taskforce. How would you approach this task?

3. You are an ADN-prepared staff nurse at an acute care facility who has enrolled in an RN-BSN program. One of the key messages presented by the RN-BSN program is the importance of evidence-based nursing prac-tice. In your first course in the program, you are asked to identify an evidence-based topic for development. The faculty members instruct you to select a topic that will be functional in your workplace. Which types of activities would you carry out to aid in the selection of this topic?

Suggested Readings

Harvey, G., Loftus-Hills, A., Rycroft-Malone, J., Titchen, A., Kitson, A., McCormack, B., & Seer, K. (2002, March). Getting evidence into practice: The role and function of facilitators. *Journal of Advanced Nursing, 37*(6), 577–588.

Hewitt-Taylor, J. (2002, December). Evidence-based practice. *Nursing Standard, 17*(14–15), 47–52, 54–55.

McCormack, B., Allison, K., Gill, H., Rycroft-Malone, J., Titchen, A., & Seers, K. (2002, April). Getting evidence into practice: The meaning of "context." *Journal of Advanced Nursing, 38*(1), 94–104.

Newhouse, R. P. (2006, July/August). Examining the support for evidence-based nursing practice. *Journal of Nursing Administration, 36*(7–8), 337–340.

Rycroft-Malone, J. (2003, July). Consider the evidence. *Nursing Standard, 17*(45), 21.

Rycroft-Malone, J. (2004). The PARIHS framework: A framework for guiding the implementation of evidence-based practice. *Journal of Nursing Care Quality, 19*(4), 297–304.

Rycroft-Malone, J., Kitson, A., Harvey, G., McCormack, B., Seers, K., Titchen, A., & Estabrooks, C. (2002). Ingredients for change: Revisiting a conceptual framework. *Quality and Safety in Health Care, 11*(2), 174–180.

References

Agency for Healthcare Research and Quality (AHRQ). (2000). *Outcomes research fact sheet, AHRQ Publication No. 00-P011*. Retrieved December 17, 2008, from http://www.ahrq.gov/clinic/outfact.htm

Brockopp, D. Y., & Hastings-Tolsma, M. T. (2003). *Fundamentals of nursing research* (3rd ed.). Sudbury, MA: Jones and Bartlett.

Bucknall, T. (2007). A gaze through the lens of decision theory toward knowledge translation science. *Nursing Research, 56*(4S), S60–S66.

Burns, N., & Grove, S. K. (2009). *The practice of nursing research: Appraisal, synthesis, and generation of evidence* (6th ed.). St. Louis, MO: Saunders Elsevier.

Cannon, S., & Boswell, C. (In press). Challenges and opportunities for teaching research. In L. Caputi (Ed.), *Teaching nursing: The art and science* (2nd ed.). Glen Ellyn, IL: College of DuPage Press.

Carroll, D. L., Greenwood, R., Lynch, K. E., Sullivan, J. K., Ready, C. H., & Fitzmaurice, J. B. (1997). Barriers and facilitators to the utilization of nursing research. *Clinical Nurse Specialist, 11*(5), 207–212.

Ciliska, D., Cullum, N., & Marks, S. (2001). Evaluation of systematic reviews of treatment or prevention interventions. *Evidence-Based Nursing, 4*(4), 100–104.

Cronenwett, L. R. (2002, February 19). Research, practice and policy: Issues in evidence-based care. *Online Journal of Issues in Nursing* [On-line serial], 7(2). Retrieved July 23, 2009, from http://www.nursingworld.org/MainMenu Categories/ANAMarketplace/ANAPeriodicals/OJIN/Columns/Keynotesof Note/EvidenceBasedCare.aspx

Davies, B. L. (2002). Sources and models for moving research evidence into clinical practice. *Journal of Obstetric, Gynecologic, & Neonatal Nursing, 31*(5), 558–562.

Dawes, M., Davies, P., Gray, A., Mant, J., Seers, K., & Snowball, R. (2005). *Evidence-based practice: A primer for health care professionals* (2nd ed.). Edinburgh, Scotland: Elsevier Churchill Livingstone.

DiCenso, A., Cullum, N., & Ciliska, D. (1998). Implementing evidence-based nursing: Some misconceptions. *Evidence-Based Nursing, 1*(1), 38–40.

DiCenso, A., Guyatt, G., & Ciliska, D. (2005). *Evidence-based nursing: A guide to clinical practice*. St. Louis, MO: Elsevier Mosby.

Estabrooks, C. A. (1998). Will evidence-based nursing practice make practice perfect? *Canadian Journal of Nursing Research, 30*(11), 15–36.

Fain, J. A. (2009). *Reading, understanding, and applying nursing research: A text and workbook* (3rd ed.). Philadelphia: F. A. Davis.

Ferguson, L., & Day, R. A. (2005). Evidence-based nursing education: Myth or reality? *Journal of Nursing Education, 44*(3), 107–115.

Fineout-Overholt, E., & Melnyk, B. (2005). Building a culture of best practice. *Nurse Leader, 3*(6), 26–30.

Finkelman, A., & Kenner, C. (2007). *Teaching IOM: Implications of the Institute of Medicine reports for nursing education*. Silver Springs, MD: American Nurses Association.

Fonteyn, M. (2005). The interrelationship among thinking skills, research knowledge, and evidence-based practice. *Journal of Nursing Education, 44*(10), 439.

Gennaro, S., Hodnett, E., & Kearney, M. (2001). Making evidence-based practice a reality in your institution: Evaluating the evidence and using the evidence to change clinical practice. *American Journal of Maternal/Child Nursing, 26*(5), 236–244.

Institute of Medicine (IOM). (2003). *Health professions education: A bridge to quality.* Washington, DC: National Academies Press.

Jolley, S. (2002). Raising research awareness: A strategy for nurses. *Nursing Standard, 16*(33), 33–39.

Kitson, A. L. (2007). What influences the use of research in clinical practice? *Nursing Research, 56*(4S), S1–S3.

Magee, M. (2005). *Health politics: Power, population, and health.* Bronxville, NY: Spencer Books.

Malloch, K., & Porter-O'Grady, T. (2006). *Introduction to evidence-based practice in nursing and health care.* Sudbury, MA: Jones and Bartlett.

Melnyk, B. M. (2003). Finding and appraising systematic reviews of clinical interventions: Critical skills for evidence-based practice. *Journal of Pediatric Nursing, 29*(2), 125, 147–149.

Melnyk, B. M. (2004). Integrating levels of evidence into clinical decision making. *Journal of Pediatric Nursing, 30*(4), 323–325.

Melnyk, B. M., & Fineout-Overholt, E. (2005). *Evidence-based practice in nursing and healthcare: A guide to best practice.* Philadelphia: Lippincott Williams & Wilkins.

Newhouse, R. P., Dearholt, S. L., Poe, S. S., Pugh, L. C., & White, K. M. (2007). *Johns Hopkins Nursing evidence-based practice: Model and guidelines.* Indianapolis, IN: Sigma Theta Tau International.

Omery, A., & Williams, R. P. (1999). An appraisal of research utilization across the United States. *Journal of Nursing Administration, 29*(12), 50–56.

Oncology Nursing Society. (2005). *EBP process* [ONS Web site]. Retrieved October 29, 2005, from http://onsopcontent.ons.org/toolkits/evidence/Process/index.shtml

Polit, D. F., & Beck, C. T. (2008). *Nursing research: Generating and assessing evidence for nursing practice* (8th ed.). Philadelphia: Lippincott Williams & Wilkins.

Porter-O'Grady, T. (2006). A new age for practice: Creating the framework for evidence. In K. Malloch & T. Porter-O'Grady (Eds.), *Introduction to evidence-based practice in nursing and health care* (pp. 1–29). Sudbury, MA: Jones and Bartlett.

Pravikoff, D. S., Tanner, A. B., & Pierce, S. T. (2005). Readiness of U.S. nurses for evidence-based practice. *American Journal of Nursing, 105*(9), 40–51.

Rolston-Blenman, B. (2009). Nurses roll up their sleeves at the bedside to improve patient care. *Nurse Leader, 7*(1), 20–25.

Rutledge, D. N., & Grant, M. (2002). Introduction. *Seminars in Oncology Nursing, 18*(1), 1–2.

Titler, M. G., Everett, L.Q., & Adams, S. (2007). Implications for implementation science. *Nursing Research, 56*(4S), S53–S59.

Vratny, A., & Shriver, D. (2007). A conceptual model for growing evidence-based practice. *Nursing Administration Quarterly, 31*(2), 162–170.

Webster's II new college dictionary. (1999). Boston: Houghton Mifflin.

Yoder, L. (2005). Evidence-based practice: The time is now! *Medsurg Nursing, 14*(2), 91–92.

Yoder, L. (2008). Evidence-based design. *Nursing Management, 39*(12), 26–29.

Chapter 2

Overview of Research

Sharon Cannon and Margaret Robinson

Chapter Objectives

At the conclusion of this chapter, the learner will be able to

1. Discuss the evolution of evidence-based practice and nursing research
2. Identify the value of using models and frameworks in nursing research
3. Differentiate between basic and applied research
4. Delineate sources for nursing research

Key Terms

➤ Applied research
➤ Basic research
➤ Best practices
➤ Bundling

➤ National Center for Nursing Research (NCNR)
➤ National Institute of Nursing Research (NINR)
➤ National Institutes of Health (NIH)

Introduction

The roots of research utilization can be traced back to the time of Florence Nightingale in the mid-1800s. Over the past 150 years, nursing research has encompassed a variety of models, settings, and foci. The following historical perspective illustrates the trajectory of nursing research.

Historical Perspective

Evolution from Nightingale to Present Time

Florence Nightingale's work on sanitation in the 1800s was one of the early efforts at linking environmental variables to clinical outcomes. In the early 1900s, the focal point of nursing research was on nursing education. In the 1940s, the concentration shifted to the availability and demand for nurses in time of war. A major milestone occurred in 1952 when the first edition of nursing research was published. In the 1970s, clinical outcomes again reemerged as a focus for nursing research, and the Nursing Studies Index by Virginia Henderson was produced. Today, through evidence-based practice (EBP), the focus is on the application of research findings to clinical decision making in an effort to improve individual patient outcomes.

? Think Outside the Box

Explore the various approaches used to generate knowledge in your practice area. For example, which information has been used to determine the method of catheterizing a laboring mother? Which information serves as the basis for the range of blood sugars used in elderly patients who are newly diagnosed with diabetes?

Florence Nightingale's *Notes on Matters Affecting the Health, Efficiency and Hospital Administration of the British Army* (1858) was one of the first published works that outlined the clinical application of nursing research ("Florence Nightingale Museum Trust," 2003; Riddle, 2005). Florence Nightingale created a polar-area diagram (or coxcomb) to display data related to the causes of mortality in the British Army during the Crimean War (**Figure 2-1**). This early pie chart used color graphics to depict deaths secondary to preventable disease, war injuries, and all other causes. Using these data, Nightingale calculated the mortality rate for contagious diseases such as

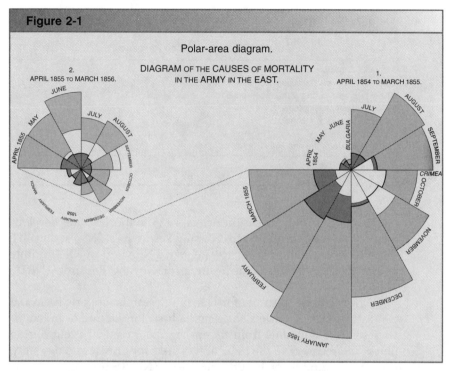

Figure 2-1

Polar-area diagram.

2.
APRIL 1855 TO MARCH 1856.

DIAGRAM OF THE CAUSES OF MORTALITY
IN THE ARMY IN THE EAST.

1.
APRIL 1854 TO MARCH 1855.

Source: Riddle, L. (2005). *Polar-area diagram: Biographies of women mathematics.* Available at: http://www.agnesscott.edu/lriddle/women/nightpiechart.htm. Accessed January 21, 2006.

cholera and typhus. Her statistical analysis demonstrated the need for sanitary reform in military hospitals.

The American Nursing Foundation, established in 1955, was devoted exclusively to the promotion of nursing research:

> The primary objectives of the foundation were to increase public knowledge and understanding of professional nursing, practical nursing and the arts and sciences on which the health of the American people depended. The foundation was to conduct studies, surveys and research; provide research grants to graduate nurses; make grants to public and private nonprofit educational institutions; and publish scientific, educational and literary works. (Kalisch & Kalisch, 1986, p. 651)

Federal support for nursing research began in 1946, with the creation of the Division of Nursing within the Office of the Surgeon General. In 1955, the National Institutes of Health (NIH) established the Nursing Research Study Section. A 1983 study entitled *Nursing and Nursing Education: Public Policy and Private Actions*, published by the Institute of Medicine, recommended that nursing research be included in the mainstream of health-related research. With growing public support,

Table 2-1
Areas of Focus for Nursing Research
Chronic illnesses Quality and cost-effectiveness of care Health promotion and disease prevention Management of symptoms Adaptation to new technologies Health disparities Palliative care at the end of life
Source: NINR, 2006b.

the Health Research Extension Act of 1985 authorized the development of the National Center for Nursing Research (NCNR) at the NIH. The NIH Revitalization Act of 1993 elevated NCNR to an NIH Institute and established the National Institute for Nursing Research (NINR, 2006a).

"The National Institute for Nursing Research supports basic and clinical research to establish a scientific basis for the care of individuals across the lifespan—from the management of the patient during illness and recovery to the reduction of risks for disease and disability, and the promotion of healthy lifestyles" (NINR, 2006b, p. 1). The strategic planning process at NINR identified areas of focus for prospective nursing research (**Table 2–1**). In April 1993, the Board of Directors of the American Nurses Association (ANA) adopted a position statement that acknowledged that "research based practice is essential if the nursing profession is to meet its mandate to society for effective and efficient patient care" (ANA, 1993, p. 1). It went on to identify the role of nursing research for the ADN-, BSN-, MSN-, and doctoral-prepared practitioner. The position statement outlined a process whereby clinicians identify relevant clinical problems for investigation and researchers design studies to address these problems (**Table 2–2**).

? Think Outside the Box

Discuss the barriers you might encounter when trying to implement evidence-based practice and research utilization in your area.

Early nursing research focused on the development of the profession of nursing, not the clinical practice of nursing. In 1970, a study conducted by Lysaught "revealed that little nursing research has been conducted on the actual effect of nursing interventions and that

Table 2-2

Research Roles at Various Levels of Nursing Education

Associate Degree

Helping to identify clinical problems in nursing practice
Assisting with the collection of data within a structured format
Using nursing research findings appropriately in clinical practice in conjunction with nurses holding more advanced credentials

Baccalaureate Degree

Identifying clinical problems requiring investigation
Assisting experienced investigators to gain access to clinical sites
Influencing the selection of appropriate methods of data collection
Collecting data and implementing nursing research findings

Master's Degree

Collaborating with experienced investigators in proposal development, data collection, data analysis, and interpretation
Appraising the clinical relevance of research findings
Creating a climate in the practice setting that promotes scholarly inquiry, scientific integrity, and scientific investigation of clinical nursing problems
Providing leadership for integrating findings into clinical practice

Source: ANA, 1993.

nursing had few definitive guidelines for its practice. The study recommended that investigation of the impact of nursing care on the quality, effectiveness and economy of health care be conducted" (Polit & Hungler, 1978, p. 11). Thus began a new era in which clinical practice emerged as a priority for nursing research.

In the 1980s, clinical pathways were introduced into nursing practice. Clinical pathways are a plan of care developed by a multidisciplinary team that outlines the sequential care that should be provided to a predictable group of patients. Early clinical pathways focused on high-volume admissions in the acute care setting, such as elective surgeries and routine obstetrical care. Clinical pathways should incorporate the applicable research. However, the intent of a clinical pathway is to manage the progression of an individual patient through a clinical event. These pathways emerged in response to shifting payment methods for health care and focused on the critical path whose steps must be accomplished for the patient to have a cost-effective and timely discharge. Measures of success were, generally, a reduction in the total cost to provide care and a reduction in the average length of stay for each patient. In the late 1990s, a growing concern arose that many hospitals had adopted clinical pathways without strong evidence that they were clinically or economically effective.

The emergence of EBP takes the application of research one step further to focus on outcomes-based practices. The emphasis is now on the assessment and evaluation of clinical practices that have demonstrated their ability to improve morbidity and mortality for patients. Frequently, multiple interventions have been identified that together enhance the clinical outcome; this practice has come to be known as bundling. A bundle is a group of interventions related to a disease or care process that, when executed together, result in better outcomes than when the interventions are implemented individually. Evidence suggests that consistently implementing these practices with all patients who have a specific disease or procedure can improve patient outcomes (Institute for Healthcare Improvement, 2006). In 2005, the Institute for Healthcare Improvement introduced care bundles for the prevention of central-line infection and ventilator-acquired pneumonia as part of the 100,000 Lives Campaign. In this case, the outcomes-based practices focus on a single aspect of care that is known to have serious complications.

Blending evidence-based research and applying it to clinical practice and patient outcomes was a goal of the work of the Institute of Medicine in its landmark publication *To Err Is Human: Building a Safer Health System* (1999). In the preparation of this report, research in human factors was applied to health care in an attempt to understand where and why systems or processes break down. Specifically, the report's authors looked at how practices in healthcare settings could be made safer so as to prevent adverse outcomes for patients.

In 2004, the Institute of Medicine expanded on its original work to look at the work environment of nurses in its publication *Keeping Patients Safe: Transforming the Work Environment of Nurses*. This report further described the need for bundles of mutually reinforcing patient safety defenses as part of the effort to reduce errors and increase patient safety. It described "bundles of changes" that are needed within four aspects of care—(1) leadership and management, (2) the work force, (3) the work process, and (4) organizational culture—to strengthen patient safety.

? Think Outside the Box

Which model and/or frameworks do you tend to use in your practice of nursing care?

Purpose of Nursing Research

The major rationale for conducting research is to build a body of nursing knowledge, thereby promoting improvement in patient outcomes. This is accomplished by using results of research in the provision of nursing care that is based on scientific data rather than on a hunch, gut feeling, or "the way I was taught." As a profession, nursing must hold its members accountable for providing safe, cost-effective, and efficient care. EBP that incorporates research findings is a model for nurses to use in their practice.

Theory, Research, and Practice

Parker (2006) defines theory as "a notion or an idea that explains experiences, interprets observation, describes relationships and projects outcomes" (p. 4). Theories are considered to be an abstract explanation. Fain (2009) defines research as "a systematic inquiry into a subject that uses various approaches (quantitative and qualitative methods) to answer questions and solves problems" (p. 5). Research can be more readily considered a specific explanation.

When considering the relationship between theory and research, one could conclude that theory gives direction to research, which in turn guides practice. As a result, many nursing research projects include a nursing theory/theoretical framework and concepts to guide the research and provide implications for nursing practice.

The evolution of the relationship of theory to research to practice has been ongoing since the days of Florence Nightingale. The current emphasis in research is on translational research and implementation science. These changes move theory into a new dimension for application to practice. If translational research is seen as a method to move a theory into another dimension, and if implementation science is perceived as supporting evidence-based practice and research utilization, then the relationship to practice is further enhanced and becomes stronger. Thus implementing research (evidence) and theory into practice (translation) optimizes EBP.

As stated in Chapter 1, it is beyond the scope of this text to examine theory in depth. Sometimes a theory is not identified for a research or evidence-based project; however, a theory is still important. The researcher or nurse using evidence to guide nursing care must, at the very least, incorporate a model, framework, plan, or system that gives direction to the project. Van Achterberg, Schoonhoven, and Grol (2008) connect models to research and theories for implementation of EBP.

Models and Frameworks

Nursing research provides a way to explain and predict the care that nurses provide, including the underlying rationale. As a result, models of nursing care and their frameworks provide ample opportunities for the generation of new nursing knowledge. As Malloch and Porter-O'Grady (2006) indicate, "Professional Care Models give nurses responsibility and authority to provide patient care. In addition, nurses are accountable for coordinating care and ensuring that continuity of care is provided across the continuum. Patients' unique needs are addressed to achieve outcomes" (p. 236).

Webster's II New College Dictionary (1999) defines a model as "a preliminary pattern serving as the plan from which an item not yet constructed will be produced; a tentative description of a theory or system that accounts for all its known properties" (p. 704). Many nursing care models and research models are problem-solving processes that begin with a question. Nurses ask clinical questions on a daily basis and often conduct research on an informal basis. When a nurse observes the same phenomena occur with multiple patients having the same diagnosis over time, a pattern emerges. The nurse has, through experience, validated his or her observations, just not in a formal, structured research model. As Burns and Grove (2009) state, "A framework is an abstract, logical structure of meaning. It guides the development of the study and enables you to link the findings to the body of knowledge used in nursing" (p. 126). When a theory is not used, a care model, plan, or system is needed in evidence-based practice and research. A model, plan, or system then functions as a framework.

Validation of Best Practices

"Best practice" is a term used by many different types of professionals in many different settings. The definition of "best practices" varies depending on the meanings assigned to the words "best" and "practices." In this book, *best practices* is defined as those nursing actions that produce the most desirable patient outcomes through scientific data.

? Think Outside the Box

Most of the research projects associated with evidence-based practice tend to be examples of applied research. Brainstorm about some possible projects that would be classified as basic research.

For best practices, research utilization supports decision making for nursing practice through a problem-solving process. Reaffirmation through scientific data validates the desired outcomes and reinforces best practices. This is an excellent example for reality testing. There may be times when a nurse thinks or feels that the result of an action is accurate, when it actually is not. Burns and Grove (2001) cite an example related to patient consumption of oxygen. The nurse's sense might be that getting a patient up to the bedside commode results in more oxygen consumption than when the patient uses a bedpan. However, research has shown this to not be accurate. Thus reality can be tested through scientific inquiry, which leads to validated best practice.

Fineout-Overholt and Melnyk (2005) suggest that "best practice" is a term used by more than healthcare providers. According to these authors, "without well-designed research, best practices cannot claim universal application" (p. 27); consensus builds best practices that are achieved through evidence.

Simpson (2005) suggests that through EBP, nurses could overlook the truth about nursing practice. Nurses need to look at what practice is and what is really done. Perhaps, research and practice need to merge to have a major impact on practice. Through this merger, practice and research would combine to actually become a validated best practice.

Basic versus Applied Research

Basic research can be defined as research to gain knowledge for knowledge's sake (Brockopp & Hastings-Tolsma, 2003; Burns & Grove, 2009; Fain, 2009). Sometimes basic research is also called bench research, such as laboratory experiments intended to elucidate cell structure. Simply stated, basic research is often useful later when, for example, a researcher addresses how a new drug being tested affects a cell's structure. Fain (2009) indicates that basic research is conducted with little concern for how it might ultimately be applied to practice.

? Think Outside the Box

Using Florence Nightingale's ideas, apply these ideas to research and evidence-based practice.

In contrast, applied research directly impacts practice and modifies current practice. Most nursing research is applied research that assists in decision making related to nursing care. This can also include the development of new approaches for care. Modification, development, and evaluation of nursing care of best practice form the heart of EBP. Applied research builds a body of knowledge for nursing practice and guides the nurse in providing patient care. An example of applied research in nursing would be a study that generates new information about the use of soap and water versus hand cleansing gels in preparation for a sterile dressing change. An applied research project might indicate that soap and water is more effective in preventing potential wound infections. The nurse would then use the applied research results in preparation for doing a sterile dressing change.

As can be seen, basic research differs from applied research primarily in terms of its focus and intent. Basic science (also known as bench science) is conducted in a laboratory and seeks to add to the knowledge base. Applied research is grounded in the practice area and its application to practice. Fain (2009) suggests that while basic research and applied research are quite different, they can be considered to form a continuum where basic research is required for interpretation of findings of applied studies. One might say that basic research in nursing is building a body of knowledge (theory) and that applied research is the application of the theory to the clinical arena (practice).

Sources for Nursing Research

Most nursing research comes from two primary sources: academia and healthcare settings. One might expect that nurses doing research in academic settings would focus only on educational research and that those conducting research in health care would focus only on practice settings. Although that distinction may hold true in some cases, most often both arenas produce research for both education and practice, because they are closely aligned with each other. This intertwining is most evident in the nursing position papers published by two major nursing organizations.

Academia

A major thrust of research in education is the evaluation of programs, technologies, and instructional design. Research in education flourished from the mid-1980s until about 2001, when funding for nursing education withered. An Act of Congress specified that no funding from the National Center for Nursing Research (NCNR) could be distributed for research in nursing education (Diekelmann, 2001). As a result, nurse educators had to seek funding outside the discipline, where the competition was intense. Consequently, little nursing education research was conducted. Nurse-educator researchers turned to research in clinical practice. Although that effort translated into some positive gains for clinical practice, it drastically affected the research needed to support innovative programs, teaching/learning activities, and other aspects of nursing education.

Since 2000, when the National League for Nursing (NLN) was reorganized, increased emphasis and financial support have been directed toward research in nursing education. In its reorganization, the NLN recognized the need for a "quality nursing education that prepares the nursing workforce to meet the needs of diverse populations in an ever changing healthcare environment ... and change the landscape related to funding for nursing education research ... to lead in promoting evidence-based teaching in nursing ..." (NLN, n.d., p. 1). This commitment to nursing education research is also expressed in the NLN's mission and goal statements. Nurse educators have recognized the need to continue seeking external funds from outside the discipline. Grant funding has also come from several governmental agencies and foundations. The current impetus for obtaining funding from outside sources is a direct result of the nursing shortage and reports on health care generated by agencies such as the Institute of Medicine (IOM). Because the nursing shortage appears destined to last for years to come, research in nursing education has a promising future. The relationship with EBP will likely remain in the forefront when such research in nursing education is carried out.

? Think Outside the Box

There are many nursing theories available within the literature. Search the literature to find evidence of nursing research utilization of a selected theory.

Healthcare Settings

According to Cronenwett (2002), in 1999 Marita Titler observed that outcomes achieved in a research study might not be replicated with multiple caregivers in the natural clinical setting. The variable demands on the bedside nurse and multiple comorbidities that exist in the hospitalized patient can make it difficult to replicate findings. Cronenwett (2002) has noted that "evidence for practice mounts slowly over time, as scientists discover first what works in controlled environments and second what works in daily clinical practice" (p. 3). Today, it is our challenge to move from a focus solely on research development to the use of valid and reliable evidence in clinical practice. Nurses have been identified as champions in the adoption of EBP. It is equally important that healthcare institutions implement mechanisms that diffuse available evidence into the practice environment.

Summary Points

1. Florence Nightingale's work emphasized clinical applications of nursing research through the creation a polar area diagram.
2. From 1900 to 1940, nursing research focused on nursing education.
3. In the 1950s, the first issue of Nursing Research was published with the notion to share research information with colleagues. Also, the American Nursing Foundation was established to promote nursing research.
4. The 1960s focused on models and frameworks of nursing practice.
5. In the 1970s, Virginia Henderson introduced the Nursing Studies Index.
6. In the 1980s, the Institute of Medicine recommended that nursing research be included in health-related research. In addition, the National Center for Nursing was established.
7. In the 1990s and 2000, both the National League for Nursing and American Nurses Association developed position papers on research-based practice.
8. In 2004, the Institute of Medicine published *Keeping Patients Safe: Transforming the Work Environment for Nurses*, which focused on the need for bundles of mutually reinforcing patient safety defenses as part of the effort to reduce errors and increase patient safety.
9. Models and frameworks of professional practice are validated through research.
10. EBP incorporates research as a professional care model.
11. Basic research is gaining knowledge for knowledge's sake.
12. Applied research directly impacts practice.
13. Sources for research in nursing can be found in academic and healthcare settings.

RED FLAGS

- Research projects should be grounded by a model or framework to anchor the concepts identified within the project.
- Assumptions about best practices must be based on scientific evidence, rather than just on everyday consensus of opinion or intuition.

Case Scenario

Incorporation of EBP into bedside nursing generally requires a change in nursing practice. Change theory models point out that each change process inevitably has potential barriers to effective implementation of the desired change. To more effectively implement EBP, one must identify these barriers to implementation of change. Funk, Thompson, and Bonnes (2005) conducted a nursing research project in an attempt to better understand barriers to implementation of nursing research among inpatient nursing units at a large university-affiliated Magnet hospital:

> The purpose of this study was to examine the effect of multifaceted organizational strategies on registered nurses' (RNs) use of research findings to change practice in an academic hospital. The specific aims were to (1) identify nurses' attitudes and perceptions about organizational culture and research utilization, (2) identify perceived barriers and facilitators to nurses' use of research in practice, and (3) determine which factors are correlated with research utilization. (Funk et al., 2005, p. 121)

Survey tools, including the BARRIERS to Research Utilization Scale and the Research Factor Questionnaire, were used to gather data. The majority of respondents (83%) were registered nurses who held a baccalaureate or advanced degree in nursing. The results demonstrated an improvement in nurses' perception after implementation of multifaceted interventions. The authors also identified journal club participation as a major strategy to facilitate the use of research in clinical nursing practice.

Case Scenario Questions

1. How might the findings vary in an academic teaching facility that was not a Magnet hospital?

2. How might the findings vary in a community-based hospital setting?

3. How might the findings vary in an outpatient or procedural-based nursing practice?

4. How might the findings vary in a hospital setting that has primarily associate-degree nursing graduates?

5. What would you anticipate would be the findings in your own clinical practice environment?

6. If you implemented a journal club, do you believe that would increase the use of research findings in your clinical practice area?

Multiple Choice Questions

1. The research role of the baccalaureate degree nurse includes

   A. Identifying clinical problems that require investigation, assisting experienced investigators to gain access to clinical sites, and collecting data.

   B. Creating a climate in the practice setting that promotes scholarly inquiry, scientific integrity, and scientific investigation of clinical nursing problems.

   C. Collaborating with experienced investigators in proposal development, data collection, data analysis, and interpretation of results.

   D. Providing leadership in integrating research into practice.

2. Potential areas of nursing research identified by the National Institute for Nursing Research include

   A. Stem cell research.

   B. Application of pharmaceuticals in clinical practice.

   C. Chronic illness, health promotion, disease prevention, and end-of-life care.

   D. Healthcare literacy.

3. The first issue of Nursing Research was published in

   A. 1858.

   B. 1952.

   C. 1985.

   D. 1992.

4. The Nursing Studies Index, the first annotated index of nursing research, was the work of

   A. Florence Nightingale.

   B. Virginia Henderson.

   C. Marita Titler.

   D. Dorothea Orem.

5. The American Nurses Association position statement acknowledges that

   A. Researchers identify clinical problems and study them.

   B. Faculty members identify clinical problems and study them.

   C. Clinicians identify clinical problems and researchers design them.

   D. Faculty members and researchers identify clinical problems and study them.

6. Clinical pathways are developed by

   A. Nursing teams.

   B. Physician teams.

   C. Educator teams.

   D. Multidisciplinary teams.

7. A bundle is a group of interventions related to a disease or care process that

    A. Results in better outcomes than when the interventions are implemented together.

    B. Results in diverse outcomes when the interventions are implemented individually.

    C. Results in confusing information about a single disease or care process.

    D. Provides insufficient evidence to alter clinical practice related to individualized interventions.

8. Professional care models give nurses

    A. Accountability.

    B. Authority.

    C. Responsibility.

    D. All of the above.

9. Best practice is an excellent example of which kind of testing?

    A. Cognitive

    B. Reality

    C. Didactic

    D. Evaluation

10. Basic research is also known as bench research and is defined as research to gain knowledge for

    A. Use in academia.

    B. Use in clinical practice.

    C. Knowledge's sake.

    D. Use in biochemistry.

11. Applied research builds a body of knowledge for nursing practice because it is the basis of

    A. Evidence-based practice.

    B. Clinical pathways.

    C. Nursing process.

    D. Nursing diagnosis.

12. Sources for nursing research come primarily from two sources:

    A. Business and occupational settings.

    B. Academic and healthcare settings.

    C. Both urban and rural settings.

    D. Pharmaceutical and business settings.

13. Best practices in nursing can be defined as

    A. A well-written plan of nursing care.

    B. A systems approach to nursing care.

    C. Nursing actions that produce desirable patient outcomes.

    D. A way for nurses to justify their care.

14. The Institute of Medicine's publication *Keeping Patients Safe* focuses on
    A. Building a safer health system.
    B. Processes to report medication errors.
    C. Transforming the work environment for nurses.
    D. Healthcare reform.

15. Theories are
    A. A guide for research and practice.
    B. Considered to be a specific explanation of an idea.
    C. Not essential to research or EBP.
    D. Static and do not change over time.

Discussion Questions

1. Identify potential opportunities for you to use EBP in your current clinical setting.
2. Identify barriers to implementing EBP in your clinical setting.
3. Identify three clinical problems requiring investigation in your nursing practice. What steps might you take to begin to explore these identified problem areas?

Suggested Readings

Booth, W. C., Colomb, G. G., & Williams, J. M. (2003). *The craft of research* (2nd ed.). Chicago: University of Chicago.

Dimsdale, K., & Kitner, M. (2004). *Becoming an educated consumer of research: A quick look at the basic methodologies of research design.* Retrieved June 29, 2009, from http://www.air.org/publications/documents/Becoming%20an%20Educated%20Consumer%20of%20Research.pdf

Gerrish, K., & Lacey, A. (2006). *The research process in nursing* (5th ed.). Oxford, UK: Blackwell.

Johnson, B., & Webber, P. (2005). *An introduction to theory and reasoning in nursing* (2nd ed.). Philadelphia: Lippincott Williams & Wilkins.

Kilbom, J., & Cogdill, S. (2004). Writing abstracts. *St. Cloud State University and LEO: Literacy Education Online.* Retrieved June 29, 2009, from http://leo.stcloudstate.edu/bizwrite/abstracts.html

Shirey, M. R. (2006, July/September). Evidence-based practice: How nurse leaders can facilitate innovation. *Nursing Administration Quarterly, 30*(3), 252–265.

van Meijel, B., Gamel, C., van Swieten-Duijfjes, B., & Grypdonck, M. H. F. (2004, October). The development of evidence-based nursing interventions: Methodological considerations. *Journal of Advanced Nursing, 48*(1), 84–92.

References

American Nurses Association (ANA). (1993). *Position statement: Education for participation in nursing research.* Retrieved January 14, 2006, from http://nursingworld.org/readroom/position/research/rseducat.htm

Brockopp, D. Y., & Hastings-Tolsma, M. T. (2003). *Fundamentals of nursing research* (3rd ed.). Sudbury, MA: Jones and Bartlett.

Burns, N., & Grove, S. K. (2001). *The practice of nursing research: Conduct, critique, and utilization* (4th ed.). Philadelphia: W. B. Saunders.

Burns, N., & Grove, S. K. (2009). *The practice of nursing research: Appraisal, synthesis, and generation of evidence* (6th ed.). St. Louis, MO: Saunders Elsevier.

Cronenwett, L. R. (2002, February 19). Research, practice, and policy: Issues in evidence-based care. *Online Journal of Issues in Nursing, 7.* Retrieved July 23, 2009, from http://www.nursingworld.org/MainMenuCategories/ANAMarketplace/ANAPeriodicals/OJIN/Columns/KeynotesofNote/EvidenceBasedCare.aspx

Diekelmann, N. (2001). Funding for research in nursing education. *Journal of Nursing Education, 40*(8), 339–341.

Fain, J. A. (2009). *Reading, understanding, and applying nursing research* (3rd ed.). Philadelphia: F. A. Davis.

Fineout-Overholt, E., & Melnyk, B. (2005). Building a culture of best practice. *Nurse Leader, 3*(6), 26–30.

Florence Nightingale Museum Trust. (2003). *The passionate statistician.* Retrieved August 19, 2009, from http://www.florence-nightingale.co.uk/cms/index.php/florence-royal-commission

Funk, R., Thompson, C., & Bonnes, D. (2005). Overcoming barriers and promoting the use of nursing research in practice. *Journal of Nursing Administration, 35*(3), 121–129.

Institute for Healthcare Improvement (IHI). (2006). *100K lives campaign.* Retrieved June 29, 2009, from http://www.ihi.org/IHI/programs/campaign/campaign.htm

Institute of Medicine (IOM). (1999). *To err is human: Building a safer health system.* Washington, DC: National Academies Press.

Institute of Medicine (IOM). (2004). *Keeping patients safe: Transforming the work environment of nurses.* Washington, DC: National Academies Press.

Kalisch, P. A., & Kalisch, B. J. (1986). *The advance of American nursing* (2nd ed.). Boston: Little, Brown.

Malloch, K., & Porter-O'Grady, T. (2006). *Introduction to evidence-based practice in nursing and health care.* Sudbury, MA: Jones and Bartlett.

National Institute of Nursing Research (NINR). (2006a). *A brief history of the NINR.* Retrieved February 26, 2006, from http://ninr.nih.gov/ninr/about/history.html

National Institute of Nursing Research (NINR). (2006b). *Mission statement.* Retrieved February 26, 2006, from http://ninr.nih.gov/ninr/research/diversity/mission.html

National League for Nursing (NLN). (n.d.). *NLN mission statement.* Retrieved February 20, 2006, from http://www.nln.org/aboutnln/ourmission.htm

Parker, M. E. (2006). *Nursing theories and nursing practice* (2nd ed.). Philadelphia: F. A. Davis.

Polit, D. F., & Hungler, B. P. (1978). *Nursing research: Principles and methods.* Philadelphia: J. B. Lippincott.

Riddle, L. (2005). *Polar-area diagram: Biographies of women mathematicians.* Retrieved January 21, 2006, from http://www.agnesscott.edu/lriddle/women/nightpiechart.htm

Simpson, R. L. (2005, December). Leader to watch. *Nurse Leader,* 3(6), 10–14.

Webster's II new college dictionary. (1999). Boston: Houghton Mifflin.

van Achterberg, T., Schoonhoven, L., & Grol, R. (2008). Nursing implementation science: How evidence based nursing requires evidence-based implementation. *Journal of Nursing Scholarship,* 40(4), 302–309.

Chapter 3

Ethics and Nursing Research

Jane Sumner

Chapter Objectives

At the conclusion of this chapter, the learner will be able to

1. Explain why ethical theories used in nursing practice are important for nursing research

2. Acknowledge how international and national codified ethical principles have influenced ethical nursing research

3. Discuss the impact of the history of human experimentation on nursing research today

4. Delineate the ethical implications in each step of the research process

5. Identify specific ethical issues when various research methodologies are utilized

Key Terms

➤ Code of ethics

➤ Deontology

➤ Ethical theories

➤ Ethics

➤ Honesty

➤ Human experimentation

➤ Informed consent

➤ Institutional review board (IRB)

➤ Respect and justice

➤ Teleology

➤ Trustworthiness

➤ Vulnerable subjects

Introduction

Nurses practice within a unique social world with its own norms, controls, rules, and regulations. Nurses, under the mandate of caring, are required to do no harm to patients. Nurse researchers are further constrained by this principle. The following statement encapsulates all the principles important for ethical nursing research. The most important and critical principle is the protection of the rights of all and any individuals participating in biomedical research.

> No one shall be subjected to torture or to cruel, inhuman or degrading treatment or punishment. In particular, no one shall be subjected without his free consent to medical or scientific experimentation. (United Nations Organization, 2002)

Nurse researchers, acting as social scientists, examine the human condition in relation to health and illness. They, too, are governed by all the ethical principles encompassed within biomedical research. Both the International Council of Nurses (ICN) and the American Nurses Association (ANA) have developed ethical codes that control the practice of the nursing profession. As the ANA (2001) made clear in its opening preamble to the Code of Ethics for Nurses, nurses have a "professional mandate to society for effective and efficient care" (p. 1). This is doubly true for the nurse researcher, whom the Code identifies as having to be qualified to conduct research, regardless of the particular role (i.e., principal investigator, clinical research coordinator, or member of an institutional review board). This means the researcher must understand all the elements required to maintain the highest ethical standards. The nurse researcher must understand what is morally and ethically appropriate to study and disseminate so as to protect the vulnerable—a group that includes everyone who participates as a subject and who trusts the nurse researcher will be ethical. "All research has ethical dimensions, and all research must be ethical" (Cipriano Silva, 2006, p. 178).

Nursing research, which lies within the domain of social science, is critical for the development of nursing knowledge. As a social science, nursing research is concerned with the human condition and, as such, is directed and controlled by all international ethical codes. The pursuit of nursing research requires participants to respect the specific ethical constraints and standards that are discussed in this chapter. The chapter discusses the ethical issues in each step of the research process:

- The research environment that ensures integrity of all human research projects
- Development of a researchable topic
- Development of research question(s)
- Participant recruitment
- Informed consent
- Data collection
- Data analysis
- Results dissemination and publication
- Issues related to protection of vulnerable populations, including confidentiality, honesty, and trustworthiness of the researcher
- Issues specific to quantitative and qualitative research
- External pressures that may influence the research project
- Emerging issues

Universal ethical theories and their relevance to nursing research are presented, as well as theories that underpin all the health disciplines. A brief review of the history of human experimentation and the need for ethical practice is provided as well.

Ethical Theories

Ethics is described as "a philosophical study of morality" (Deigh, 1995, p. 244), but the line between morality and ethics is often blurred. Not infrequently, little distinction is made between the two. However, the original meanings of the words "moral" and "ethics" may assist in separating the two. Moral is a "custom" (from the Latin *mos, moris*), which suggests that it is not a constant, but rather will change over time. With this premise, then, one can argue that the norms of a society, which are based on a moral perspective that everyone agrees to and is expected to live by, have the potential to change over time. Ethics comes from the Greek *ethos*, meaning "character," which can be applied to both the individual and the individual's behavior. When combined, "custom" and "character" lead to a "right way" to lead one's life.

"In relation to social research [ethics] refers to the moral deliberation, choice and accountability on the part of researchers throughout the research process" (Edwards & Mauthner, 2002, p. 14). Ethics are the standards by which a society lives and acts, and they have embedded within them various principles. The principles most relevant to nursing are (1) the value of life, (2) goodness or rightness, (3) justice or fairness, (4) truth telling or honesty, and (5) individual freedom (Thiroux, 1980).

The value of life refers to recognition of the importance of life, preserving life when appropriate but also accepting the reality of death. Issues that arise within this principle and that nurses confront include abortion, assisted suicide, and euthanasia.

Goodness or rightness is more difficult to pin down. Immanuel Kant (1724–1804) indicated that goodness means that we promote goodness over badness, that we cause no harm, and that we prevent badness or harm. Florence Nightingale supported this perspective when she said, "Hospitals should do the sick no harm" (Tschudin, 1992, p. 54).

Justice or fairness does not occur if we are not good. After all, doing good includes treating all equally and with equal distribution.

Truth telling or honesty, Tschudin (1992) suggested, may be the most difficult principle to live by, partly because truth is interpreted differently by different people. Truth is conveyed in communication that involves at least two participants, both of whom are speaker and listener, and who may hear things differently from the intention of the speaker. However, Tschudin cites Benjamin and Curtis (1986), who stated that "a person of integrity . . . is one whose responses to various matters are not capricious or arbitrary, but principled. One of the qualities most of us admire in others and try to cultivate in ourselves is personal integrity" (p. 59).

Finally, regarding the principle of individual freedom, "We need to use freedom to preserve life, do right and be good, act justly and tell the truth" (Tschudin, 1992, p. 59). Both societal and individual freedoms exist, ensuring just action and the doing of right and good. Societal pressures or limitations on freedoms may constrain the individual from acting justly and doing good.

Tschudin (1992) points out that ethics are identified as either normative or descriptive. Normative ethics are prescriptive ethics; they relate to the standards that have been laid down and are generally accepted in any society as the guidelines for what one should do. From normative ethics emerges the code by which a profession lives, which is particularly true in nursing. In contrast, descriptive (or scientific) ethics arise from what people do. Tschudin (1992) suggests that a code of ethics subscribed to by physicians tends to derive from scientific ethics as these clinicians investigate illness with the aim of curing of it. Regardless of which type of ethical theory is accepted by a group or profession (i.e., physicians or nurses), the principles of goodness, justice, and truth are indissolubly entwined together. These values, along with individuals' behavior, underpin their specific code of ethics.

? Think Outside the Box

Consider the various ethical theories. Which one seems to align with your nursing practice and why?

Utilitarianism (Teleology)

Aristotle is regarded as a teleologist, although he does not necessarily take a wholly utilitarian perspective (utilitarianism is identified somewhat more narrowly than teleology). The teleology theory is closely associated with Jeremy Bentham and John Mill, two English philosophers. Simply put, it relates to the means justifying the ends and consequences of the actions, which may be either good or bad. Mills emphasized the duty of "good action" on the basis of happiness, or the greatest happiness that required the right action. Three propositions form the basis of utilitarianism:

1. Actions are judged right or wrong based on the "virtue" of their consequences.
2. In assessing the consequences, all that is of concern is the amount of happiness that results.
3. When calculating happiness or unhappiness, no one person's reaction is more important than the reaction of anyone else (Rachels, 1995).

According to the views espoused by advocates of utilitarianism, the only thing that matters in the final analysis is the consequences. Rachels (1995) states that utilitarianism, with its adherence to the principle of utility, is the standard for judging right and wrong and firmly "rejects corruption" (p. 115). This perspective reduces—if not eliminates—feelings, desires, and "intuition" (p. 115) from rational and moral decision making.

While this ethical theory is applied in healthcare delivery, it is perhaps somewhat difficult to apply and of limited use, except in weighing all the consequences of an action before it occurs, and in making the decision whether the end truly justifies the means. In many instances, this would not be the case if one is to do no harm to the patient. However, if adherence to the principle of utility is applied, then it can be assumed that reason will trump feelings and emotions. For nurses, who often reside in lower positions in the power hierarchy, utilitarian-based decisions may prove hard to accept when imposed from above.

The implication for nursing is that all nursing actions should be focused on doing the right thing or good (beneficence), rather than on doing harm (maleficence). In relation to nursing research, Edwards and Mauthner (2002) describe ethical theory as the situation in which the right thing is that research produces new knowledge, providing the human subject is not put at increased risk during the process of conducting the research.

Deontology

In deontology, the theory focuses on the intrinsic nature or "rightness" of the action itself, and some actions are seen as right and others as wrong. With "right" action, the individual is obligated to act regardless of the consequences. Kant is believed to be the first to put duty at the forefront of moral behavior (Norman, 1998). In particular, Kant believed that because humans are "rational" entities, they are entitled to be treated with dignity, they always have value, and they must be never used as means—they are always ends. With this thinking comes responsibility, and Kant made clear his position that individuals must take responsibility for their actions.

Kant also defined "oughts" of reasoned behavior as "act only according to that maxim by which you can at the same time will that it should become a universal law" (Kant, 1785, cited by Rachels, 1995, p. 110). The limitation of this perspective is that a universal law should be upheld without exception, which makes difficult or impossible the context for the behavior. The obligated duties of deontology are as follows:

- Duties of fidelity
- Duties of reparation
- Duties of gratitude
- Duties of justice
- Duties of beneficence
- Duties of self-improvement
- Duties of nonmaleficence (Ross, cited by Norman, 1998)

If one understands the meanings of these duties, then it is not difficult to accept why deontology is more easily accepted within the healthcare delivery system, and particularly in the nursing profession, with its strong sense of duty and obligation to the patient.

Embedded in this ethical theory is the freedom of the individual but also consideration for the common good. "A right action is only right if it is done out of a sense of duty, and the only good thing without any qualification is a person's goodwill: the will to do what one knows to be right" (Tschudin, 1992, p. 51). Nursing has as its mandate the obligation to protect the vulnerable patient—and therein lies the cause for justice. Edwards and Mauthner (2002) describe this theory as "actions governed by principles" (p. 20), to include honesty, respect, and justice. For the nurse researcher, the obligation is to protect the human subject through demonstration of respect and honesty.

Values Theories

Principles of ethics not uncommonly used in health care include (1) respect, (2) autonomy, (3) beneficence (or nonmaleficence), and (4) justice. All ethics codes related to human experimentation stress respect for persons, both from the perspective of individual autonomy and by emphasizing the rights of those with diminished autonomy to the same protections. Autonomy refers to the ability to make careful choices. In relation to research, a potential subject should receive all the information required to make an informed decision.

Beneficence refers to the practice of maximizing benefits while minimizing risks. In relation to research, as stated by the Council of International Organizations of Medical Sciences (CIOMS, 2002), "this principle gives rise to norms requiring that the risks of research be reasonable in light of the expected benefits . . . the research design be sound . . . investigators competent to perform the research and to safeguard the welfare of the research subjects." Another term for beneficence is nonmaleficence, or the doing of no harm to the individual. Beneficence is identified as an obligation, and every effort must be made to ensure the well-being of the research subject. *The Belmont Report* (National Institutes of Health [NIH], 1979) indicated that the principle of beneficence applies to society at large as well as to specific investigators. Thus there are obligations inherent in all human research projects that have implications measured in terms of long-term effects for the society at large.

Finally, the principle of justice is particularly applicable to the "vulnerable," but is more widely viewed as the "ethical obligation to treat each person in accordance with what is morally right and proper, to give each person, what is due to him or her"(CIOMS, 2002). *The Belmont Report* (NIH, 1979) describes what is due as "(a) to each person an equal share, (b) to each person according to individual need, (c) to each person according to individual efforts, (d) to each person according to societal contribution, and (e) to each person according to merit." "Equal" in this instance implies equity, although clearly at times not everyone will be equal. Nevertheless, there should be equity or justice in distribution of whatever is distributed. The implication of "distributive justice," to which both CIOMS and The Belmont Report refer, is that the issues of vulnerability of human subjects must be addressed as the same for everyone.

In human studies, nursing and medical practitioners are tending to vulnerable populations simply by means of the illnesses that brought patients to the attention of healthcare providers. CIOMS (2002) describes vulnerability as a "substantial incapacity to protect one's own interests owing to such impediments as lack of capability to give informed consent, lack of alternative means of obtaining medical care or other expensive necessities, or being a junior or subordinate member in a hierarchical group." Human subjects are therefore vulnerable before they are invited to participate in research projects, and this imposes further ethical obligations on the researcher to protect them.

Virtues Theory

Virtues are regarded as character traits. Norman (1998) cites Hume's (1751) list of virtues, which gives insight into these traits:

- Qualities useful to others: benevolence, justice, and fidelity
- Qualities useful to their possessor: discretion, industry, frugality, strength of mind, and good sense
- Qualities agreeable to their possessor: cheerfulness, magnanimity, courage, and tranquility
- Qualities agreeable to others: modesty and decency (p. 55)

Rachels (1995) adds "courage, self-control, generosity, and truthfulness" (p. 159) to this list, and suggests that moral philosophers can frame these virtues within the larger question of "what is the right thing to do" (p. 160) for the moral agent in "habitual action"(p. 163). Nevertheless, these characteristics, while important, do not offer a complete ethical theory. They assist in explaining how they can influence moral reasoning and behaviors. Rachels indicates that they may provide moral motivation, but it is important to realize that emotion may be an influence and that care is required to maintain impartiality. The virtue characteristics clearly play a role in determining how ethical theories are interpreted and utilized, but the theory itself does not depend on virtues themselves.

Historical Overview

The twentieth century has seen an explosive increase in human research, with a concomitant need for ethical oversight and controls. Significant medical breakthroughs, however, have occurred throughout history as a result of experimenting on other human beings. For example, in 1789, Edward Jenner first inoculated his son, aged 1 year, with swinepox against smallpox in England. This vaccination method proved to be ineffective, and later Jenner used cowpox on other human subjects. This approach was successful and led the way for effective inoculation against smallpox, a lethal disease (Reich, 1995). Despite his undoubted achievement, Jenner's work raises a number of key ethical issues:

- No consent was obtained from the subject.
- No understanding was established as to whether the agents used (i.e., swinepox and cowpox) were safe for human use.
- Research was performed on a minor who would have had no understanding of what was happening, although the argument could be made that because the researcher was the father of the child, it was a nonissue. However, this practice would be deemed unacceptable today.

Nevertheless, throughout Western European history, there is evidence of the relevance of ethical behaviors in human research. Moses Maimonides (1135–1204), a Jewish physician and philosopher, "instructed colleagues always to treat patients as ends in themselves, not as means for learning new truths" (Reich, 1995, p. 2248). Claude Bernard, writing in France in 1865, stated, "Morals do not forbid making experiments on one's neighbor or one's self . . . the principle of medical and surgical morality consists in never performing on man an experiment which might be harmful to him to any extent, even though the result might be highly advantageous to science, i.e., to the health of others" (Reich, 1995, p. 2249).

However, recognition of the need for regulated ethical constraints emerged as a result of horrific episodes during the twentieth century. The most egregious documented atrocities were probably the Nazi experiments that were conducted mainly on prisoners during World War II. These experiments included "putting subjects to death by long immersion in subfreezing water, deprivation of oxygen to learn the limits of bodily endurance, or deliberate infection by lethal organisms in order to study the effect of drugs and vaccines" (Reich, 1995, p. 2253). In addition, "Nazi experimental atrocities included investigation of quicker and more effective means of inducing sexual sterilization (including clandestine radiation dosing and unanesthetized male and female castration and death)" (Reich, 1995, p. 2258).

In addition to these appalling events, highly unethical human research studies were performed in the United States. The most infamous was the Tuskegee Syphilis Study, which involved African American males suffering from secondary syphilis; the treatment of penicillin (the recommended and available medication) was deliberately withheld from these patients so that the progression of the disease could be studied. The Tuskegee study, which was initiated in the mid-1930s, was not halted until 1972, when a newspaper published an account of it. At no time were the human subjects fully informed about the study, and in some instances they appear to have been deliberately misinformed. Among the many sad aspects of the study was the fact that subjects more than likely, in all innocence, infected others, because their syphilis was not being treated. Therefore, maleficence was directed not only toward the study subjects, but also toward their families, which compounded the researchers' ethical lapses.

Instances of human drug testing or usage with inadequate ethical oversight have also occurred. Thalidomide, a widely used sedative in the 1950s (though not in the United States), was given to some pregnant women to control morning sickness. When the tragic malformations of their fetuses were made public, thalidomide was removed from the market for this particular use. Thalidomide was one of a group of drugs for which it is evident that there was already knowledge about the potential for teratogenicity (malformation of fetuses). Yet because this drug had been "widely praised, advertised, and prescribed on the grounds that it was unusually safe" (Dally, 1998, p. 1197), it was never properly tested for safety before human use. Instead, because of the highly effective advertising campaign conducted by the drug's manufacturer, the medical community ignored the evidence and went on using thalidomide. This case highlights another aspect of the relevance of stringent ethical controls in human research studies.

More recently, the inadequate design of medical research study at Johns Hopkins School of Medicine led to the death of one of the subjects. In this instance, prior to the initiation of the study on the inhalation of the drug hexamethonium, a limited and sketchy review of the literature was performed using only a medical index Web site. Such reviews are limited in terms of how far back they can search. The failure to explore the full history of the drug resulted in a healthy 24-year-old female losing her life: A review of the literature from an earlier period would have revealed potential hazards in association with this drug and its proposed route of administration. This case points to the importance of the careful design and organization of a study before it is initiated. Fault lay at many levels, not the least of which was the researcher but also perhaps with Johns Hopkins' research review board (Perkins, 2001).

Interestingly, the World Medical Association in 1964 first made ethical principles for medical research involving human subjects public in the Declaration of Helsinki. Specifically, in section B, Basic Principles for All Medical Research, item #11 states, "Medical research involving human subjects must conform to generally accepted scientific principles, be based on a thorough knowledge of the scientific literature, [and] other relevant information . . ." (http://www.wma. net/e/policy/b3.htm). Clearly, in the Johns Hopkins study, the study design did not adhere to international standards.

? Think Outside the Box

Consider several examples of human experimentation that have occurred during the history of medical research. Have these projects resulted in beneficial outcomes for society? Can human experimentation be justified when the greater good of society is at stake? Defend your thoughts.

Codifying Research Ethics

The core ethical issue is the need for voluntary consent of the potential research subject so that a fully informed individual participates. Many efforts have been to address this issue, but perhaps the most significant arose from the Nuremberg Trials, in which the Nazi war crimes were investigated. The result was the Nuremberg Code of 1946, in which it is stated, "the voluntary consent of the human subject is absolutely essential. . . . This means that the person involved should have legal capacity to give consent . . . the research subject should be so situated as to be able to exercise free power of choice" and human subjects "should have sufficient knowledge and comprehension of the elements of the subject matter involved as to make an understanding and enlightened decision" (Reich, 1995, p. 2253).

In the United States during the 1960s, different agencies within the federal government began more stringently regulating funded research on human subjects. On July 1, 1966, the National Institute of Health, through the Public Health Service, assigned "responsibility to the institution receiving the grant for obtaining and keeping documentary evidence of informed patient consent" (Reich, 1995, p. 2254). It also mandated "review of the judgment of the investigator by a committee of institutional associates not directly associated with the project" (Reich, 1995, p. 2254). Finally, the "review must address itself to the rights and welfare of the individual, the methods used to obtain informed consent, and risks and potential benefits of the investigation" (Reich, 1995, p. 2254).

In 1973, Congress formally recognized the importance of ethical standards in human research when it created the National Commission for the Protection of Human Subjects of Biomedical and Behavioral Research, whose "mission is to protect the rights and welfare of research human subjects." Research oversight by the federal government continues with a constant updating of regulations, which can be found in the Code of Federal Regulations, Title 45 and 21—specifically in the Protection of Human Subjects Rule (Department of Health and Human Services [DHHS], 2005). Federal efforts to improve the safeguards to human subjects in research continue apace, culminating most recently with Health Insurance Portability and Accountability Act (HIPAA).

ICN has followed suit, making the need for protection of human rights very clear in its own Code of Ethics, which focuses on four principal elements: (1) the nurse and people; (2) nurses and practice; (3) nurses and the profession; and (4) nurses and coworkers. Ethical behaviors within these relationships are expected at all times, not just in areas of research. The second statement in the "nurses and people" element of the ICN Code of Ethics (2006) reads as follows: "In providing care, the nurse promotes an environment in which the human rights, values, customs and spiritual beliefs of the individual, family and community are respected" (p. 2). As a social science, nursing research must demonstrate ethical values that reflect the values of the profession at any one time (Jeffers, 2005). Human rights, equity, and justice are stressed specifically in relation to educators and researchers. The "nurses and the profession" element of the ICN's Code of Ethics states that the researcher must "conduct, disseminate and utilize research to advance the profession" (p. 7). Although ethics is not named directly here, its importance is inherent in the entire document.

ANA (2001) has it own Code of Ethics for Nurses, in which specific vulnerable populations are identified. These populations include children, the elderly, prisoners, students, and the poor. The Code was published in 1994, copyrighted in 1997, and updated and republished in 2001. It also indicates that the nurse clinician identifies clinical problems that need examining and the researcher designs the study in association with the clinician. What is clear in this statement is that research topics in nursing should be focused on practice, which in itself should provide an ethical underpinning for nursing research.

Environment for Ethical Research

Most nurse researchers are associated with institutions having ethical regulations already in place that the researcher is required to follow. This offers protection to the institution, the researcher, and the human subjects. The research institution housing the project typically has an office for reviewing all research proposals, usually called the institutional review board (IRB). The issues that receive the most intense IRB scrutiny relate to thorough evaluation by the research team of the risks and benefits of the project, the provision of sufficient protection for human subjects, and the implementation of sufficient monitoring of the project once approval is given to proceed (Rothstein & Phuong, 2007). In addition, this office is most helpful in ensuring that the researcher submits all the required paperwork, including the proposal for the study, the consent form that study participants will sign, the budget, and whatever tools the researcher will be using in data gathering (i.e., surveys or instruments, or interview guides in the case of qualitative studies).

DHHS has developed a Code of Federal Regulations that controls the IRB offices in various types of healthcare organizations. The membership of the IRB must have at least five members of different backgrounds who also have the competence to review research proposals. It is expected that the membership will have cultural and gender diversity, as well as an awareness of local community mores. Thus, not only will there be healthcare professionals on the board, but there will also be members who are "unaffiliated" with the institution; at least one member must have scientific interests, and one may not (Rothstein & Phuong, 2007). The members are expected to be knowledgeable about all federal guidelines and regulations. When reviewing a proposal, an IRB member may not have involvement with the project (DHHS, 2005). Unfortunately, there have been instances when the IRB members have had some sort of conflict of interest or lack of objectivity that renders the board less capable of being just, fair, and protective of human subjects (Rothstein & Phuong, 2007).

The IRB members meet once a month to review all proposals, which they have already carefully scrutinized, and they may request further information to make informed decisions. When the IRB is satisfied that the researcher will provide full protection of the human subjects, the researcher is given permission to proceed and the project is given an identifying number. The researcher must report progress back to the IRB every 12 months. However, the IRB members expect the researcher to follow the protocol exactly as laid out in the proposal. If the project has more than one researcher, all must be listed on the protocol and, if requested by the institution, the curriculum vitae (CV) of each must also be attached. The issues of specific concern for ensuring ethical research are that the risks to the subjects are minimized (or are at least reasonable, providing the expected outcomes or benefits can be attained); subject selection is equitable; informed consent is sought from participants; and issues relating to data collection and storage, privacy, and confidentiality are managed according to regulations (DHHS, 2005).

The researcher is expected to be competent to perform the research. Lenz and Ketefian (1995) indicate that in 1989, the Institute of Medicine's Committee on the Responsible Conduct of Research was concerned that there was "a lack of formal training in scientific ethics and the responsible conduct of science as a deficit in the training of scientists and clinicians" (p. 217). Although baccalaureate degree programs and higher levels of nursing education include courses on research, it is not until a student is writing either a master's thesis or a doctoral dissertation that he or she begins to understand the process that enables the research to be ethical and legal.

According to Ketefian and Lenz (1995), "Scientists have traditionally valued their independence in the conduct of their research. In the main, society and academic institutions have to be willing to give certain freedoms and latitude . . . in return, increased accountability is . . . demanded" (p. 268). However, an institution does not want its reputation sullied by sloppy, illegal, or unethical research. Research trustworthiness, reliability, and usefulness are utterly dependent on the credibility of the researcher, the work, and the institution. The rules and regulations are the most rigorous when an institution receives federal funding. In such cases, the IRB office is insistent on all requirements being met. Ultimately, the research has to be honest.

Although multiple brakes are now applied in an attempt to prevent unethical research from occurring, some continue to have concerns that there is still the potential for inadequate protection of human subjects. Wood, Grady, and Emanuel (2002) believe that the review process is "bureaucratic and inefficient" (p. 2) and suggest that IRB members are overworked, frightened by the possibility of federal audits, and not always understanding "ambiguous regulations" (p. 2). They continue: "Federal regulators are aggravated by the limited scope of their authority and variable adherence to regulations" (p. 2), and their concerns are not limited to these particulars. For the nurse researcher, however, adherence to the ethical standards for human subject protection applied by the organization for which the researcher works and the codes of ethics developed by ICN and ANA is crucial regardless of external concerns.

Evidence-Based Practice and Ethical Implications

In the clinical environment, considerable effort is being made to implement evidence-based nursing practice. Such practice is derived from several elements, including experiential knowledge on the part of the nurse (i.e., knowing what works in practice and why); having clinical judgment and skills of critical inquiry; knowing the individual patient both as a human being and in terms of his or her pattern of responses to what is occurring; and knowledge of current scientific research findings (Borsay, 2009; Redman, 2007; Tanner, 2006). Evidence-based practice is designed to reduce unthinking, ritualistic practices in nursing care (Siedlecki, 2008).

Quality improvement (QI) is constantly performed in healthcare organizations: Data are gathered in order to improve patient outcomes through "local innovations in and assessment of the processes and systems of care delivery" (Redman, 2007, p. 217). This process is designed for rapid implementation of change. It is different from the slower rigorous, empirical research approach, which is more deliberative and follows a "fixed protocol with a clearly defined method and . . . a period of analysis after completed data collection" (Lynn et al., 2007, p. 668). Quality improvement is not empirical research. There is some concern, however, related to the ethics of human subject protection in QI practices (Grady, 2007; Lynn et al., 2007). To date, there has been no standard established regarding whether there should be a separate IRB process for QI.

Changes that are derived from QI are not regarded as the strongest evidence in EBP. Rather, EBP is dependent on generalizable scientific evidence (Batalden & Davidoff, 2007). The research utilized in evidence-based nursing practice utilizes well-tested scientific study data and the study has undergone the ethical scrutiny required.

Developing a Researchable Topic

Although nurse researchers may have curiosity about and interest in many topics they believe have the potential for expanding the body of nursing knowledge, some topics may not be realistically researchable for a number of reasons. The critical factor relates to protection of the vulnerable subject. As nurses, we are deeply and intimately involved with human beings at their most vulnerable, and the research topic may well pose a further threat to those individuals' vulnerability. When developing a researchable topic, the nurse researcher is called upon to utilize "ethical sensitivity" so as to decide what is appropriate, to have the "ability to perceive rightness and wrongness" (Weaver, 2007, p. 142), and to know what one is doing that affects the welfare of another person either directly or indirectly.

Issues related to the researcher also determine whether a topic is researchable. Volker (2004) indicates that attempting to research certain topics could put the researcher at risk "for loss of professional license, legal actions, imprisonment and peer ostracism" (p. 119). The types of topics that pose a threat to the researcher, according to Volker (2004), include those examining "social deviance, [those impinging] on powerful social interests, or [those examining] a deeply personal sacred value held by study participants" (p. 117). Nurses should not be studying illegal activities as a general rule, of course. The example Volker uses—patient requests to assist them with suicide—is an issue that nurses confront in their practice, however; thus it should be examined. The ANA's 1994 statement on assisted suicide states, "Nursing has a social contract with society that is based on trust, and therefore patients must be able to trust that nurses will not actively take human life" (p. 4). Volker is not saying that the topic of assisted suicide cannot be examined, but rather that careful vigilance must be taken to ensure the study design is meticulously developed to protect both the researcher and the researched. The ANA Code of Ethics also makes it very clear that the nurse researcher "has a duty to question and if necessary to report or refuse to participate in research they deem morally objectionable" (ANA, 1994).

In legally sensitive research projects, further measures can be sought that protect the researcher against "compelled disclosure" (Anderson & Hatton, 2000, p. 249) or breaking confidentiality covenants (Volker, 2004) and that offer additional protection for the study subjects. In particular, a Certificate of Confidentiality may be issued by DHHS in such cases. Federal law states that a Certificate of Confidentiality

> may authorize persons engaged in biomedical, behavioral, clinical, or other research (including research on the use and effect of alcohol and other psychotic drugs) to protect the privacy of individuals who are the subject of such research by withholding from all persons not connected with the conduct of such research the names or other identifying characteristics of such individuals. Persons so authorized to protect the privacy of such individuals may not be compelled in any Federal, State, or local civil, criminal, administrative, legislative, or other proceedings that identify such individuals. (Public Health Service Act, 42 USC~163, 1988)

Volker (2004) makes it clear that "researchers who engage in socially sensitive research must be prepared for scrutiny by diverse professional and lay parties who have varying agendas and interests" (p. 123). Research projects are usually undertaken in institutions that have a well-developed ethical structure and that are highly conscientious in following federal guidelines and regulations, so as to protect the vulnerable patients under their care. As a consequence, the researcher, as he or she develops the project, has resources immediately available for advice and consultation, including the IRB, professional colleagues, attorneys, and an ethics committee.

? **Think Outside the Box**

Vulnerable populations are always with us. Can you think of some additional ones that are emerging in the current healthcare environment? Explain why you see these groups as vulnerable. Which issues need to be considered when determining the vulnerability of a group of people?

The topic that the nurse researcher chooses should be one of real interest to him or her. The researcher should be willing to allocate the preparatory time and effort to ensure that the project meets all of the institution's ethical guidelines. Ethical behavior requires intellectual honesty of the researcher—giving credit due to others, not stealing ideas from others without acknowledgment, and not initiating data collection before institutional approval has been given. Plans for seeking funding for the study, the study design, methodology, data collection, and the dissemination of results (even if insignificant) at the conclusion of the study are also critical parts of developing the topic for research.

In discussing the Canadian system of protecting human subjects, Pilkington (2002) makes it clear that if a research project is not scientifically valid, then it is unethical to involve human subjects. It is the responsibility of the IRB (known as a "research ethics board" in Canada) to ensure that a study is scientifically valid. In defining whether a research project is scientifically valid, Pilkington (2002) states bluntly, "If a study does not hold substantial promise of answering a significant question(s), thereby generating valuable knowledge, then there is no justification for exposing persons to the actual or potential risks and inconvenience of participation" (p. 197). Scientific validity, therefore, influences how a researchable topic is developed to be an ethical research study.

Developing Researchable Questions

Although the nurse researcher may have a burning interest in a particular topic, developing the question(s) appropriately is most important when gearing up for a formal study. This development is necessary to narrow the topic down to a specific focus, clarify the methodology, determine whether the topic has embedded in it useful questions that will give shape to the study, and ensure that significant research results will emerge and add to the body of nursing knowledge. The questions have to be broad enough to obtain results, yet not so broad so as to yield diffuse and possibly meaningless results.

Thorough reading on the subject can assist in developing questions that meet these criteria. This preliminary investigation can help identify the gaps in the literature and hone the researcher's thinking about what it is specifically that he or she wants to investigate. Communication with both clinician colleagues and fellow nurse researchers can also assist in refining the questions.

Whether the questions are worded as statements, which is more common in qualitative studies, or framed as a hypothesis and a null hypothesis depends on the type of study and the chosen methodology. If the questions are not synchronous with the study, then results are more likely to be unreliable and of little use.

The ethical component of this endeavor derives from ANA's demand for effective and efficient care of the patient. If the research design is faulty at any level—and specifically the question development level—then one must ask if the results will improve the efficiency and effectiveness of patient care.

Participant Recruitment and Informed Consent

Vulnerable populations are always a concern for all research regulatory bodies, but there are some populations who are particularly vulnerable—the very young, the frail elderly, prisoners, the mentally incompetent, and women. In addition, issues related to socioeconomic status, education, and language may contribute to a specific population's vulnerability (Anderson & Hatton, 2000; Rogers, 2005). The researcher must be sensitive to these issues as well as to the points specifically outlined in federal regulations. This can make recruitment more difficult and the need for true informed consent crucial. Very specific regulations can be found in the *Belmont Report* (NIH, 1979), the International Ethical Guidelines for Biomedical Research Involving Human Subjects (CIOMS, 2002), and the DHHS's *Protection of Human Subjects* document (2005), including sections relating the protections needed for specific vulnerable populations.

The key ethical issue embedded in informed consent is that the individual always has the freedom of choice to participate or not participate, and may withdraw from the study at any time. This freedom of choice is built on a series of components:

- The language is simple enough to be clearly understood.
- The potential subject adequately comprehends the project.
- The subject has had to time to think about the study and its potential risks and benefits, and to discuss it with family members.
- The consent is not coerced.
- The written consent is documented.

CIOMS (2002) discusses "inducements" to participation, which can be identified as coercion and, therefore, are not appropriate. Several authors have expressed concern over how to achieve the consent and indicate that, in fact, obtaining consent should be a continuous process throughout a research project. In other words, the researcher should regularly check in with the subject to ensure that he or she is still a willing and informed participant (Edwards & Mauthner, 2002; Miller & Bell, 2002). The only payment or compensation allowed includes the costs of transportation or loss of earnings due to participation in the research project. It is unethical to offer more financial incentives, as they may encourage a potential subject to consent against his or her better judgment. It is also unethical for the researcher to receive compensation from a pharmaceutical company to conduct a study.

Research using children participants encompasses all the usual ethical issues relating to informed consent, privacy, and confidentiality, but includes several other factors that may compound the issues: Children exist in a natural power hierarchy with adults, but are able to communicate and understand according to their interpretation of the world around them (Kirk, 2007). Children must believe they are part of the project, but researchers must be alert to the specific child's "agenda" and continually check back with the child to ensure that he or she wants to continue to participate. Parents are also involved with providing informed consent, but researchers must ensure that children do understand what they are getting into and that their consent is given freely. In some instances, only one parent's consent is required, although two parents' consent is preferable. On occasion, a child and parents may not agree on continued participation; in general, it is the child's decision that is accepted in such cases.

The success of the study may depend on the warmth, interest in the child, and rapport established by the researcher, so that the child trusts the researcher. These characteristics have been demonstrated to be critical in longitudinal studies with children (Ely & Coleman, 2007), particularly when ill children are subjected to discomforting treatments. A slightly different issue arises with teenagers who, while still legally minors, have the right to give informed consent without parental consent (Roberson, 2007). Parents still have legal responsibility "to ensure the child [receives] appropriate medical care, [but] there is also the ethical need to 'respect the rights and autonomy of every individual, regardless of age'" (Kunin, 1997, cited by Roberson, 2007, p. 191).

Recruiting the desired composition and number of participants may require establishing multiple research sites, which can create some problems for the researcher, even as it confers some distinct advantages to the study: Such studies are "likely to produce generalizable, high quality results . . . [increase the] likelihood of attracting funding . . . [provide access to] a broader range of practice settings and patient with a wider range of diagnoses . . . [and] expedite data collection" (Twycross & Corlett, 2007, p. 35). Multisite research enables experts to work together and perhaps close the theory–practice gap. Of course, there are some notable difficulties in conducting multisite studies, including those related to establishing and maintaining collaborative, trusting relationships with one's colleagues; meeting face-to-face; overcoming organizational cultural differences; and having to gain IRB approval at each site.

Data Collection and Data Analysis

Protection of vulnerable human subjects remains the critical ethical issue with data collection and analysis. First and foremost, the privacy and confidentiality of the subjects must be protected, which means that the data must be locked securely in a safe place at all times. Data may include audiotapes, surveys, or videotapes, among other media.

Videorecording is becoming more popular for data collection because of 'its inherent accuracy and reliability as a record of events and detailed, nuanced levels of observation and analysis permitted" (Broyles, Tate, & Happ, 2008, p. 59). Additional ethical issues must be addressed when such data collection methods are used, however—namely, privacy; participant burden and safety; storage, location, and condition of storage of recordings; maintenance of the recordings in storage; access to recordings; use of the recordings as part of a presentation; and whether the actual taping will interfere with clinical care. The IRB will make decisions on all these issues and may require that faces be blurred and/or eyes are covered with a black box in the final recording.

Each institution has specific guidelines about how long data files must be kept. Lutz (1999) has raised the issue of premature destruction of original data, predominantly in studies on particularly vulnerable populations (e.g., battered women). According to this author, such destruction could occur if the researcher were concerned about court subpoenas that could compromise the participants' safety. However, premature destruction could lead to institutional accusations of scientific misconduct, which suggests that the researcher has a fine line to walk between ethical and unethical actions.

Ethical analysis and interpretation depend on the honesty and trustworthiness of the researchers. Although healthcare organizations make every effort to ensure ethical behaviors within their research environments, ultimately it rests with the researchers to ensure that the project is indeed conducted ethically in all areas, including analysis, interpretation, and dissemination of results. The opposite of ethical behavior is scientific misconduct, which brings dishonor to both the individual and the institution, and renders the research project meaningless. In addition, concern for the welfare of the vulnerable human subjects is negated when misconduct occurs. Scientific misconduct, an extremely serious issue, is defined by DHHS as follows:

> Fabrication, falsification, plagiarism or other practices that seriously deviate from those that are commonly accepted within the scientific community for proposing, conducting or reporting research. It does not include an honest error or honest differences in interpretations or judgments of data. (Commission on Research Integrity, 1995, p. 1)

Lutz (1999) has cited Macrina (1995), who states that falsification involves results being manipulated or tampered with, fabrication refers to "totally unfounded results" (p. 90) being produced, and plagiarism is "theft of another person's ideas" (p. 90). History makes evident that falsification, fabrication, and plagiarism are unconscionable and utterly unethical.

Publication

At the end of the research project, when it is time to publish the results, journals accept only peer-reviewed manuscripts as a further ethical dimension (Ketefian & Lenz, 1995). Peer referees are required to evaluate the scientific merit of the research study as well as the manuscript's acceptability for a particular journal. To warrant publication, the research findings are expected to contribute new knowledge to the practice of nursing (Driever & Pranulis, 2003). Without that expectation, the research is inappropriate, if not unethical. Those who review manuscripts for publication must have the knowledge and expertise to evaluate the work appropriately (Pilkington, 2002).

An emerging literature is focusing on issues related to publication. Conn (2008) discusses how pressure may be put on the author to change results because the manuscript reviewers resist "unexpected outcomes" (p. 161) and want revisions that are not consistent with the results. The authors may need to make changes, but those changes should not come at the expense of reliable data results. Freda and Kearney (2005) discuss how editors can face ethical issues when articles have been published in more than one journal; when data are published in more than one journal with no changes; or when there is evidence of author misconduct, demand for credit for someone "undeserving" of credit, lack of IRB approval, or misconduct related to lack of informed consent or an undeclared conflict of interest.

A recent study by Henley and Dougherty (2009) revealed another potential problem related to publication of research results: discrepancies in the quality of the reviews submitted by many persons who serve as peer reviewers. According to these authors, "Peer review is the mainstay of the editorial process" (p. 18). The key issues of concern within a paper were poor reviews related to the study's theoretical framework (47.2%), literature review (35.15%), discussion and interpretation of results (22%), and data analysis/presentation (21.9%). In terms of usefulness of the written comments to the author, 14.4% of peer reviews were deemed poor. Finally, in terms of usefulness to the editor, 12.2% of peer reviews were poor or inadequate. These authors recommended formal training and a probationary period for all potential reviewers.

A further ethical issue relates to who should be listed as first author when multiple researchers participated in the study. Generally, the principal investigator is listed as first author. However, in the case of multiple authors, negotiation determines the first author named on various publications. Ketefian and Lenz (1995) point out that listing authors in order of their extent of effort made is the most ethical way of recognizing authorship. These authors also suggest that it is unethical to publish the same manuscript or article in multiple journals. It is appropriate to publish several articles on the same study, provided that each manuscript is written with a different focus. In addition, all contributions and funding sources for an article must be acknowledged.

? **Think Outside the Box**

Determine if your school or hospital has an institutional review board (IRB). Which criteria do the board members use when approving a research project?

Issues in Quantitative and Qualitative Research

There is concern in qualitative research about the increased risk for ethical lapses inherent with this research methodology. As Birch and Miller (2002) state, this "type of research relationship may involve acts of self-disclosure, where personal, private experiences are revealed" (p. 92) and is never value free or "value neutral" (Christians, 2003, p. 213). The researcher must be aware of this potential and approach this type of research by making every attempt to acknowledge any personal biases.

In qualitative research, interviews are commonly used to gather data, resulting in face-to-face exposure for both the researcher and the researched. The dialogue serves as the research data that are then analyzed and interpreted. The vulnerable patient immediately becomes more vulnerable as the researcher delves into his or her lived experience. Anonymity and confidentiality are inevitably compromised in the interaction between researcher and human subject, which means there is an even greater need for data security and constant awareness on the part of the researcher of these issues. Honesty and trustworthiness of the research are even more important in such cases. Firby (1995) has stated, in relation to an IRB giving permission for a qualitative research project, "We should not simply assume that because research has been accepted by a committee it is morally justifiable in its methods" (p. 41). The moral obligation of nursing is to do good, and to do no harm. Therefore, qualitative nursing research must meet that obligation.

In contrast to qualitative research, quantitative research, which initially arose from the objective methodology of the Enlightenment's scientific paradigm, is supposed to be value neutral. The quantitative researcher is less likely to engage in face-to-face self-disclosure, which protects both him or her and the subject. The facts are supposed to speak for themselves. However, the researcher must be alert to the potential for his or her biases to influence the interpretation of data. Nevertheless, there remains the ethical principle of justice and the need for informed consent for human participants in such studies.

External Pressures

Conducting research studies is never easy, but various pressures making it more difficult may push the researcher toward unethical behaviors. According to Lutz (1999), these pressures include limited funding, the competition for achieving tenure for faculty, and "increasing emphasis on producing research reports" (p. 92).

The Health Insurance Portability and Accountability Act (HIPAA) is designed to protect patients against unauthorized disclosure of their health and medical records. At the same time, it adds another source of pressure for nurse researchers, as passage of HIPAA has led to some new concerns related to health research. According to Erlen (2005), these regulations were written for healthcare delivery organizations, and not for universities per se; nevertheless, the latter organizations have had to develop their own policies and procedures that meet the requirements of HIPAA. At times it has proven difficult to draw "clear boundaries," and universities have tended to err on the side of caution by providing for additional protection of human subjects, privacy, confidentiality, and informed consent. This has meant additional training for anyone who wishes to engage in research. The institution's IRB office sets the policy for how the researchers of that institution can proceed while adhering to HIPAA regulations.

HIPAA and its ramifications are key ethical considerations for the nurse researcher. With the drive for evidence-based research to underpin practice, the nurse researcher needs to be aware that study data and their interpretation must be shared, but within the constraints of HIPPA. To meet these criteria, data must contain no identifiers of an individual in a sample. Thus subjects may be given a code number or letter. Only the researcher maintains a list linking the sample identifiers with their associated codes, and this document must be kept secure at all times.

Emerging Issues

Although nurses generally have not been involved in animal, genetic, or biological material research in the past, this situation is changing and is likely to continue to do so as more transdisciplinary, translational research occurs. The issues of concern with animals include ensuring that the least harm and suffering is inflicted, using animals only when absolutely necessary, using the fewest animals possible, and, when seeking IRB permission, ensuring that someone on the board understands the implications of animal research. In relation to genetic and biological materials research, the same moral and ethical obligations apply as when dealing with any human subjects (Cipriano Silva, 2006).

An environment that has been neglected as a site for study in the past, but is likely to draw increasing attention from researchers in the future because of the aging of the U.S. population, is the community-based care facility (i.e., nursing home). All of the usual ethical research issues apply in this setting, but some additional concerns may arise relating to ensuring the quality of life, safety, and satisfaction of those residing in nursing homes, and ensuring that the study will not impose an undue burden on the participants. Proxies may be required to give consent for resident participation if the resident is mentally incompetent or extremely frail; however, use of proxies requires that the proxy holder have the authority to give this type of consent, and he or she must be adequately informed of the study's focus. In a study by Cartwright and Hickman (2007), it was discovered that community-based facility administrators had limited understanding of the protections established by an IRB that gives consent to a study, although most seemed aware of federal and state statutory requirements in terms of informed consent. In an attempt to overcome these deficits,

Cartwright and Hickman developed a Bill of Rights for Community-Based Research Partners that could prove valuable for similar institutions.

Conclusion

The lessons learned from the history of human experimentation have led to the development of ethical codes, both nationally and internationally. These controls are crucial for the protection of vulnerable human subjects. Indeed, ensuring adequate protection of human subjects requires that particular care be taken in each step of the research process. The obligations inherent within nursing demand the "moral deliberation, choice and accountability" (Edwards & Mauthner, 2002, p. 14) of the nurse researcher. Nurses in their practice are tending to humans at their most vulnerable, and this level of understanding adds to the responsibility of the nurse researcher. Achieving valid research that enhances nursing knowledge is dependent on adherence to the highest ethical standards. The key components necessary to ensure that these ethical standards are met, as described in this chapter, should provide a useful guide for all nurses embarking on a research project.

Summary Points

1. History provides many lessons on the importance of protection of vulnerable human subjects. These history lessons have led to the development of national and international ethical codes of conduct.
2. Both the International Council of Nurses (ICN) and the American Nurses Association (ANA) acknowledge the obligations of the nursing profession to the vulnerable human and, as such, stress ethical standards in nursing research.
3. Ethical theories guide the standards of nursing research.
4. Some populations are more vulnerable than others (e.g., children); as such, they must be provided with the utmost protection during research.
5. Each step of the research process involves meeting ethical standards.
6. The privacy and confidentiality of the human subject must always be guaranteed.
7. Informed consent must be given by a human subject participant who truly understands to what he or she is consenting.
8. The honesty and trustworthiness of the nurse researcher are crucial in ensuring valid—and valuable—results are derived from any study.

RED FLAGS

- Every study must address the ethical aspects of that study. Documentation of this focus may be demonstrated through a statement reflecting IRB approval of the study.
- Every study must speak to how the subjects will be protected from harm— physical and/or psychological—during the research process.

Critical Discussion: Ethical Issues in Nursing Research

1. You are not the principal investigator in a research study of incarcerated women who are HIV positive or have AIDS, but you are one of the researchers who has received permission to interview some of the women who volunteered to participate. One woman gives you inappropriate information about another prisoner, whom she states propositioned her for sex; the interviewee claims this prisoner has AIDS. As you leave the prison, the warden asks you to relate what happened during this interview. Discuss your responsibilities as a researcher in this sensitive study. A number of critical elements must be taken into account: the interviewee divulging information about another prisoner's possible HIV/AIDS status and behaviors, confidentiality and protection of human subjects, the warden's request, and your ethical responsibility to the study and to your institution.

2. You are the principal investigator studying young teenagers (10–14 years old) who are receiving aggressive treatment for life-threatening cancers. One 11-year-old boy has had many bouts of chemotherapy, which have made him acutely ill. His parents would like the child to participate in the study, but he refuses. What he shares could potentially be of use in treating other young teenagers. Clearly, there are some issues of consent here. Discuss what you should do.

3. You are one of a group of nurse researchers who are participating in a multinational study. The sample will include people of many different ethnic groups, all of whom speak different languages, and will include women and children. You understand the process of IRB review in your own institution, but many other issues arise when one is participating in international studies. Among the issues of concern here are the need for an interpreter, confidentiality, local permission requirements, management of the study in the foreign country, recruitment of persons into the study, and protection of human subjects in a different country. How can these issues be resolved so that the study may be conducted?

Multiple Choice Questions

1. When developing a nursing research project, why is it important to remember the ethical constraints?

    A. The study will not be approved by the institutional review board without these constraints.
    B. The protection of human subjects underlies all human research projects.
    C. The results will not be trustworthy and replicable.
    D. The nurse researcher will not be able to get funding for the project and, therefore, will not be able to complete the project.

2. The atrocities performed on prisoners in Nazi Germany violated which ethical principles?

    A. Value of life, justice, and respect
    B. Beneficence, nonmaleficence, and value of life
    C. Autonomy, nonmaleficence, and respect
    D. Justice, autonomy, and nonmaleficence

3. Protection of vulnerable individuals is a critical ethical component in human research studies. How did Edward Jenner fail to meet this standard when he tested swinepox on his one-year-old son?

    A. He thought the new knowledge overrode any concern he should have for the rights of his son.
    B. He did not know any better.
    C. He ignored the point that he could not get informed consent from his son, who was particularly vulnerable.
    D. Give that smallpox was such a lethal disease at that time, it was better for Jenner to ignore his son's vulnerability so to gain new knowledge.

4. The Tuskegee Syphilis Study lasted many years, and none of the human subjects were properly informed about the study's conduct. Which ethical principle was egregiously ignored in this study?

    A. Autonomy
    B. Respect
    C. Nonmaleficence
    D. Justice

5. Why does an ethical research environment assist with ensuring scientific integrity?

    A. Within this environment, expectations for scientific integrity are laid out.
    B. Federal regulations related to ethical standards are adhered to, increasing the likelihood of integrity.
    C. The researcher always works within an ethical environment, which encourages the practice of ethical research behaviors.
    D. Scientific integrity ensures funding, which means that the study will be completed.

6. Why do federal regulations specify that the makeup of the institutional review board should reflect cultural and gender diversity and an awareness of local mores?

A. This practice ensures that all research projects presented to the IRB will receive fair examination and not be denied without discussion.

B. Gender studies have not been common until recently, and females react differently to different treatments.

C. Awareness of local customs and culture means that both IRB members and researchers understand issues of concern in a non-American population.

D. There is now great interest in researching healthcare issues in persons of different cultures.

7. Why is it important that the researcher be competent to conduct research?

A. It is not ethically appropriate for an incompetent person to conduct research.

B. An incompetent researcher will not be able to get informed consent from the vulnerable subject, which is unethical.

C. An incompetent researcher should always work with someone who is competent, so that he or she can learn the process.

D. Research is a complicated process that has to be learned.

8. What is the issue of greatest concern when developing a research project?

A. The competence of the researcher to do the research

B. The availability of funding

C. The protection of the vulnerable subject

D. Informed consent

9. A Certificate of Confidentiality may be required to protect both the researched and the researcher. Why?

A. The nurse researcher will not lose his or her license to practice and do research because of the sensitive topic being researched.

B. If the research topic is particularly sensitive, this certificate protects patients from divulging issues uncomfortable to them.

C. The certificate protects the researcher and the researched from being coerced by governmental authorities to reveal sensitive information.

D. The certificate means that no information is shared with those who should not be informed.

10. Why do research questions have to be developed carefully?

A. The wrong question for the study means the wrong answer.

B. Carefully developed and refined questions focus the research project.

C. Without careful development of the questions, the research results will be meaningless.

D. It is unethical not to develop questions carefully.

11. Informed consent is a crucial issue in research projects because
    A. Research results will be more meaningful.
    B. The researcher will be adhering to international codes of ethics from which federal regulations are drawn.
    C. The project will be rejected by the IRB, because the subject is not informed about the study.
    D. The consenting subject will understand what the research is about and will have the choice to participate (or not).

12. Scientific misconduct on the part of the researcher is very serious. What constitutes scientific misconduct?
    A. Lying about the project to subjects when seeking informed consent
    B. Fabrication, falsification of data, and plagiarism
    C. Attributing only partial authorship to other contributors when they have done most of the work
    D. Making false claims about a project being funded when the researcher is talking about his or her work

13. HIPAA, which was designed to protect all humans and their medical records in this era of electronic paperless records, has imposed another restraint on conducting research. Why?
    A. It is more difficult to obtain IRB permission to conduct a research project.
    B. With paperless medical records, there are no data to analyze, even when interview data and surveys are involved.
    C. The regulations protect against unauthorized disclosure; although IRB permission includes this protection, additional care is taken under HIPAA.
    D. HIPAA ensures that highly sensitive data (e.g., HIV/AIDS status) is not disclosed.

14. Privacy and confidentiality are always issues in human subject research. What are the important steps to ensure that they are protected?
    A. The researcher does not talk about what the subject shares until the project's results are published in a peer-reviewed journal.
    B. All data are kept securely locked in a safe place and destroyed when the study is completed.
    C. Care with replication studies must be taken so that original data are not shared in the second study.
    D. All data are kept securely locked in a safe place and may be destroyed only according to IRB instructions.

15. Both the International Council of Nurses and the American Nurses Association make it clear that the ethical standards of the profession require the same obligations from the nurse researcher. Why?

A. For the protection of vulnerable clients and patients
B. For the protection of the nurse researcher
C. Because of an obligation inherent within the nursing profession
D. Because practice on which these ethical standards are built focuses nursing research

Discussion Questions

1. Several nurses are working together to develop a research project. Only one is doctorally prepared; the others have either a master's degree or a baccalaureate degree. The preparatory work is to be shared equally among all the nurses. As the project evolves, it turns out that those who do not have a doctorate do all the work. At a meeting, the doctorally prepared nurse insists that she be listed as the principal investigator for the grant to be submitted and as the first author on all publications. She bases her request on a belief that the reviewers of the grant would "pay more attention to the application" if the principal investigator has a doctoral degree. Discuss the ethical issues embedded in this situation.

2. The protection of human subjects lies at the heart of any research project. Part of this protection entails the need to obtain informed consent. A female nurse wants to do a qualitative study investigating what it means for males to live with diabetes mellitus and the resultant impotence. Qualitative research usually involves interviewing the human subject— and sexual impotence is a particularly sensitive subject. How should the nurse explain the study to her potential sample to ensure that the consent is truly informed and that the subjects will not drop out of the study because of extreme discomfort during the interview? What are the ethical issues involved?

3. Codes of ethics in human research, developed partly as a result of the atrocities of the mid-twentieth century, continue to be refined. The dictionary definitions of "moral" and "ethics" suggest that the meanings of these terms can and will change, and the evolving codes support this idea. Yet codes of ethics are based on some universal theories and values theories. Discuss why, despite the universality of these theories, the codes continue to evolve.

Suggested Readings

American Association of Critical Care Nurses (AACN). (2005). *Ethics in critical care nursing research.* Retrieved July 22, 2009, from http://classic .aacn.org/AACN/research.nsf/0/daddec18fb7e925788256826007dec91 ?OpenDocument

Department of Health and Human Services (DHHS). (1998). *Sponsor–investigator–IRB interrelationship.* Retrieved July 22, 2009, from http:// www.fda.gov/ScienceResearch/SpecialTopics/RunningClinicalTrials /GuidancesInformationSheetsandNotices/ucm115972.htm

Department of Health and Human Services (DHHS). (2005). *Protection of human subjects rule, 45 C.F.R. §.* Retrieved June 29, 2009, from http:// www.hhs.gov/ohrp/humansubjects/guidance/45cfr46.htm

Goldman, E. (2001, May). *Vulnerable subjects.* Retrieved June 29, 2009, from http://poynter.indiana.edu/sas/res/vs.pdf

Im, E-O., & Chee, W. (2002, July/August). Issues in protection of human subjects in Internet research. *Nursing Research, 51*(4), 266–269.

International Council of Nurses (ICN). (2006). *The ICN code of ethics for nurses.* Retrieved July 22, 2009, from http://www.icn.ch/icncode.pdf

Lanter, J. (2006). Clinical research with cognitively impaired subjects. *Dimensions of Critical Care Nursing, 25*(2), 89–92.

Levine, C., Faden, R., Grady, C., Hammerschmidt, D., Eckenwiler, L., & Sugarman, J. (2004). The limitations of "vulnerability" as a protection for human research participants. *American Journal of Bioethics, 4*(3), 44–49.

National Institutes of Health (NIH). (1979). *The Belmont report: Ethical principles and guidelines for the protection of human subjects of research.* Retrieved March 3, 2006, from http://www.nihtraining.com/ohsrsite /guidelines/belmont.html

Rogers, B. (2005). Research with protected populations: Vulnerable participants. *AAOHN Journal, 53*(4), 156–157.

Smith, L. (2001, May/June). Ethics and the research realist. *Nurse Educator, 26*(3), 108–110.

United Nations Organization. (2002). International covenant on civil and political rights, article 7. Universal declaration of human rights. In Council for International Organizations of Medical Sciences (CIOMS). *International ethics guidelines for biomedical research involving human subjects.* Retrieved March 3, 2006, from http://www.cioms.ch/guide-lines_nov_2002_blurb.htm

World Medical Association (WMA). (1964–2004). *World Medical Association: Declaration of Helsinki: Ethical principles for medical research involving human subjects.* Retrieved June 29, 2009, from http://www.wma.net/e/policy/b3.htm

References

American Nurses Association (ANA). (1994). *Position statement: Assisted suicide.* Washington, DC: Author.

American Nurses Association (ANA). (2001). *Code of ethics for nurses.* Retrieved July 22, 2009, from http://www.nursingworld.org/ethics/ecode.htm

Anderson, D. G., & Hatton, D. C. (2000). Accessing vulnerable populations for research. *Western Journal of Nursing Research, 22*(2), 244–251.

Batalden, P. B., & Davidoff, F. (2007). What is "quality improvement" and how can it transform healthcare? *Quality and Safety in Health Care, 16*(1), 2–3.

Benjamin, M., & Curtis, J. (1986). *Ethics in nursing* (2nd ed.). New York: Oxford University Press.

Birch, M., & Miller, T. (2002). Encouraging participation: Ethics and responsibilities. In M. Mauthner, M. Burch, J. Jessop, & T. Miller (Eds.), *Ethics in qualitative research* (pp. 91–106). London: Sage.

Borsay, A. (2009). Nursing history: An irrelevance for nursing practice? *Nursing History Review, 17*(1), 14–27.

Broyles, L. M., Tate, J. A., & Happ, M. B. (2008). Videorecording in clinical research: Mapping the ethical terrain. *Nursing Research, 57*(1), 59–63.

Cartwright, J. C., & Hickman, S. E. (2007, October). Conducting research in community-based care facilities: Ethical and regulatory implications. *Journal of Gerontological Nursing, 33*(10), 5–11.

Christians, C. G. (2003). Ethics and politics in qualitative research. In N. K. Denzin & Y. S. Lincoln (Eds.), *The landscape of qualitative research: Theories and issues* (2nd ed., pp. 208–244). Thousand Oaks, CA: Sage.

Cipriano Silva, M. (2006). Ethics of research. In J. Fitzpatrick & M. Wallace (Eds.), *Encyclopedia of nursing research* (2nd ed., pp. 177–180). New York: Springer.

Commission on Research Integrity. (1995). *Integrity and misconduct in research* (Department of Health and Human Services, Publication No. 1996–746–425). Washington, DC: U.S. Government Printing Office.

Conn, V. S. (2008). Staying true to the results. *Western Journal of Nursing Research, 30*(2), 161–162.

Council for International Organizations of Medical Sciences (CIOMS). (2002). *International ethics guidelines for biomedical research involving human subjects.* Retrieved March 3, 2006, from http://www.cioms.ch/guidelines_nov_2002_blurb.htm

Dally, A. (1998). Thalidomide: Was the tragedy preventable? *Lancet, 351*(9110), 1197–1199.

Deigh, J. (1995). Ethics. In R. Audi (Ed.), *The Cambridge Dictionary of Philosophy* (pp. 244–249). Cambridge, UK: Cambridge University Press.

Department of Health and Human Services (DHHS). (2005). *Protection of human subjects rule, 45 C.F.R. § 46.* Retrieved July 27, 2009, from http://www.hhs.gov/ohrp/humansubjects/guidance/45cfr46.htm

Driever, M. J., & Pranulis, M. F. (2003). New challenges for issues in clinical nursing research. *Western Journal of Nursing Research, 25*(8), 937–947.

Edwards, R., & Mauthner, M. (2002). Ethics and feminist research: Theory and practice. In M. Mauthner, M. Burch, J. Jessop, & T. Miller (Eds.), *Ethics in qualitative research* (pp. 14–31). London: Sage.

Ely, B., & Coleman, C. (2007). Recruitment and retention of children in longitudinal research. *Journal for Specialists in Pediatric Nursing, 12*(3), 199–202.

Erlen, J. A. (2005). HIPAA: Implications for research. *Orthopedic Nursing, 23*(2), 139–142.

Firby, P. (1995). Critiquing the ethical aspects of a study. *Nurse Researcher, 3*(1), 35–41.

Freda, M. C., & Kearney, M. H. (2005). Ethical issues faced by nursing editors. *Western Journal of Nursing Research, 27*(4), 487–499.

Grady, C. (2007). Quality improvement and ethical oversight. *Annals of Internal Medicine, 146*(9), 680–681.

Henley, S. J., & Dougherty, M. C. (2009). Quality of manuscript reviews in nursing research. *Nursing Outlook, 57*(1), 18–26.

Hume, D. (1751). *An enquiry concerning the principles of morals.* Oxford, UK: Oxford University Press.

Institute of Medicine (IOM). (1989). *The responsible conduct of research in the health sciences.* Washington, DC: National Academies Press.

International Council of Nurses (ICN). (2006). *The ICN code of ethics for nurses.* Retrieved July 22, 2009, from http://www.icn.ch/icncode.pdf

Jeffers, B. R. (2005). Research environments that promote integrity. *Nursing Research, 54*(91), 63–70.

Kant, I. (1785). Fundamental principles of the metaphysics of morals. In J. Rachels (1995), *The elements of moral philosophy* (2nd ed., pp. 107–131). New York: McGraw-Hill.

Ketefian, S., & Lenz, E. R. (1995). Promoting scientific integrity in nursing research. Part II: Strategies. *Journal of Professional Nursing, 11*(5), 263–269.

Kirk, S. (2007). Methodological and ethical issues in conducting qualitative research with children and young people: A literature review. *International Journal of Nursing Studies, 44*(7), 1250–1260.

Kunin, T. F. (1997). Ethical issues in longitudinal research with at-risk children and adolescents. Cited in A. J. Roberson (2007), Adolescent informed consent: Ethics, law, and theory to guide policy and nursing research. *Journal of Nursing Law, 11*(4), 191–196.

Lenz, E. R., & Ketefian, S. (1995). Promoting scientific integrity in nursing research. Part I: Current approaches in doctoral programs. *Journal of Professional Nursing, 11*(5), 213–219.

Lutz, K. F. (1999). Maintaining client safety and scientific integrity in research with battered women. *Image: Journal of Nursing Scholarship, 31*(1), 89–93.

Lynn, J., Baily, M. A., Bottrell, M., Jennings, B., Levine, R., Davidoff, F., et al. (2007). The ethics of using quality improvement methods in health care. *Annals of Internal Medicine, 146*(9), 666–673.

Macrina, F. L. (1995). *Scientific integrity: An introductory text with cases.* Washington, DC: ASM Press.

Mill, J. A. (1967). *Utilitarianism.* London: Longmans.

Miller, T., & Bell, L. (2002). Consenting to what? Issues of access, gate-keeping and informed consent. In M. Mauthner, M. Burch, J. Jessop, & T. Miller (Eds.), *Ethics in qualitative research* (pp. 53–69). London: Sage.

National Institutes of Health (NIH). (1979). *The Belmont report: Ethical principles and guidelines for the protection of human subjects of research.* Retrieved March 3, 2006, from http://www.nihtraining.com/ohsrsite/guidelines/belmont.html

Norman, R. (1998). *The moral philosophers: An introduction to ethics* (2nd ed.). Oxford, UK: Oxford University Press.

Perkins, E. (2001). Johns Hopkins tragedy: Could librarians have prevented a death? *Information Today, 18*(8), 51, 54. Retrieved July 27, 2009, from http://www.infotoday.com/newsbreaks/nb0108061.htm

Pilkington, F. B. (2002). Scientific merit and research ethics. *Nursing Science Quarterly, 15*(3), 196–200.

Public Health Service Act, 42 USC~163. (1988). Cited in D. L. Volker (2004), Methodological issues associated with studying an illegal act: Assisted dying. *Advances in Nursing Science, 27*(2), 117–128.

Rachels, J. (1995). *The elements of moral philosophy* (2nd ed.). New York: McGraw-Hill.

Redman, R. W. (2007). Knowledge development, quality improvement, and research ethics. *Research and Theory for Nursing Practice: An International Journal, 21*(4), 217–219.

Reich, W. T. (Ed.). (1995). *Encyclopedia of bioethics.* New York: Simon & Schuster Macmillan, pp. 2248–2259.

Roberson, A. J. (2007). Adolescent informed consent: Ethics, law, and theory to guide policy and nursing research. *Journal of Nursing Law, 11*(4), 191–196.

Rogers, B. (2005). Research with protected populations: Vulnerable participants. *AAOHN Journal, 53*(4), 156–157.

Ross, W. D. (1954). *Kant's ethical theory.* Oxford, UK: Oxford University Press.

Rothstein, W. G., & Phuong, L. H. (2007). Ethical attitudes of nurse, physician and unaffiliated members of institutional review boards. *Journal of Nursing Scholarship, 39*(1), 75–811.

Siedlecki, S. L. (2008). Making a difference through research. *AORN Journal, 88*(5), 716–729.

Tanner, C. A. (2006). Thinking like a nurse: A research-based model of clinical judgment in nursing. *Journal of Nursing Education, 45*(6), 204–211.

Thiroux. J. P. (1980). *Ethics, theory and practice.* Encino, CA: Glencoe.

Tschudin, V. (1992). *Ethics in nursing: The caring relationship.* Oxford, UK: Butterworth Heinemann.

Twycross, A., & Corlett, J. (2007). Challenges of setting up a multi-centered research study. *Nursing Standard, 21*(49), 35–38.

United Nations Organization. (2002). International covenant on civil and political rights, article 7. Universal declaration of human rights. In Council for International Organizations of Medical Sciences (CIOMS), *International ethics guidelines for biomedical research involving human subjects.* Retrieved March 3, 2006, from http://www.cioms.ch/guidelines_nov_2002_blurb.htm

Volker, D. L. (2004). Methodological issues associated with studying an illegal act: Assisted dying. *Advances in Nursing Science, 27*(2), 117–128.

Weaver, K. (2007). Ethical sensitivity: State of knowledge and needs for further research. *Nursing Ethics, 2*(4), 141–155.

Wood, A., Grady, C., & Emanuel, E. J. (2002). *The crisis in human participants research: Identifying the problems and proposing solutions.* Retrieved July 27, 2009, from http://bioethicsprint.bioethics.gov/background/emanuelpaper.html

World Medical Association (WMA). (1964–2004). *World Medical Association Declaration of Helsinki: Ethical principles for medical research involving human subjects.* Retrieved July 27, 2009, from http://www.wma.net/e/policy/b3.htm

Chapter 4

Problem Statement, Research Question, Hypothesis

Lucy B. Trice and Kathaleen C. Bloom

Chapter Objectives

At the conclusion of this chapter, the learner will be able to

1. Discuss processes involved in identifying a researchable problem in nursing practice
2. Write an effective problem statement
3. Discuss essential characteristics needed to pose a research question
4. Identify the criteria for establishing research variables
5. Contrast the various types of hypotheses
6. Explain the differences between conceptual and operational definitions
7. Critically evaluate research questions and hypotheses found in research reports for their contribution to the strength of evidence for nursing practice

Key Terms

➤ Associative hypothesis

➤ Categorical variable

➤ Causal hypothesis

➤ Complex hypothesis

➤ Confounding variable

➤ Continuous variable

➤ Demographic variable

➤ Dependent variable

➤ Dichotomous variable

➤ Directional hypothesis

➤ Discrete variable

➤ Extraneous variable

➤ Hypothesis

➤ Independent variable

➤ Nondirectional hypothesis

➤ Null hypothesis

➤ Problem statement

➤ Research hypothesis

➤ Research question

➤ Simple hypothesis

➤ Variable

Introduction

Every research study begins with a problem the researcher would like to solve. For such a problem to be researchable, it must be one that can be studied through collecting and analyzing data. Some problems, although interesting, are by their nature not appropriate research problems because they are not researchable. Problems involving moral or ethical issues are not researchable, as the solutions to these problems are based on an individual's values. For example, one could not research a question such as "Should marijuana use be legalized?" because the answer to the question depends on one's values rather than on a clearly right or wrong answer. This is not to say that marijuana use cannot be studied. One could study people's opinions regarding marijuana use. For example, one might ask the question, "Do cancer patients hold more favorable opinions regarding legalization of marijuana use than the general public?" The need to avoid moral/ethical questions as a research topic applies to both quantitative and qualitative studies.

Other factors influence whether a problem is researchable using quantitative methods. For a problem to be considered researchable by quantitative methods, the variables to be studied must be clearly defined and measurable. This clarity is necessary to apply statistical measures that will identify relationships among the variables. Qualitative studies are not subject to the same restriction, as the purpose of these studies is to describe in detail the phenomenon of interest as it is perceived by the study subjects. In other words, qualitative studies are descriptive in nature and are not concerned with relationships among variables.

Identifying Researchable Problems

There are a number of sources from which researchable problems can arise. Personal experience, whether as a healthcare professional or as a consumer of health care, is a rich source. For example, reviewing procedure manuals might raise the question, "Does one procedure for giving mouth care apply to all patients?" In considering such diverse groups of patients as those with endotracheal or nasogastric tubes in place; those with full-blown AIDS, often accompanied by buccal mucosal lesions; and cancer patients on chemotherapy, one might ask, "Does one size fit all, or should separate procedures be established for each case?" Thus, as Macnee and McCabe (2008) point out, practice experience is a major source for identifying gaps in knowledge that would benefit from research.

Burns and Grove (2007) suggest that the nursing literature could also be a valuable source for researchable problems, particularly for the novice researcher. For example, the researcher might identify a topic of interest and then review the nursing research literature to determine which kinds of studies have been done in that area. Seeing how other researchers have approached a problem can often spark new ideas or perhaps point to studies that would benefit from replication. In addition to offering such indirect assistance in the development of a problem statement, the research literature, including unpublished dissertations and theses as well as published research articles, provides direct assistance through specific suggestions for future research in the area. These suggestions may be offered under a special heading for future research, or they may be part of the discussion of the findings.

Polit and Beck (2008) contend that social issues often give rise to topics relevant to healthcare research. For example, the feminist movement raised questions about gender equity in health care and in healthcare research. The civil rights movement led to research on minority health problems in general and to explorations of the differences in effectiveness of medical treatment in different ethnic groups.

? Think Outside the Box

Using the following examples, develop problem statements, research questions, and/or hypotheses for each one. (1) Which information has been used to determine the method of catheterizing a laboring mother? (2) Which information serves as the basis for the range of blood sugars used within newly diagnosed elderly diabetics? (3) Which items need to be included into the formation of a problem statement, research question, and hypothesis?

Table 4-1		
Funding Priorities of NINR, 2006–2010		
1. Promoting health and preventing disease		
2. Improving quality of life		
3. Eliminating health disparities		
4. Setting directions for end-of-life research		
Source: NINR, n.d.		

The research priorities of the profession, and particularly of the funding bodies interested in healthcare research, are also a primary source for generating researchable problems. For example, the National Institute of Nursing Research (NINR, n.d.) has as its mission "to promote and improve the health of individuals, families, communities, and populations . . . across the lifespan" (p. 7). The priorities identified by the NINR reflect both the interests of the nursing profession and the interests of the major federal funding agency dedicated to nursing (**Table 4-1**). These priorities are updated on a regular basis and are published on the NINR Web site (http://www.ninr.nih.gov).

Determining Significance of the Problem

Once the problem of interest has been identified, before going any further the researcher must determine the significance of the problem to nursing as well as the feasibility of studying the problem. Significance refers to whether a problem is worth studying. A number of authors agree on the criteria that can be used to determine the significance of a problem to nursing (Burns & Grove, 2007; LoBiondo-Wood & Haber, 2006; Polit & Beck, 2008):

- Will nursing's stakeholders (patients, nurses, healthcare community) benefit from the findings of the study?
- Will the findings be applicable to practice, education, or administration?
- Will the findings extend or support current theory, or generate new theory?
- Will the findings support current nursing practice or provide evidence for changing current practice and/or policies?

Some authorities recommend that two additional criteria be considered when determining the significance of a problem:

■ Will the findings address nursing research priorities? (Burns & Grove, 2007)

■ Will the results of the proposed study build on previous findings? (Burns & Grove, 2007; Polit & Beck, 2008)

If the research problem does not meet the majority of these criteria, it should be reworked or, if that is not possible, simply abandoned. The single most important of these criteria is perhaps the first one: Will nursing's stakeholders (patients, nurses, healthcare community) benefit from the findings of the study? If this question cannot be answered with a resounding "yes," then the problem is probably not worth studying. Nursing is a discipline that takes pride in research aimed at benefiting patients and changing practice for the better. In the move to evidence-based practice (EBP), benefit to patients and applicability to practice—and especially support for current practice or evidence for changing current practice—are paramount in assessing the significance of a research problem. According to Farrell (2006), "Practices are sorely needed that are based on sound evidence" (p. 119).

Examining Feasibility of the Problem

Feasibility refers to whether the study can be done. It includes considerations such as cost of the study, availability of study subjects, time constraints, availability of facilities and equipment, cooperation of others, interest of the researcher, and expertise of the researcher (Burns & Grove, 2001, 2009; LoBiondo-Wood & Haber, 2006; Polit & Beck, 2008).

Cost

EBP has emerged from the desire of the majority of healthcare providers (both institutions and individuals) to do what is right for the patient and what will result in more good than harm (Craig & Smyth, 2002). The evidence for EBP is gathered through research (DiCenso, Guyatt, & Ciliska, 2005; Schmidt & Brown, 2009)—and all research studies cost money to some degree. It is the researcher's task to obtain support for the research from the institution in which it will be conducted as well as from potential funding bodies, both within the institution itself and in outside agencies. When seeking this support, the researcher must present a clear picture of the value of the research in terms of patient outcomes versus the costs involved. The current economic climate, which emphasizes the link between outcomes value and resources expenditure, demands nothing less (Malloch &

Porter-O'Grady, 2006). In the final analysis, the deciding factor with regard to feasibility of a particular study may be how much the study will cost versus the funds and other necessary support that are available to the researcher.

Availability of Subjects

The type and number of study subjects will vary depending on the purpose and design of the study. Larger numbers of participants are generally needed for quantitative studies if the findings are to be considered significant, whereas smaller numbers of subjects are appropriate for studies using a qualitative design. Clearly, a sufficient number of subjects must be available for the study to be feasible.

Time Constraints

Studies done in connection with the pursuit of academic degrees (e.g., research projects, theses, dissertations), of necessity, have a time frame for their completion. The same is true for studies supported by grant monies, as well as studies for which grant monies are being sought. For a study to be considered feasible, it must have the possibility of being completed within the applicable time constraints.

Availability of Facilities and Equipment

The need for special facilities and equipment can add greatly to the cost of a study. Although not all studies require specialized equipment or facilities, for those that do, both the cost and the availability of these items must be taken into consideration when determining the feasibility of the study.

Cooperation of Others

All studies require a certain amount of cooperation from others. The researcher may need referrals from others to obtain research subjects, for example, or to arrange for use of laboratories or other kinds of facilities. Student researchers in particular often need assistance with data entry in quantitative studies, data transcription in qualitative studies, and statistical analysis. These types of assistance are frequently offered to student researchers without a fee; however, obtaining the assistance requires cooperation from those providing these services. The study subjects themselves must also cooperate in a sense, if the data are to be collected in a timely manner. Thus cooperation of these important others is an essential ingredient of a feasible study. Securing that cooperation falls squarely on the shoulders of the researcher. In their discussion of obtaining cooperation from various others, Burns and Grove (2001) contend that researchers need to maintain objectivity throughout the course of the study, avoiding a tendency to take themselves too seriously; "a sense of humor is invaluable" (p. 426).

Interest of the Researcher

Conducting research, although often rewarding when the final results are in, is nevertheless hard work. To embark on a study that is not of fairly profound interest to the researcher is foolhardy at best, and at worst it can lead to failure to complete the study. If the researcher is not interested in doing the research, then carrying out the study is not generally feasible.

Expertise of the Researcher

Ideally, the researcher should have prior knowledge and experience in the field of study in question. This is not to say that a study would be considered infeasible solely because it is a new area of study for the researcher. Certainly, seasoned researchers frequently "branch out" into new areas of study. When less experienced researchers are involved, however, Polit and Beck (2008) caution that difficulties may arise in developing and carrying out a study on a topic that is totally new and/or unfamiliar.

Addressing Nursing Research Priorities

If the body of knowledge that deals with the practice of nursing is to be expanded, the major focus of nursing research should be on issues that influence patient outcomes. Further, it is through this type of research that we will gather the evidence to document the quality and effectiveness of nursing care (Moorhead, Johnson, Maas, & Swanson 2008). The specific areas of focus, in terms of patient outcomes, vary widely. As noted elsewhere, doing research can be costly in terms of dollars, so it behooves the researcher to attempt to match his or her research interests not only with those of the institution where the individual works, but also with the priorities established by funding agencies. The major federal funding agency dedicated to nursing is NINR. Other funding bodies with research priorities relevant to nursing include the Agency for Healthcare Research and Quality; private organizations such as the Kellogg Foundation and the Helene Fuld Health Trust; professional organizations such as the American Nurses Foundation and Sigma Theta Tau International; and nursing specialty organizations such as the Association of Perioperative

Registered Nurses and the American Association of Critical Care Nurses, to name a few. Taking care to address the funding priorities of a particular organization enhances the possibility of obtaining from that organization the funding needed to complete the research project.

Problem Statement

The problem statement presents the idea, issue, or situation that the researcher intends to examine in the study. The statement should be broad enough to cover the concern prompting the study, yet narrow enough to provide direction for designing the study. It can be conceptualized in the form of a declarative sentence or a question. In some cases, the term "research question" is used interchangeably with "problem statement."

? **Think Outside the Box**

Formulate a conceptual and operational definition for catheterization, laboring mother, blood sugar, and newly diagnosed elderly diabetic.

The problem statement is the foundation of the study, and as such is usually preceded by several paragraphs of background information that set the stage for the proposed study. These paragraphs identify the significance of the problem, present justification that the problem is researchable, and provide supporting documentation from the literature. This general discussion of the problem culminates in the problem statement. The problem statement is often further clarified by including the purpose and goal(s) of the study, all of which are derived from the problem statement.

Research Question

Although the terms "research question" and "problem statement" are sometimes used interchangeably, the research question is often more specific than the problem statement. Additionally, research questions (rather than hypotheses) are frequently used to guide studies that are exploratory in nature and aimed at describing variables or perhaps identifying differences between groups in relation to these variables. Research questions also guide studies that examine relationships among the variables being studied but do not test the nature of these relationships. Studies designed to test the nature of the relationships among variables are generally guided by hypotheses rather than research questions (Burns & Grove, 2009; Fain, 2004).

Research questions can be used to guide both quantitative and qualitative studies. Quantitative studies are often initiated to answer several questions derived from the problem of interest, each focused on a specific variable to be measured in the population. For example, McCaffrey, Ruknui, Hatthakit, and Kasetsomboon (2005) were interested in the effects of yoga on hypertension. Specifically, they were looking at the stress scores, blood pressure, and body mass index (BMI) of individuals who participated in yoga versus individuals who did not. The following research questions might be used to guide this study:

1. Does yoga affect the blood pressure in persons who practice yoga?
2. Does yoga affect the stress level in persons who practice yoga?
3. Does yoga affect the BMI in persons who practice yoga?

Each of these questions is narrowly focused, dealing with one independent variable (participation in yoga) and one of the dependent variables (blood pressure, stress, and BMI, respectively).

Qualitative studies, by their nature, explore phenomena about which little is known. Burns and Grove (2007) point out that the research questions guiding these types of studies are limited in number and generally broad in scope, and they include variables or concepts that are more complex than those guiding quantitative studies. For example, Gullick and Stainton (2008) investigated the living experience of chronic obstructive pulmonary disease (COPD) in individuals with severe emphysema. Using a qualitative approach (namely, phenomenology), they conducted in-depth interviews with 15 patients and 14 family members of those patients. The research question guiding this study might be stated as follows: What are the essential themes common to the experience of living with COPD among individuals with severe emphysema? The concepts in this question are much broader than those cited for the earlier quantitative example.

Components of the Problem Statement

A well-written problem statement for a quantitative study, whether written as a declarative statement or a question, has two components: the population of concern and the variable(s) to be studied. For example, a researcher might be interested in investigating the use of pet therapy in nursing home residents to increase morale. The population in this case would be nursing home residents. Depending on the specific concern under investigation, the researcher could also narrow the population by age (e.g., nursing home residents between the ages of 75 and 85 years) or other characteristics, such as the ability to follow simple directions (e.g., nursing home residents between the ages of 75 and 85 years who are able to follow simple directions). The variables of interest would be pet therapy and morale.

Strictly speaking, the term "variable" refers to measurable qualities or characteristics of people, things, or situations that can change, vary, or fluctuate. For example, blood pressure, pulse rate, anxiety level, and degree of pain are all characteristics of people that can vary from one person to another. The presence (or absence) of a parent in a hospitalized child's room during painful procedures is a situation that can vary from one hospitalized child to another. Variables are the foundation of quantitative studies; they constitute what is being studied in the designated population.

Researchers often want to know what causes or influences a particular phenomenon or, in some cases, what alleviates or diminishes that phenomenon. For example, one might want to know if a hospitalized child's anxiety level during a painful procedure would be lessened if a parent were present during the procedure. In this case, there are two variables of interest: the child's anxiety level and the presence of a parent during the painful procedure. The researcher is investigating the effect that the presence of a parent has on the child's anxiety level during a painful procedure. Because the variable "presence of a parent" is having an effect on the variable "child's anxiety level," it is termed the independent variable. By the same token, the variable being affected (i.e., child's anxiety level) is termed the dependent variable. In a study investigating more than one variable, the variable(s) that is (are) acting on, influencing, or causing an effect on the other variable(s) is (are) called the independent variable, and the variable(s) being acted on is (are) called the dependent variable(s) (Burns & Grove, 2009; LoBiondo-Wood & Haber, 2006; Polit & Beck, 2008).

Other types of variables that can affect the outcome of the study but are not the variables the researcher is investigating are referred to as extraneous variables. In the example cited earlier, the age of the child could affect his or her anxiety level, regardless of whether a parent is present in the room, and therefore would be considered an extraneous variable. The researcher could control for the variable of age by limiting the study population to a particular age group. Another variable that might affect the child's anxiety level, regardless of whether a parent is present in the room, is the nature of the painful procedure. The procedure could be specified to control for this variable. With any study, it is important to identify and control for extraneous variables; otherwise, the study results may be confusing and inaccurate.

Most studies have extraneous variables of one sort or another. It is important for the researcher to recognize and control for these variables, either in the study design or through statistical procedures, to preserve the validity of the study results. If a study cannot control for an extraneous variable, the variable is then termed a confounding variable.

The term "demographic variable" refers to characteristics of the subjects in the study. Data on these characteristics are usually collected during the study and are then used to describe the study group. Many different kinds of demographic information can be collected, including details about age, gender, ethnicity, educational level, marital status, and number of children. The types of demographic data collected depend on the purpose of the study; however, at a minimum, data on age, gender, and ethnicity should be gathered.

? Think Outside the Box

Why is it necessary to have a problem statement, research question, or hypothesis? What benefit does it provide? Is one better than others? Which restrictions arise related to the use of the problem statement, research question, or hypothesis?

If a variable can take on a wide range of values (from 0 to 100 or larger), it is often referred to as a continuous variable. A continuous variable is not limited to whole-number values. Examples of continuous variables include age, weight, salary, and blood pressure. In contrast, variables that can take on only a finite number of values, usually restricted to whole numbers, are referred to as discrete variables. For example, respiratory rate would be considered a discrete variable, as it can take on only whole-number equivalents; although variation in respiratory rate can occur from person to person, a finite number of these variations are compatible with life.

Categorical and dichotomous variables are similar because they represent characteristics that can be measured only in the sense that they are either present or not present. These kinds of variables are often assigned a number for identification, but the number does not represent a quantity. For example, ethnicity might be divided into white, African American, Hispanic, Native American, Pacific Islander, and Asian American, with each classification assigned an identifying number. The assigned number, however, would have no meaning other than identifying the occurrence of each race, perhaps to facilitate counting the number of occurrences of that particular race in the study. In this case, race would be considered a categorical variable, with each race included in the study representing a category. If only two categories are possible for a categorical variable, it may be referred to as a dichotomous variable. For example, gender is considered a dichotomous variable, as two categories are possible—male and female.

Writing the Problem Statement

As noted previously, problem statements for quantitative studies may be written in the form of a declarative statement or a question (**Table 4-2**). The two components that must be included in every problem statement are the population of interest and the variable(s) to be measured. For example, if we were interested in studying the effect of presence of a parent on anxiety level in children undergoing painful procedures, we might construct a problem statement in the form of a question: "Does the presence of a parent affect the anxiety level in children ages 3–5 years undergoing initiation of intravenous therapy?" Alternatively, the same problem could be stated as a declarative statement: "The presence of a parent affects the anxiety level in children ages 3–5 years undergoing initiation of intravenous therapy." Both statements contain a population of interest (children ages 3–5 years undergoing initiation of intravenous therapy) and two variables (presence of a parent—independent variable; anxiety level of the child—dependent variable). The only difference between the two is the form of the statement—one is presented as a question and the other as a declarative statement.

Table 4-2

Problem Statements	
Declarative Statement Format	**Question Format**
Music therapy affects the level of anxiety during cesarean section.	Does music therapy affect the level of anxiety during cesarean section?
There is a relationship between participation in pet therapy and attitude in nursing home residents.	Is there a relationship between participation in pet therapy and attitude in nursing home residents?
Peer support increases adherence to weight-loss diets in diabetic women.	Does peer support increase adherence to weight-loss diets in diabetic women?
There is a relationship between osteoporosis and self-esteem.	Is there a relationship between osteoporosis and self-esteem?
The number of medication errors made by nurses increases when the number of medications per patient is greater than three.	Does the number of medication errors made by nurses increase when the number of medications per patient is greater than three?

Hypotheses

A research question asks whether a relationship exists between variables in a particular population. In contrast, a hypothesis stipulates or predicts the relationship that exists. For example, if the research question is "Does the presence of a parent in the room affect the anxiety level in children ages 3–5 years undergoing initiation of intravenous therapy?", then we might develop several hypotheses:

1. The presence of a parent in the room affects the anxiety level in children ages 3–5 years who undergo initiation of intravenous therapy.
2. The presence of a parent in the room reduces the anxiety level in children ages 3–5 years who undergo initiation of intravenous therapy.
3. The presence of a parent in the room has no effect on the anxiety level in children ages 3–5 years who undergo initiation of intravenous therapy.
4. The presence of a parent in the room increases the anxiety level in children ages 3–5 years who undergo initiation of intravenous therapy.

The advantage of a hypothesis over a research question is that the hypothesis puts the question into a form that can be tested. It is the nature of hypotheses to predict relationships among or between variables. For a hypothesis to be testable, it must stipulate a relationship between at least two variables in a given population.

Within EBP, the research question format incorporates the population of interest, the intervention, a comparison of interest, outcomes, and timing to ensure clarity of the subject. This process can also be applied to developing one or more hypotheses for a research study. Each hypothesis should contain the population of interest, the independent variable(s), the dependent variable(s), and the comparison of interest, all of which should lead to the outcome of the study.

Hypotheses and Qualitative Studies

Hypotheses are used in quantitative studies but are not appropriate for qualitative studies. By their nature, they present the researcher's opinion in the form of a prediction about the outcome of the study. In qualitative studies, however, researchers focus on the viewpoints of the subjects participating in the study rather than on their own. Thus the participants' viewpoints, rather than the researcher's hypothesis, guide the qualitative study. Generally, the purpose of qualitative studies is to explore new concepts and ideas about which little is known, or to discover new meanings for concepts. In keeping with this purpose, researchers using qualitative methods take great care to set aside their preconceived notions about the phenomena under investigation. A hypothesis would be a disadvantage in a qualitative study, because it would predict the outcome of the study and potentially bias the results. Thus, while qualitative studies may generate hypotheses that can then be tested using quantitative methods, they are not themselves guided by research hypotheses.

Types of Hypotheses

A testable hypothesis, also called the research hypothesis, predicts the relationship between two or more variables in a population of interest. All four of the hypotheses in the previous example could be considered testable.

Hypotheses may be directional, nondirectional, or null:

▪ A directional hypothesis predicts the path or direction the relationship will take. In the preceding example, both hypothesis 2 and hypothesis 4 are directional hypotheses. Hypothesis 2 predicts a decrease in anxiety with the presence of a parent, and hypothesis 4 predicts an increase in anxiety with the presence of a parent.
▪ A nondirectional hypothesis predicts a relationship but not the path or direction of the relationship. Hypothesis 1 in the previous example is a nondirectional hypothesis; it states that the presence of a parent affects the anxiety level in children ages 3–5 years but does not stipulate the direction of the effect.
▪ A null hypothesis, also called a statistical hypothesis, predicts that no relationship exists among or between the variables in the study. When inferential statistics are used to analyze data, the assumption is that the null hypothesis is actually being tested. Because this is understood, many researchers do not state the null hypothesis when reporting their findings in the literature. In the previous example, hypothesis 3 is stated in the null form.

Hypotheses may also be classified as simple or complex: A simple hypothesis specifies the relationship between two variables, whereas a complex hypothesis specifies the relationships between and among more than two variables. In the previous example, all four of the hypotheses could be classified as simple hypotheses. In each case, there are only two variables—the presence of a parent and the anxiety level in children ages 3–5 years. An example of a complex hypothesis might be "Religious beliefs, presence of social support, and ethnic background affect the perception of pain in patients who are terminally ill with cancer." Here there are four variables—religious beliefs, the presence of social support, ethnic background, and perception of pain. Complex hypotheses may also be termed multivariate hypotheses for the simple reason that they contain more than two variables.

? Think Outside the Box

Describe a problem in which a null hypothesis would be used and state the null hypothesis.

In addition, hypotheses may be categorized as associative or causal. These terms reflect the relationship between or among the variables in the hypothesis. For example, in an associative hypothesis, the hypothesis is stated in a way indicating that the variables exist side by side, and that a change in one variable is accompanied by a change in another. However, there is no suggestion that a change in one variable causes a change in another—merely that the variables change in association with each other (Reynolds, 1971).

In contrast, a causal hypothesis is stated in a way indicating that one variable causes or brings about a change in one or more other variables (Burns & Grove, 2009). As one might expect, the variable inducing the change is referred to as the independent variable, and the variable being changed is the dependent variable. Causal hypotheses may also be called directional hypotheses. Continuing with the example of the presence of a parent in the room with a child during a painful procedure and its effect on the child's anxiety level, two of the hypotheses can be termed causal—hypothesis 2 and hypothesis 4. Hypothesis 2 predicts a decrease in anxiety (dependent variable) with the presence of a parent in the room (independent variable), and hypothesis 4 predicts an increase in anxiety (dependent variable) with the presence of a parent in the room (independent variable).

Defining Variables for the Study

The variables to be studied in quantitative research projects are generally defined in two ways—conceptually and operationally. The conceptual definition is a broad, more abstract definition that is generally drawn from relevant literature, particularly the theoretical literature; the researcher's clinical experience; or, in some cases, a combination of these sources. The conceptual definition is similar to a dictionary definition in that it provides the general meaning associated with the variable, but it is more in-depth and broader in scope. Although considered the starting point, conceptual definitions rarely give direction regarding how the variable will actually be measured for the study. The operational definition, by contrast, stipulates precisely how the variable will be measured, including which tools will be used, if applicable. If a conceptual definition is abstract, an operational definition is concrete. This concreteness is necessary to allow for precise measurement of the variable(s) of interest in the study.

Evidence-Based Practice Considerations

Stommel and Wills (2004) point out that the ability to apply research findings to practice is an expected competency of advanced practice nurses. However, if we accept that it is the desire of all practitioners of nursing to provide "only that care that makes a positive difference in the lives of those whom they serve" (Porter-O'Grady, 2006, p. 1), then it is clear that all professional nurses—from the new graduate to the seasoned veteran—should have the ability to apply research findings to practice. Inherent in this ability is an understanding of how the research process unfolds and what constitutes good research.

Further, Melnyk and Fineout-Overholt (2005) maintain that "the goal of EBP is to use the highest quality of [research] knowledge in providing care to produce the greatest impact on patients' health status" (p. 75). To accomplish this, practitioners—and particularly staff nurses who are at the bedside caring for patients on a daily basis—must have the tools to critically analyze research so as to make appropriate EBP decisions. To critically analyze research, these staff nurses must possess a working knowledge of the language of research; recognize a researchable problem statement; distinguish between and among variables, identifying independent versus dependent variables; determine the population of interest; and above all, recognize a well-conducted study, one whose findings are worth consideration for applying to practice. In its purest and best form, EBP happens at the bedside. The burden of implementation rests squarely on the shoulders of the staff nurse.

For more information on EBP, visit the following site: http://nursing.asu.edu/caep/resources/index.htm.

Summary Points

1. Every study begins with a problem the researcher would like to solve.
2. There are many sources for researchable problems, including personal experience, the nursing literature, social issues, and the research priorities of funding bodies.

3. The significance of the problem to nursing and the feasibility of studying the problem are important aspects to consider before embarking on any research project.
4. The problem statement presents the issue or situation to be examined and should identify the population of interest as well as the variables that will be studied.
5. Variables may be classified in a variety of ways: (a) independent versus dependent, (b) continuous versus discrete, (c) extraneous, (d) confounding, (e) categorical, and (f) dichotomous.
6. The problem statement may be written as a question or as a declarative sentence.
7. Hypotheses predict the relationship between or among variables.
8. Hypotheses may take many forms: (a) directional versus nondirectional, (b) simple versus complex, (c) associative versus causal, and (d) null.
9. Variables to be studied are generally defined both conceptually and operationally.
10. For nurses to pursue evidence-based practice, they must understand the research process and all of its components.

RED FLAGS

- Quantitative studies address research problems, research questions, and/or hypotheses.
- Qualitative studies do not use hypotheses, but rather explore research problems and research questions. If a qualitative study discusses a hypothesis, thought should be given to its focus and validity.
- A hypothesis must have at least one independent variable and one dependent variable; it is usually stated in a declarative statement format rather than as a question.
- Key variables within a study should have at least the operational definition provided for consideration.

Multiple Choice Questions

1. Most research studies begin with

    A. An investigation of social injustices.

    B. An examination of the National Institute of Nursing Research's funding priorities.

    C. A problem the researcher would like to solve.

    D. An interest in health disparities.

2. To be considered researchable, a problem

    A. Should include an ethical dimension.

    B. Must deal with patient outcomes rather than social issues.

    C. Has to be clearly defined.

    D. Must be amenable to study by collecting and analyzing data.

3. Which of the following questions is important to ask when determining the significance of the research problem?

    A. What will it cost to complete the study?

    B. Is there an available pool of subjects?

    C. Does the researcher have the necessary expertise?

    D. Will the findings be applicable to nursing practice?

4. Which of the following elements would be inappropriate in a researchable problem?

    A. An ethical issue

    B. A population divided by race

    C. More than one variable

    D. Clear definitions for all components

5. Which of the following best represents a well-constructed problem statement?

    A. Does peer pressure affect the use of tobacco in adolescent females?

    B. What affects pain perception in the hospital?

    C. This study will examine the relative efficacy of injectable versus oral pain medication.

    D. Do cancer patients ever feel lonely?

6. What are the two essential parts of the research problem statement?

    A. The problem and the outcome

    B. The variable and the population

    C. The theory and the concepts

    D. The intervention and the outcome

7. Your problem statement is "In the hospital setting, the presence of social support from family affects the pain perception of patients with spinal cord injury." Which of the following is (are) the dependent variable(s)?

    A. Type of spinal cord injury
    B. Social support from family and pain perception
    C. Social support from family
    D. Pain perception

8. Your hypothesis is "Nursing home residents ages 65–90 years who have Alzheimer's disease die at an earlier age than those who do not have Alzheimer's disease." Which answer best represents the independent variable?

    A. Age at death
    B. Having Alzheimer's disease
    C. Dying at an early age
    D. Living in a nursing home

9. What is a confounding variable?

    A. A variable that describes the characteristics of the study subjects
    B. A variable that can take on a wide range of values
    C. A variable restricted to whole-number values
    D. An extraneous variable that cannot be controlled

10. Which of the following best represents a categorical variable?

    A. Ethnic origin
    B. Age at death
    C. Systolic blood pressure
    D. Weight

11. The research question is "Does music therapy increase satisfaction during cesarean delivery?" Which of the following best represents a null hypothesis drawn from this research question?

    A. Music therapy affects satisfaction during cesarean delivery.
    B. Music therapy is not related to satisfaction during cesarean delivery.
    C. Music therapy increases satisfaction during cesarean delivery.
    D. Music therapy decreases satisfaction during cesarean delivery.

12. Which of the following hypotheses represents a complex hypothesis?

    A. Music therapy affects satisfaction during cesarean delivery.
    B. Patients with spinal cord injuries who have regular support from family members experience fewer symptoms of dysreflexia.
    C. Social support, balanced diet, and regular exercise decrease the incidence of postpartum depression.
    D. Exposure to pet therapy increases appetite in elderly patients.

13. Which of the following statements best describes the difference between a research question and a hypothesis?

A. One is a declarative sentence; the other is a question.
B. One questions a relationship; the other predicts a relationship.
C. One assumes a relationship; the other denies that one exists.
D. One is researchable; the other is statistical.

14. Which of the following pairs of hypotheses are similar to each other?

A. Simple and complex
B. Associative and causal
C. Directional and causal
D. Null and complex

Both predict that one variable brings about a change in another variable

15. A conceptual definition of a variable is one that is

A. Broad and abstract.
B. Narrow and abstract.
C. Concrete and continuous.
D. Narrow and concrete.

Discussion Questions

1. You are a nurse who works in a primary care clinic that treats patients with chronic diseases. Many of the elderly patients have diabetes, and you have noticed that some of them have more difficulty following their medical regimens than other patients. You want to develop a research study to investigate this problem. How would you go about doing so? What would be a possible problem statement?

2. You are a BSN student enrolled in a research course. The instructor has given you the following problem statement: "Do dietary knowledge and eating habits affect participation in regular exercise among hypertensive adult women?" Develop four hypotheses that might be drawn from this problem statement: a null hypothesis, a directional hypothesis, a non-directional hypothesis, and an associative hypothesis. Can all of these hypotheses be developed? If any of them cannot be developed, why not?

3. Read the following abstract and then provide the following information:
   A. Identify the population of interest.
   B. Identify the variables.
   C. Construct a research question that could have guided this study.
   D. Construct a null hypothesis.
   E. Construct a directional hypothesis.

   Abstract: To compare patients with diabetes and new-onset foot ulcers treated in Veterans Health Administration (VHA) and non-VHA settings.

   Methods: The treatment of patients with new-onset diabetic foot ulcers was prospectively monitored in three VHA and three non-VHA hospitals and outpatient settings until ulcer healing, amputation, or death.

   Results: Of the 302 individuals enrolled in this study, 47% were veterans receiving VHA care. There were no significant differences between veterans and nonveterans in terms of baseline wound classification, diabetes severity, or comorbid conditions. Veterans received significantly fewer sharp debridements, total-contact casts, and custom inserts than their nonveteran counterparts, and they had significantly more X-rays, local saline irrigations, IV antibiotics, and prescriptions for bed rest. The percentage of amputations was higher in veterans but did not achieve statistical significance.

   Conclusions: Many commonly held stereotypes of veteran men were not found. Veterans and nonveterans with foot ulcers were similar in terms of health and foot history, diabetes severity, and comorbid conditions. There was considerable variation in treatment of diabetic foot ulcers between VHA care and non-VHA care, yet this variation did not result in statistically significant differences in ulcer outcomes (Reiber et al., 2001).

Suggested Readings

Beitz, J. (2006). Writing the researchable question. *Journal of Wound, Ostomy, & Continence Nursing, 33*(2), 122–124.

Fineout-Overholt, E., Melnyk, B., & Schultz, A. (2005). Transforming health care from the inside out: Advancing evidence-based practice in the 21st century. *Journal of Professional Nursing, 21*(6), 335–344.

Hudson-Barr, D. (2005). From research idea to research question: The who, what, where, when and why. *Journal for Specialists in Pediatric Nursing, 10*(2), 90–92.

Law, R. (2004). From research topic to research question: A challenging process. *Nurse Researcher, 11*(4), 54–66.

Library of Washington. (n.d.). *The basics in research 101.* Retrieved June 29, 2009, from http://www.lib.washington.edu/uwill/research101 /basic03.htm

References

Burns, N., & Grove, S. K. (2001). *The practice of nursing research: Conduct, critique, and utilization* (4th ed.). Philadelphia: W. B. Saunders.

Burns, N., & Grove, S. K. (2007). *Understanding nursing research: Building an evidence-based practice* (4th ed.). Philadelphia: W. B. Saunders.

Burns, N., & Grove, S. K. (2009). *The practice of nursing research: Appraisal, synthesis, and generation of evidence* (6th ed.). Philadelphia: W. B. Saunders.

Craig, J. V., & Smyth, R. L. (2002). *The evidence-based practice manual for nurses.* London: Churchill Livingstone.

DiCenso, A., Guyatt, G., & Ciliska, D. (2005). *Evidence-based nursing: A guide to clinical practice.* St. Louis, MO: Mosby.

Fain, J. A. (2004). *Reading, understanding, and applying nursing research* (2nd ed.). Philadelphia: F. A. Davis.

Farrell, M. P. (2006). Living evidence: Translating research into practice. In K. Malloch & T. Porter-O'Grady (Eds.), *Introduction to evidence-based practice in nursing and health care* (pp. 107–124). Sudbury, MA: Jones and Bartlett.

Gullick, J., & Stainton, M. C. (2008). Living with chronic obstructive pulmonary disease: Developing conscious body management in a shrinking life-world. *Journal of Advanced Nursing, 64*(6), 605–614.

LoBiondo-Wood, G., & Haber, J. (2006). *Nursing research: Methods and critical appraisal for evidence-based practice* (6th ed.). St. Louis, MO: Mosby.

Macnee, C. L., & McCabe, S. (2008). *Understanding nursing research: Reading and using research in evidence-based practice* (2nd ed.). Philadelphia: Lippincott Williams & Wilkins.

Malloch, K., & Porter-O'Grady, T. (2006). *Introduction to evidence-based practice in nursing and health care.* Sudbury, MA: Jones and Bartlett.

McCaffrey, R., Ruknui, P., Hatthakit, U., & Kasetsomboon, P. (2005). The effects of yoga on hypertensive persons in Thailand. *Holistic Nursing Practice, 19*(4), 173–180.

Melnyk, B. M., & Fineout-Overholt, E. (2005). *Evidence-based practice in nursing and healthcare: A guide to best practice.* Philadelphia: Lippincott Williams & Wilkins.

Moorhead, S., Johnson, M., Maas, M., & Swanson, E. (2008). *Nursing outcomes classification (NOC)* (4th ed.). St. Louis, MO: Mosby.

National Institute of Nursing Research (NINR). (n.d.). NINR mission. Retrieved June 29, 2009, from http://www.ninr.nih.gov/AboutNINR/NINRMissionand StrategicPlan

Polit, D., & Beck, C. (2008). *Nursing research: Generating and assessing evidence for nursing practice* (8th ed.). Philadelphia: Lippincott Williams & Wilkins.

Porter-O'Grady, T. (2006). A new age for practice: Creating the framework for evidence. In K. Malloch & T. Porter-O'Grady (Eds.), *Introduction to evidence-based practice in nursing and health care* (pp. 1–29). Sudbury, MA: Jones and Bartlett.

Reiber, G., Smith, D., Carter, J., Fotieo, G., Deery, H., Sangeorzan, J., et al. (2001). A comparison of diabetic foot ulcer patients managed in VHA and non-VHA settings. *Journal of Rehabilitation Research & Development, 38*(3), 309–317.

Reynolds, P. (1971). *A primer in theory construction.* Indianapolis, IN: Bobbs-Merrill.

Schmidt, N. A., & Brown, J. M. (2009). *Evidence-based practice for nurses: Appraisal and application of research.* Sudbury, MA: Jones and Bartlett.

Stommel, M., & Wills, C. (2004). *Clinical research: Concepts and principles for advanced practice nurses.* Philadelphia: Lippincott Williams & Wilkins.

Chapter 5

Literature Review: Searching and Writing the Evidence

Dorothy Greene Jackson

Chapter Objectives

At the conclusion of this chapter, the learner will be able to

1. Define the concept of literature review
2. Discuss the purpose of a literature review
3. Recognize the importance of collaboration with a library specialist
4. Relate the literature review to the research process
5. Identify steps for conducting a literature review using electronic retrieval methods
6. Differentiate research articles from non-research articles
7. Identify guidelines for evaluating research articles
8. Identify steps for writing a literature review
9. Relate the literature review to evidence-based nursing practice

Key Terms

➤ Database

➤ Literature review

➤ Research article

➤ Search engine

Introduction

This chapter provides practical guidelines for conducting and writing a literature review for an evidence-based proposal in nursing. Guidelines and tips are given for selecting appropriate databases for electronic retrieval of research review articles. Steps are given for the process of writing and organizing data based on evidence and issues in nursing practice.

Definition and Purpose of the Literature Review

The literature review is a written, analytic summary of research findings on a topic of interest. It is a comprehensive compilation of what is known about the phenomenon. The review is guided by the researcher's curiosity about a particular subject and gaps in the knowledge about the subject area.

The literature review is intended to assess the evidence regarding the research topic by identifying and synthesizing studies that examine the subject of interest. The main purpose of the literature review is to identify what is known and unknown about an area that has not been totally resolved in practice. A second purpose is to determine how an issue can be resolved and managed based on research evidence. The literature review provides the background and the context within which the research is conducted. It lays out the foundation of the study. Specifically, a good review of the literature does the following:

- Identifies a research problem and indicates how it can be studied
- Helps clarify and determine the importance of a research problem
- Identifies what is known about a problem and identifies gaps (what is unknown) in a particular area of knowledge
- Provides examples based on documented studies for resolving a nursing issue
- Provides evidence that a problem is of importance
- Identifies theoretical frameworks and conceptual models for organizing and conducting research studies
- Identifies experts in the field of interest
- Identifies research designs and methodologies for conducting like studies
- Provides a context for interpretation, comparison, and critique of study findings (Norwood, 2000; Polit & Beck, 2008)

The Literature Review and the Research Process

The literature review usually happens early during the research process. In qualitative research, however, this step may come at the end of the study. Initially, the researcher has a hunch or curiosity about something observed in practice. Soon this idea is translated into a research problem or research question. Shortly thereafter, the review of the literature is conducted to see what has happened in other situations where the problem has occurred. In terms of its placement in a research article, the review of the literature usually follows the statement of the research problem or the research question.

The reason the review comes early in the research process is because it sets the stage (lays the foundation) for the rest of the study. As mentioned earlier, the review of the literature provides the theoretical framework for how the current study will be structured, helps to frame the research question into a research hypothesis, and identifies what will be studied and measured in the study.

For example, suppose there is a unit in a local 340-bed hospital in which no nurse has resigned or left the staff in 15 years. This unit exists in a setting where the nursing shortage is rampant and the attrition rate is at an all-time high. A newly hired nursing administrator becomes curious about this unit. She calls the director of the unit to visit and discuss the reason turnover is so low on this unit. From the conversations with several other staff members of this unit, the administrator formulates in her mind the theory that a good manager is the most important link to the low attrition rate on the unit. Although a low attrition rate does not seem to be a problem requiring research, this idea can be translated so that some insight is gained to answer the administrator's question, "Is the staff's perception of the nurse manager associated with the attrition or retention rate on a unit?" Searching the literature for studies about managers and retention or attrition can further illuminate this research question. The literature review may then describe what has been found to be true from other similar settings by conducting a survey of nurses who have worked in the same facility or unit for at least 15 years. The new administrator could use this survey or questionnaire to conduct a small research study on her hospital's unit.

This hypothetical example illustrates the importance of the literature review and demonstrates how it fits within the rest of the research process. The idea for the study came from the review of the literature.

Differentiating a Research Article from a Non-Research Article

Many good sources of very valuable information that may contribute to nursing practice exist. However, for the purposes of illuminating the value of evidence-based knowledge, this chapter focuses on data from original research. Oftentimes it is difficult to locate original research, especially when little research has been published in a particular area. If that is the case, the lack of previous studies serves as an opportunity, as it can stimulate the development of research data for that particular issue.

The importance of research derives from the fact that it has been conducted using a consistently acceptable scientific method known and respected by the research world. It is not just someone's opinion, but rather has been examined critically. Research articles consistently contain components that are required by a scientific decision-making process. Table 5-1 describes components of a research article.

Sometimes it is easy to choose non-research information for conducting research. For example, reports from state agencies, various nursing organizations, or Web sites may present information that is very important to a body of knowledge, yet has not been critically

---

Table 5-1

Components of a Research Article

- **Title:** The title describes what the study was about.
- **Abstract:** The abstract is a brief summary of the problem of interest to the researcher. It describes, in approximately 120 words, what took place in the research study and makes a brief statement about the outcome. It helps to determine relevance to the reader who is conducting a search of the literature.
- **Introduction/literature review:** This component gives the background of the research topic and explains why it is important, based on a selective review of relevant literature. It compares and contrasts other research articles and summarizes what is already known and not known about the topic.
- **Purpose of the study/hypothesis/problem statement:** The purpose explains the aim of the study. It is the hypothesis or the research question that the author wants to answer or support.
- **Methodology/procedures/research design:** This component tells what happened. It describes in detail what actions the author took to carry out the study. The method describes the procedure for how the research was conducted and how the information was analyzed or statistical testing was done. It also describes the population, including how it was selected; the setting where the research took place; the number of participants in the study; the type of study, either qualitative or quantitative; and the tools used to collect the data or the method used to attain the information in the study.
- **Major findings/results/analysis/discussion:** This component describes the outcome of the study.
- **Summary/conclusion/ideas for future studies/implications:** This component highlights major findings of the study and identifies the gaps in the study or any areas that need further research. Recommendations for policy or practice are discussed in this section.
- **Works cited/references/acknowledgments:** The reference list should be organized in a recognized literary format (such as APA) or other recognized reference formats.

examined in a research study. Some nationally conducted surveys may provide very important information, but may not be considered true research because not all the people in a particular population were included or not enough people returned the surveys. Unless all of the critical components are incorporated in the research process, the information obtained in the investigation should not be considered research. In addition, searching the literature is not considered research, but rather a mechanism for providing background information for the research project.

Conducting a Literature Review Search

The guidelines presented in this section of the chapter are targeted toward the novice researcher. It is advised that the student researcher seek the help of a professional librarian at the beginning of a research project and throughout the research process when it is necessary to access comprehensive information from appropriate sources. Most literature searches can be done by electronic retrieval. Researchers can find most of the material they need from doing their own personal searches; however, the most comprehensive searches are done with the help of professional library personnel. Many librarians are credentialed or specially trained in working with particular databases or particular aspects of data management and retrieval.

? Think Outside the Box

In your current clinical setting, which types of evidence materials are used as the foundation of policies? Discuss the appropriateness and effectiveness of these types of evidence.

Some of the special types of librarians include research, law, medical, government documents, and consumer health librarians. Many librarians play an integral role in research. Nurses should consider their own expertise when starting a research project or conducting research literature reviews.

The Importance of Library Specialists in Conducting a Literature Review

Finding pertinent articles that deal with the topic at hand may be a complex task and may require the expertise of a research librarian. Librarians are able to assist users at finding information in a timely manner. As a result of their education, training, and experience, they are well versed on the databases, including the way in which the information is catalogued and organized and the terminology needed to retrieve the information that is most relevant to the user. Their specialized knowledge may help the user conduct a more comprehensive search from multiple sources. Librarians' search expertise makes them highly skilled at weeding out irrelevant documents that otherwise might inundate the user and cause the researcher to spend unnecessary time chasing down blind alleys.

Nevertheless, with the advancement of the electronic library, conducting a search is much easier for the beginning researcher than ever before. With a little help from expert information specialists (librarians) and guidance from a good mentor, the beginning researcher can conduct literature searches and write a literature review that provides evidence supporting a meaningful research proposal or project.

The Research Idea

The first step in conducting a literature review is brainstorming about an idea or an area of interest. The nurse's practice area is probably one of the most common sources for a research idea in the nursing field. Important issues in nursing provide sage ideas for research. For example, the nursing shortage, the cost of health care, the quality of care for uninsured persons, and nursing education changes are all broad areas that may generate a researchable topic. Ideas may also come from reading professional journals or from the news media.

In addition, articles in professional journals may end with the phrase, "additional research is needed to explore the nature of. . . ." Here is a snapshot of one such article: "More research is needed on how organizational structures influence empowerment of leaders" (Force, 2005, p. 341). In this example from an article on the relationship of managers and nurse retention, the author sets forth an idea for further research. Oftentimes, the conclusion of an article marks the starting point for other research ideas.

The Research Question

Most nurses have a hunch or curiosity about some aspect of nursing science or patient care. It is helpful to formulate that idea into a question that, if answered, would contribute to the field of nursing. Formulation of a research question is covered in another section of this textbook. For the purposes of this chapter, asking a simple question based on the area of interest helps the novice researcher focus on topics and key concepts for conducting the literature search. For example, the student researcher may be curious about how long it takes the new baccalaureate-prepared nurse graduate to feel comfortable on the job. A possible question could be, "What is the role transition time for baccalaureate-prepared nurse graduates in management positions in a small hospital?"

Reading is another very important source of research ideas. In the article cited earlier, the author suggested that more research should be conducted to explore how organizational structure can influence nurse retention. The author implied that there is a gap in the literature about this idea or that more should be known about this idea. Because the focus of the article was nurse retention, examples of questions stemming from that need could be "What is the impact of the organizational structure on nurse retention?" and "What is the relationship between nurses' perception of empowerment and retention?" Of course, after undertaking further reading, the researcher may have different ideas. Thus the research question does not need to be etched in stone.

Forming an initial question is a good place to start the process of conducting the literature review search. To start the research, it is important to distinguish between databases and search engines.

Definition of Database

It is appropriate at this time to define a database and to indicate how it is different from a search engine. Let's start by saying that Google is a search engine and MEDLINE is a database. "A search engine is a collection of software programs that collect information from the Web, index it, and put it in a database so it can be searched" (Ackerman & Hartman, 2003, p. 47). The job of a search engine is to retrieve the information in a format that is accessible visually on screen at an on-site library or in downloadable, readable (full-text) written format.

In contrast, a database is an organized body of related information arranged for speed of access and retrieval ("Database," 2000; Princeton University, 2003). A database is a storage location, like a library, where information is stored, catalogued, maintained, and updated systematically.

Two main types of databases are available—bibliographic and full text. Bibliographic databases give directions on where to find the information, whereas full-text databases contain the information itself. In other words, the full-text type of database contains the article itself in a downloadable format. In recent years, more major databases have added an increased number of full-text capabilities.

Databases Useful to Nursing

The two most useful databases for nursing literature are Medical Literature Analysis and Retrieval System Online (MEDLINE®) and the Cumulative Index to Nursing & Allied Health Literature (CINAHL®) (Table 5-2). MEDLINE provides literature related to medicine, nursing, and dentistry. The focus of information in MEDLINE is biomedicine, but this database also contains the citations that are provided in CINAHL. The CINAHL database provides authoritative coverage of the literature related to nursing and allied health.

The MEDLINE database is generally considered the premier bibliographic database for providing access to the North American biomedical literature. It stores and indexes more than 4,500 journals published in more than 70 countries. The database is probably updated more frequently than any other database of its type—daily, Monday through Friday (National Library of Medicine [NLM], 1993–2006). The NLM Web site (www.nlm.nih.gov), which contains nursing and medical citations, can be accessed free of charge from the Internet. In other words, library privileges are not required, only access to the Internet. Thus this Web site is an excellent place to start a literature search.

The MEDLINE database uses a controlled vocabulary. This means that information is catalogued according to specific words or subject headings as in a dictionary. Although most people start searches using key words, this type of search does not yield the most comprehensive results. The dictionary for finding the words that most appropriately define or match the search term or concept in MEDLINE is the Medical Subject Heading (MeSH) database guide. This feature can be accessed from the NLM/PubMed Web site, adjacent to the left search boxes in most cases. PubMed is a service of the NLM that includes more than 16 million citations from MEDLINE and other life science journals dating back to the 1950s. PubMed includes links to full-text articles and other related resources (NLM).

Table 5-2
Databases Useful in Nursing
Medical Literature Analysis and Retrieval System Online (MEDLINE®)
Cumulative Index to Nursing & Allied Health Literature (CINAHL®)
Cochrane Library
Nursing & Health Sciences: A Sage Full-Text Collection
Nursing Journals (Proquest Nursing Journals)
Test and measurement databases, theses, and dissertations
PsycINFO
AID Search

This example illustrates the difference between a key word search and a subject heading search. The key words "patient visitation" might be used to locate journal articles focusing on how nurses perceive open visitation in intensive care units. When the term "patient visitation" was used to search in MEDLINE, 142 citations were retrieved (at the time of this book's writing). When the subject or controlled vocabulary term found in the MeSH database guide (dictionary) was used ("visitors to patients"), 1,278 citations were located. Knowing how a database stores information is very important in conducting effective and relevant searches. Using dates, types of nursing units, or other strategies can narrow this search.

CINAHL is probably the most popular database used by nurses. It indexes more than 1,800 journals and more than 25,000 full-text articles from 1982 to the present (CINAHL Information Systems, 2005). CINAHL houses nursing publications, including the *American Journal of Nursing* and the publications of the National League for Nursing. It also indexes journals in the allied health fields related to physical therapy, occupational therapy, cardiopulmonary technology, emergency service, physician assistant health education, radiology technology, medical laboratory technology, medical records, surgical technology, and medical assistants. Other selected journals related to biomedicine, consumer health, and librarianship health sciences are included as well (CINAHL Information Systems, 2005).

CINAHL publications can be searched using the EBSCOhost® and Ovid and are available for use only through a library. EBSCOhost provides approximately 200 full-text and secondary databases (EBSCO Publishing, 2006). It accesses databases in business, medical, public, and nursing publications.

Just as in MEDLINE, records in CINAHL are indexed by a controlled vocabulary or subject headings. Subject headings provide descriptors of the terms listed in the database. Searching by the terms or subjects used in the database yields results that are more relevant to the topic being searched. Subject headings can be viewed by clicking the CINAHL Headings button on the EBSCOhost toolbar. To begin the search, the subject heading term should be entered in the Find field. Searches using this tool can also be done by using key words. The EBSCOhost system matches articles with appropriate subject terms by a process called mapping.

CINAHL can also be accessed using the Journals@Ovid Full Text database. This database contains research articles, book and media reviews, and full-text nursing articles. Information in this database is searched by using key words.

A number of other databases are useful in nursing. They include the Cochrane Library, Nursing & Health Sciences: A Sage Full-Text Collection, Nursing Journals (Proquest Nursing Journals), PsycINFO,

---

Table 5-3

Full-Text Databases Useful in Nursing

- Academic Search™ Premier (http://www.epnet.com): Designed for academic institutions; contains full-text scholarly publications; source—EBSCOhost research database.
- AIDSinfo (http://www.aidsinfo.nih.gov): Federally approved HIV/AIDS research information for patients and healthcare providers.
- CINAHL® Plus with Full Text.
- www.epnet.com/thisTopic.php?topicID=172&marketID=1.
- Cumulative Index to Nursing and Allied Health (CINAHL).
- The Cochrane Collaboration (http://www.cochrane.org): Evidence-based medicine systematic reviews.
- Health and Psychosocial Instruments (HAPI): Evaluation and measurement instruments in health; available through Ovid Technologies.
- Health and Wellness Resource Center (http://www.gale.com/HealthRC): Informational sources, magazines, videos, journals, and newspapers on health and disease.
- Health Reference Center Academic (http://www.gale.com/customer_service/sample_searches/hrca .htm): Articles on fitness, pregnancy, medicine, nutrition, diseases, public health, occupational health and safety, alcohol and drug abuse, HMOs, prescription drugs, and more. The material contained in this database is intended for informational purposes only.
- Journals@OVIDFullText (http://www.ovid.com/site/about/terms.jsp?top=42): The second generation of *Ovid Full Text*, which combines all the capabilities of *Ovid Full Text Collections* with several important features and functions.
- MEDLINE with MeSH (http://www.ncbi.nlm.nih.gov/entrez/query.fcgi?DB=pubmed): Medical Literature Analysis and Retrieval System Online (MEDLINE®) is the U.S. National Library of Medicine's (NLM) premier bibliographic database that contains more than 16 million references to journal articles in life sciences, with a concentration on biomedicine.
- Health Sciences: A Sage Full-Text Collection (http://csa.tsinghua.edu.cn/factsheets/sagenurs-set-c .php): A searchable database of bibliographic records and full-text journal articles.
- Proquest Nursing Journals (http://www.proquest.com/products_pq/descriptions/pq_nursing_journals .shtml): Designed to meet the needs of students and researchers at academic institutions; includes information on obstetrics, nursing, geriatrics care, oncology, and more.

AID Search, tests and measurements databases, theses and dissertations, and free Internet databases (Table 5-3):

▨ Cochrane Library: A regularly updated collection of evidence-based medicine databases. These databases include systematic reviews of subjects, including economics, health interventions, controlled trials, and methodologies.

▨ Nursing & Health Sciences: A Sage Full-Text Collection: Includes full text of 24 journals published by Sage.

▨ Nursing Journals (Proquest Nursing Journals): Full-text journals.

▨ PsycINFO: Includes journals from the social sciences.

▨ AID Search: Includes journals and reports dealing with AIDS treatment and research.

▨ Tests and measurements databases.

▨ Mental Measurements Yearbook.

▨ Health and Psychosocial Instruments.

? **Think Outside the Box**

Which databases have you used in your literature searches? Discuss
the pros and cons of those databases you are familiar with using.

Basics of Searching

Any review of published articles about the topic is only as good as
what has been searched. In other words, "the first requirement for
writing a good literature review . . . is to do a good literature search"
(Kellsey, 2005, p. 526). A good place to start is to identify concepts
from the research question that can be the focus of the search. For
the research question mentioned earlier ("What is the relationship
between nurses' perception of empowerment and retention?"), concepts include empowerment and nurse retention. These words can be
used as the search terms.

Successful searching takes some planning and thought. Because
search engines locate an enormous number of documents, the results
can sometimes be overwhelming. A clear search strategy is necessary
to narrow the results to relevant, usable information. In developing
an effective search strategy, it is important to identify the main concepts from the research question or topic and determine any synonyms for these terms. For example, for the sample research question,
"What is the relationship of nurses' perception of empowerment and
retention?" the concepts are "nurses," "empowerment," and "retention." Other alternate words include "power" and "authority" (for
"empowerment") and "retaining" (for "retention").

The following steps outline the basics of conducting a search
from electronic sources. The researcher should consider the use of
MEDLINE while following these steps.

1. Select a topic of interest and identify the concepts or search terms.
   Think in terms of controlled vocabularies or subject headings for
   databases when selecting the topic. Subject headings yield more
   precise results than key words.
2. Access the NLM/PubMed Web site using the Internet browser.
3. Locate the MeSH database guide to the left of the main PubMed
   page.
4. Type the search term in the MeSH search box.
5. Select the subject heading from MeSH that matches the search
   term and place it in the PubMed search box. It will be necessary
   to switch back from the MeSH database guide to the main
   PubMed page. This can be done by selecting PubMed from the
   toolbar drop-down box.

6. Choose limit options as appropriate by date, author, and title.
7. To combine search strategies, use "and" or "or" in the search box. "And" is more restrictive (reduces the number of citations), and "or" is less restrictive.

Other Key Information

When searching for basic information, textbooks can sometimes be helpful and acceptable. A textbook often provides a foundation, a framework, or a gold standard by which other sources are measured. For example, when studying about health disparities, the book that contains the premier report is *Unequal Treatment: Confronting Racial and Ethnic Disparities in Health Care* (Smedley, Stith, & Nelson, 2003). It provides data sources, initial research findings, and suggested models that attempt to explain some of the issues surrounding this problem. From reading this book, it is possible to identify the gaps in the literature and the authors of major articles describing the research in this area. This type of information can also be used as background for the research proposal. If the requirements for the proposal include the use of recent information (not more than five years old), for example, then research journal articles should be used.

Another point to keep in mind is that the more precise the search, the fewer the number of resources that will be retrieved. The more general the search, the larger the number of articles that will be retrieved. After conducting the initial search, the researcher should review the abstracts of the articles and determine if more or less information is needed. The search should then be modified based on how the materials match the research question.

Evaluating the Literature

Evaluation of what has been published is an important and sometimes complex process. Many sources refer to this process as "critiquing the literature." The term "evaluation" is used here because it is more representative of what takes place and does not seem as overwhelming. Beginning researchers may find this an intimidating process, because they have far less experience than the authors of the original works. This should not always be the case, of course. Many times, the reader has more clinical knowledge than some of the people writing the articles. It is necessary to build on the analytical skills that most nurses have and to draw from the practice experience. The good thing about nursing is that there are enough variety and specialization in practice and academia for every nurse to have something of value to offer. Thus it is important that beginning researchers believe they have the skills necessary to raise questions about what is published.

A good place to locate information for evaluation of the literature is in the discussion section of an article, where the authors talk about the limitations of the study. Other tools to evaluate articles may be provided in the classroom setting from nursing faculty.

The evaluation process consists of a review of the components of the study and a comparison of the study with other studies related to the same research topic. The driving force behind the evaluation is the need to determine whether the study supports the research question identified and whether it identifies gaps in the literature that support the gap the beginning researcher or student has in mind.

It is generally accepted that the components of the study that should be reviewed include (1) the purpose of the study, (2) the sample size and selection, (3) the design of the study (methods used), (4) the data collection procedures, (5) the analysis of the data, and (6) the author's conclusion. The theoretical framework is also an important section to review, although it is sometimes not included owing to space constrictions imposed by the publisher. However, it remains an important part of the study, as it provides structure for conducting the study and explaining the results. The framework is not addressed in this chapter.

A discussion of the areas selected for evaluation follows. These areas correspond to the headings in "Gaps in the Literature" table (Table 5-4).

Article

When choosing articles from the literature, the researcher should be aware of the authors' credentials. It is important to identify where they work and how to contact them if you have questions about what they have written. Oftentimes, their e-mail addresses are available. Many authors are helpful and willing to give ideas to beginning researchers on request. The article usually provides some brief background about the authors that informs the reader about their credibility in writing about the research topic. It is important to document the citation of the article and contact information of the author. It may seem painstaking at the time, but it is time well spent to document all the information about how to locate the article, such as the author, date of publication, title of article, title, volume, and page numbers of the article.

Purpose

The purpose of the study explains why the study is being done. It is distinct from the problem, in that the problem addresses what the

Table 5-4

Gaps in the Literature

Article (Title, author, journal, publication date, contact information for author)	Purpose (Why study was conducted)	Sample (Number of participants, demographics, other characteristics, geographic location)	Methods (Design, instruments or questionnaires, data collection, data analysis)	Major Findings (Results, statistical significance, conclusions)	Limitations (Factors that may complicate the interpretation of the findings)	Gaps (Suggestions for further study that support the research question)

study is about (Nieswiadomy, 2008). This is an appropriate section for the researcher to determine what he or she wants to do with the findings of the study. For example, if the problem of the study is obesity in third-grade students in public schools, the purpose could be to determine if the environment of the school and the age of the children may contribute to food consumption choices. The findings could then be used to make changes in the school or to enhance healthy behaviors in the children while they are at school.

The purpose of the study is usually located in the first few paragraphs of the study. Identifying the purpose may help later in grouping similar types of studies and also in organizing the writing of the literature review.

Sample/Population

The sample is a representation of the entire population of interest. All persons in the universe could not be studied, so a representative sample is selected that may have characteristics similar to the general population being studied. For example, caregivers may be the population of interest. Because it is impossible to study all the caregivers in the world, a sample with similar experiences could be chosen. To choose a manageable sample size, the sample may be narrowed to those caregivers who care for their spouses and live in a particular county of Texas.

? **Think Outside the Box**

Select a topic. Discuss the specific steps you would use to conduct a literature review on that topic. Which words would you use to do the search, and why? Which databases would you use, and why?

The sample/population section of the study describes the study participants. The author describes demographic characteristics (e.g., age, gender, race, ethnicity, educational level, geographic location, income level) of the persons who will be in the study. The description of the sample and how it was selected helps the researcher make statements about the generalizability of the study—that is, whether similar findings would be obtained in other locations under the same or similar conditions. How the sample was selected may affect the study findings. If the participants were randomly selected using random tables or computer software, the findings are more likely to be generalizable to other similar subjects. In contrast, if the sample was selected based on who showed up at the announcement of the study (known as a convenience sample), it is less likely that the findings could be generalized to other groups.

This section can be documented by providing just a few statements, such as "persons 65 years of age and older caring for their 65-and-older spouses with Alzheimer's disease in their home in rural west Texas."

Methods

The methods section of the study describes the strategy for how the study is conducted. In quantitative research, which is the focus of this chapter, the methods section includes (1) the inclusion criteria, explaining how the participants were selected; (2) the exclusion criteria, explaining why subjects were not selected; (3) the sample size and whether it was adequate; (4) the design; (5) the instruments or surveys used; (6) data collection procedures; and (7) data analysis (Portney & Watkins, 2008).

The design describes whether the investigation was a descriptive, correlational, exploratory, or experimental study. (Research study designs are covered elsewhere in this text.) The main points of interest for the reader in the methods section should be whether the methods used to collect the data were controlled for any outside conditions that could confuse the findings of the study and whether the methods affected the accuracy of the findings. For example, if the study focuses on the relationship of weight to blood pressure, the researcher must have ensured that the weight scales and blood pressure machines were calibrated and functioning properly. The procedure for how this was done should also be described in the study. If the condition of the measuring instruments is not standardized, it will be impossible to know whether the findings were accurate. Thus the methods section of the article should include a description of the conditions under which the weights and blood pressures were measured and the person taking the measurements. If surveys or questionnaires were used, the researcher should discuss how the reliability and validity of these instruments were determined when used with other subjects.

Put simply, the design identifies the number of subjects, the number of groups, and the type of intervention, and the conditions under which the intervention was performed (Portney & Watkins, 2008). This section of the study helps the reader interpret the degree of accuracy or validity of the findings.

The analysis of the data describes the statistical tests that were used to test the research hypothesis. For example, if the study sought to determine the relationship between two variables, a correlational test would be done. If the study sought to determine the difference between two variables, the test would be a t-test. The reader should make note of the type of testing and compare it with the testing done in other studies; he or she should also determine if the appropriate test was done to match the research hypothesis.

Major Findings

The findings (or results) may overlap with the discussion section of the study, but it is most appropriate for the results to stand alone. The results section should be reported without the researcher's interpretation (Portney & Watkins, 2008). This is a factual section that may be explained with tables and charts. It is important for the reader to determine whether the results match the purpose of the study and the research question. In addition, the reader should make note of any statistically significant results and the tests that were used.

Limitations

The limitations of the study describe the elements that may have complicated the results. For example, suppose a study was done to measure improvement in test scores after an instructive video on electrical safety on small appliances in the workplace was presented to the study participants. A pre-test was given before the video was shown, and a post-test was given one week after the video presentation. If the scores were low on the post-test, a limitation could be that there was too much of a time lapse between the test, the instruction, and the post-test. Discussing this limitation of the study may suggest ways to improve the study if it is later replicated. Limitations may also help to identify gaps in the literature that could be considered in other studies.

Gaps in the Literature

This section is of greatest importance for the review of the literature; however, it cannot be given due diligence unless all the other parts of the research study are examined first. The discussion and conclusion section of the article is generally where most of the suggestions for future research are presented. Suggestions for future research usually represent gaps in knowledge about the research topic. Perhaps a particular group suffers a worse outcome than other populations, relative to a particular disease condition. The gap in the literature might then be that no studies have examined the nature of this problem.

The discussion and conclusion section is where authors most often compare their findings with other studies, offer alternative explanations, or offer support for existing practice (Portney & Watkins, 2008). This section is a reflection of the authors' interpretation and experience, biases, and interests relevant to the findings of the study at hand. The authors discuss unanswered questions and point out gaps in the knowledge on the research topic.

The reader should examine this section very carefully for missing pieces of knowledge and for what is unknown about the research area, looking for information that justifies the research being proposed. This information could be gaps related to unanswered questions regarding gender, age, ethnicity, characteristics of health-care facilities, geographic locations, differences in disease outcomes, or any combination of variables that have not been examined. These would represent gaps in the literature.

Writing the Literature Review

The literature review is not a list of article summaries, but rather a well-written synthesis of information about a topic that includes a discussion on the research that has been done, the methodologies, the strengths and weaknesses of findings, and gaps that require more knowledge. The approach to writing the review should be to convince the reader that the information supports the need for the proposed study. The format for writing the review may vary depending on the purpose of the review. If the review is conducted for a class assignment, the student should follow the grading criteria. If the review is part of a grant proposal, it is usually succinct and points out various themes, conceptual models, theories that explain the research question, and gaps in the literature that support the need for the grant.

Unfortunately, it is all too easy to get bogged down while actually writing the review. The researcher usually reads numerous articles before settling on those used in the literature review. One manageable tool of organization is an outline. Others have recommended the use of grids or matrices for organizing the review of the articles, or index cards for categorizing the materials read (McCabe, 2005; Polit & Beck, 2008). One way of developing headings for an outline is to mark notes on the articles. After reading the articles chosen for the review, it is helpful to go back and write in the margins adjacent to pertinent information in the text or to list on the first page of the article the reasons why the article was chosen (e.g., good questionnaire, clearly written design, independent and dependent variables listed and defined, similarities to another study).

? Think Outside the Box

Select a research article. Examine which aspects from the article must be documented within the summary provided for a literature review.

Answering Key Questions

A good written review should answer some basic questions. Listed here are questions developed from the information found in most published research studies. These questions are based on experiences of the author from a confluence of reading, conducting, and critiquing research reviews and information learned from graduate courses in nursing and library science.

- What was the main focus of the articles (research question, purpose, objectives)?
- Did the articles represent recent (less than five years old) as well as classic studies?
- What were the designs of most of the studies (research questions, methodology, sample size, population characteristics, pertinent conclusion)?
- Which studies did not positively support the research question?
- What were the target populations of most of the studies (e.g., nurses in emergency departments, medical–surgical units, operating rooms)?
- Which models or conceptual frameworks were used to explain the structure of the studies?
- What were the general findings and limitations in most of the studies?
- Which articles were the most similar in findings, design, or other features?
- Which gaps were identified in the articles?
- What was the overall conclusion for the literature review that supports the research question and need for your proposal?

An Outline for Writing the Review

Discussion of the preceding questions should be helpful in providing organization to the review. The following outline provides further guidance for developing headings and completing the written review. The components of the outline include (1) the purpose, (2) a description of the search strategy, (3) the themes or categories of similar types of articles, (4) limitations, (5) gaps in what is known about a research area, and (6) a discussion and conclusion. A more detailed description of an outline for organizing the writing of the review appears in Table 5-5.

Other Writing Tips

When writing a literature review for a class, it is important to follow the grading criteria and the objectives of the course. The length of

---

Table 5-5

Outline for a Literature Review

I.   Purpose of the review
II. Description of how search was conducted
     A. Databases used
     B. Key words and subject headings
     C. Rationale or criteria for articles chosen in the review
        1. Articles five years old or less
        2. Classic articles or books
III. Themes of articles
     A. Similarities in articles that support the research question
        1. Purposes, designs, target populations, tools of measurement (e.g., questionnaires, methodologies)
        2. General findings
     B. Conceptual framework, models, or theories that explain the research described in the articles
     C. Inconsistencies in articles
        1. Articles that do not provide positive support for the research question identified
IV. Limitations
     A. Components identified by the authors of the articles that were limitations in the studies
V.   Gaps in the articles
     A. Gaps identified by the authors of the articles
VI. Discussion and conclusion
     A. Summary statement of how articles support the proposal
     B. Identification of gaps perceived and how the proposal will meet the needs of some aspect of nursing practice

---

the review, in terms of the number of pages, depends on the criteria and purpose of the review. The student should follow the headings and subheadings of the writing style required by the course (e.g., American Psychological Association [APA] or other sources). Paraphrase the key points of the articles and avoid using too many direct quotes. Also, be aware that lengthy writing does not necessarily mean comprehensive writing. Being able to synthesize what is called for in the writing and to give the reader what was promised in the purpose of the writing is what is most important.

Linking the Literature Review to Evidence-Based Nursing Practice

Evidence-based practice is an important issue in nursing today. Nurses need to know why they do what they do. Although many support the idea of intuition, the profession must provide logical explanations for the actions of nursing based on scientific findings. The literature review provides the foundation for good research. To make sound decisions, today's nurses must be well read. The research presented in the literature review may provide nurses with the background they need to make informed choices in practice. The ability to critically analyze scientific literature is a skill every nurse should develop, and a skill that is central to deciding whether to incorporate new information into practice based on the strength of the evidence.

? Think Outside the Box

Discuss how you would determine the credibility of information found on the Internet.

Summary Points

1. The literature review is the foundation of the research proposal.
2. A good literature review begins with a good literature search that is assisted by a professional librarian.
3. The assistance of an expert librarian may both enhance the relevance of material found and reduce the amount of time spent conducting the search.
4. A database search using subject headings yields more precise information than a key word search.
5. The literature review identifies what is known and unknown about the research topic.
6. The review should focus original research studies dealing with the selected topic.
7. The literature reviews identifies gaps in the literature.
8. The gaps in the literature should support the research question.

RED FLAGS

- Literature summaries should provide enough information about the different sources related to sample size, methodology, and results to allow for a clear understanding of the application of that information to the current project.
- Within the literature review, the sources used should be predominantly primary sources, not secondary sources.
- The current expectation is for references to be within the five-year limit unless the article is a classical/benchmark study.
- When Internet sources are used, the credibility of the information must be reflected in the literature review.
- Gaps in the literature review should be identified.

Multiple Choice Questions

1. A literature review is

   A. Everything that is known about a subject.
   B. An analytical summary of research findings.
   C. All approved data on a research topic.
   D. A compilation of all positive results of research.

2. The purpose of the literature review is to

   A. Identify a problem that has not been resolved.
   B. Clarify the importance of a research problem.
   C. Identify gaps in the literature.
   D. All of the above.

3. The literature review should occur

   A. Near the end of the research process.
   B. Shortly before the analysis of the problem.
   C. Early in the research process.
   D. None of the above.

4. When conducting a literature review, it is advisable to

   A. Seek most information from the Internet.
   B. Gather all data from books.
   C. Gather all data from journals.
   D. Seek assistance from a librarian.

5. Evidence-based nursing literature provides the nurse with the ability to

   A. Choose only those practice activities based on evidence.
   B. Describe and analyze published research results.
   C. Use textbook information.
   D. Problem-solve all nursing issues.

6. A database differs from a search engine in the following manner:

   A. A database stores the information.
   B. A search engine takes you to the information.
   C. Databases are specialized by area of knowledge.
   D. All of the above.

7. The database that is considered the premier bibliographic database for providing access in the North Americas for biomedical literature is

   A. Google.
   B. MEDLINE.
   C. CINAHL.
   D. Yahoo!.

8. It is appropriate to use key word searches in which of the following contexts?
   A. Evidence-based medicine
   B. Ovid
   C. MEDLINE
   D. Evidence-based nursing

9. The purpose section of a research study usually
   A. Tells the geographic location of the study.
   B. Tells why the study was done.
   C. Is the methodology of the study.
   D. Tells what the study is about.

10. The gaps in the literature are
    A. Missing pieces in the knowledge of the research area.
    B. Questions about the research that have not been explained.
    C. Suggestions for future research made by the author.
    D. All of the above.

11. The main difference between a research article and a non-research article is
    A. A research article reports statistics on surveys and a non-research article does not.
    B. A research article describes research by the original author.
    C. A non-research article describes the methods of how the study was conducted.
    D. A non-research article conducts analysis and statistical testing on the data presented in the article.

Discussion Questions

1. You are interested in seeing what has been written about using dietary supplements to treat bone loss in postmenopausal women. You have been told that appropriate MeSH headings include "dietary supplements" and "osteoporosis, postmenopausal," but you want to use the MeSH database to verify these terms. You also know that you want only English-language articles, so you limit your search by using the Limits function and setting Language to English. Execute your search and examine the results. (This exercise was provided by Dr. Jeffrey Huber, personal communication, Texas Woman's University, 2003.)

2. To gain a greater understanding of evidence-based nursing, conduct a search to retrieve references to the published literature about aspirin use for prevention of myocardial infarction. Choose the full-text Nursing Collection produced by Ovid. Develop a search strategy for this topic. Review your results.

Suggested Readings

Ahern, N. R. (2005). Using the Internet to conduct research. *Nurse Researcher 13*(2), 55–70.

University of California, Berkeley Library. (n.d.). *Finding historical primary sources.* Retrieved July 11, 2009, from http://www.lib.berkeley.edu/instruct/guides/primarysources.html

University Libraries, University of Maryland. (n.d.). *Primary, secondary and tertiary sources.* Retrieved July 11, 2009, from http://www.lib.umd.edu/guides/primary-sources.html

Yale University Library. (2006). *Primary sources at Yale.* Retrieved July 11, 2009, from http://www.library.yale.edu/instruction/primsource.html

References

Ackerman, E., & Hartman, K. (2003). *Searching and researching on the Internet and the World Wide Web* (3rd ed.). Wilsonville, OR: Franklin, Beedle & Associates.

CINAHL Information Systems. (2005). *The CINAHL database*. Birmingham, AL: EBSCO Industries. Retrieved May 30, 2006, from http://www.cinahl.com/prodsvcs /cinahldb.htm

"Database." (2000). *American heritage dictionary of the English language* (4th ed.). Boston: Houghton Mifflin. Retrieved March 27, 2006, from http://dictionary .reference.com/search?q=database&r=66

EBSCO Publishing. (2006). *EBSCOhost*. Birmingham, AL: EBSCO Industries. Retrieved May 31, 2006, from http://www.epnet.com/thisMarket.php?marketID=2

Force, M. (2005). The relationship between effective nurse managers and nursing retention. *Journal of Nursing Administration, 35*(7–8), 336–341.

Kellsey, C. (2005). Writing the literature review: Tips for academic librarians. *College Research Library News, 66*(7), 526–527.

McCabe, T. F. (2005). How to conduct an effective literature search. *Nursing Standard, 20*(11), 41–47.

National Library of Medicine (NLM). (1993–2006). *PubMed*. Bethesda, MD: Author. Retrieved March 28, 2006, from http://ncbi.nlm.nih.gov/entrez/query.fcgi

Nieswiadomy, R. M. (2008). *Foundations of nursing research* (5th ed.). Upper Saddle River, NJ: Pearson Prentice Hall.

Norwood, S. L. (2000). *Research strategies for advanced practice nurses*. Upper Saddle River, NJ: Prentice Hall Health.

Polit, D. F., & Beck, C. T. (2008). *Creating and assessing evidence for nursing practice* (8th ed.). Philadelphia: Lippincott Williams & Wilkins.

Portney, L. G., & Watkins, M. P. (2008). *Foundations of clinical research: Applications to practice* (3rd ed.). Upper Saddle River, NJ: Prentice Hall Health.

Princeton University. (2003). *Wordnet* (Version 2.0). Retrieved March 27, 2006, from http://dictionary.reference.com/search?q=database&r=66

Smedley, B. D., Stith, A. Y., & Nelson, A. R. (2003). *Unequal treatment: Confronting racial and ethnic disparities in health care*. Washington, DC: National Academies Press.

Chapter 6

Sampling

Kathaleen C. Bloom and Lucy B. Trice

Chapter Objectives

At the conclusion of this chapter, the learner will be able to

1. Discuss basic concepts related to sampling
2. Contrast inclusion and exclusion criteria in the sampling process
3. Distinguish between probability and nonprobability samples
4. Identify types of sampling strategies used for qualitative and quantitative research
5. Discuss approaches to determining sample size
6. Critically evaluate sampling plans found in research reports for their contribution to the strength of evidence for nursing practice

Key Terms

➤ Accessible population

➤ Cluster sampling

➤ Convenience sampling

➤ Exclusion criteria

➤ External validity

➤ Inclusion criteria

➤ Internal validity

➤ Nonprobability sampling

➤ Population

➤ Probability sampling

➤ Purposive sampling

➤ Quota sampling

➤ Random sampling

➤ Representative sample

➤ Sample

➤ Sampling error

➤ Simple random sampling

➤ Snowball sampling

➤ Stratified sampling

➤ Systematic sampling

➤ Target population

➤ Theoretical sampling

Introduction

Keeping in mind that evidence-based practice (EBP) is about integrating the strongest research evidence with clinical expertise and patient needs (Malloch & Porter-O'Grady, 2006; Melnyk & Fineout-Overholt, 2005), it is time to examine the research design decisions made in terms of sampling. Regardless of the topic of the research, every investigator must make decisions about which subjects will provide data to answer the research question. This sampling plan is a process that involves making choices about who or what to include in the sample, how to select the sample, and how many subjects to include in the sample for a particular study. These decisions are critical in designing high-quality clinical studies to build evidence-based nursing practice.

A population is the entire set of elements that meet specified criteria. An element may be a person, a family, a community, a medical record, an event, a laboratory specimen, or even a laboratory animal. Often called the target population, this set encompasses every element in the world that met the sampling criteria, such as all pregnant adolescents, preterm infants, persons with diabetes, or children who are chronically ill. The accessible population, by comparison, is that portion of the target population that the investigator can reasonably reach. It might include pregnant adolescents enrolled in an alternative high school in the southeastern United States, persons with diabetes who are enrolled in diabetic education at a local hospital, or children with a chronic illness who are enrolled in a summer camp. The sample, drawn through a specified sampling strategy from the accessible population, consists of those elements from whom or about whom data are actually collected (Figure 6-1).

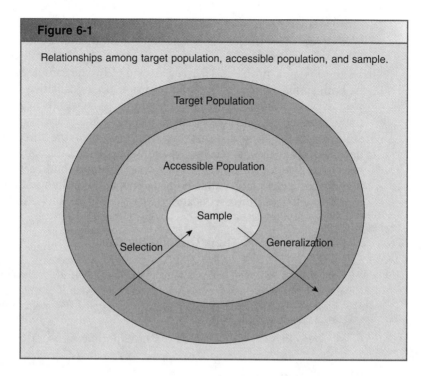

Figure 6-1

Relationships among target population, accessible population, and sample.

Why Sample?

Researchers use samples rather than populations for reasons of efficiency and cost-effectiveness. It would be almost impossible, and generally impractical, to conduct a study on the entire population, although this is the population to which the investigator would like to be able to generalize the conclusions. Sampling strategies, therefore, have been designed to select a subset of the population to represent the entire population.

The overarching concern in evaluating a sample in quantitative research is how well the sample represents the target population. A representative sample is one that looks like the target population in terms of important characteristics. Decisions with respect to sampling strategies are made in an effort to reduce sampling error. Sampling error is the difference between data obtained from the sample and data that would be obtained if the entire population were included in the study. Thus, to the extent that the sample from which data was collected possesses important characteristics of the accessible and target populations, the findings can be used to develop EBP with these populations.

The major concern in evaluating a sample in qualitative research is how well the sample represents the phenomenon of interest. In other words, the sample must be appropriate to provide information on the research problem. The data provided by the sample needs to be both sufficient and relevant. For example, in a qualitative study on parents' and children's reactions to the terrorist attacks that took place on September 11, 2001, researchers sought to interview parents and children in the Boston area, from which two of the three planes departed (Beauchesne, Kelley, Patsdaughter, & Pickard, 2002). The researchers performed the interviews in the one-month period following the attacks and found both parents and children willing and eager to talk about the events and their reactions, feelings, and fears.

? Think Outside the Box

Examining the following examples, which type of sampling techniques could you use to access the target population for each:
- Which information has been used to determine the method of catheterizing for a laboring mother?
- Which information serves as the basis for the range of blood sugars used within elderly persons who are newly diagnosed with diabetes?

As has been discussed in other chapters, two key elements in evaluating quantitative research are issues related to the internal and external validity of the findings. Internal validity refers to the extent to which the results of the study present an accurate picture of the real world. In other words, did the independent variable make a difference in the outcome, or were there other factors at work? The choice of a sampling strategy is designed to reduce sampling bias, one of the threats to internal validity. Sampling bias is evident when groups of people are either underrepresented or overrepresented in a sample. When assessing the sample in a study, the researcher should ask, "Did any characteristics of the sample influence the outcomes of the study?" Another threat to internal validity is changes in the world or within research participants themselves during the course of the study. Imagine, for example, the effects of the events on and after September 11, 2001, or in the aftermath of Hurricane Katrina, on emotional, mental, and physical health and how they might affect study outcomes.

External validity, in contrast, refers to issues with generalizability of the findings from the research beyond the sample and situation that were studied. In other words, to whom and under which circumstances could the findings from this study be applied? When assessing the sample in a study, the researcher should ask, "How well does this group reflect the population as a whole?"

Internal and external validity do not apply in the same way to qualitative research. In qualitative studies, the sample is evaluated as to whether it is representative of the phenomenon of interest, rather than representative of the population as a whole. When assessing the sample in a qualitative study, the researcher should ask, "Did the sample chosen have the ability to talk about a phenomenon or an experience from the perspective of someone who was affected by it?"

Who to Sample?

The responsibility of the investigator is to specify the sampling criteria or the characteristics necessary to be part of the research sample. It is these criteria that determine the target population. Sampling criteria may be very broad or very specific. These criteria are established to minimize bias or to control for irrelevant variability in the sample. Choosing a sample based on carefully selected criteria increases the strength of the evidence, thereby enhancing the ability to generalize the findings.

The researcher must make two different types of decisions—who should be considered for inclusion in the sample and who should be excluded from the sample. Inclusion criteria (sometimes called eligibility criteria) are those characteristics that must be met to be considered for participation in the study. Here, the investigator specifies what the sample will look like and which characteristics all study participants will have in common.

Exclusion criteria are not the polar opposite of the inclusion criteria, but rather those characteristics that, if present, would make persons ineligible to be in the sample, even though they might meet all of the inclusion criteria. These exclusions limit the representativeness of the sample and, therefore, the generalizability of the findings. As such, exclusion criteria should be specified after careful consideration. They should represent only those conditions or characteristics that might potentially make a difference in the outcome.

The specification of inclusion and exclusion criteria should not be taken lightly. Each criterion should be based on sound reasoning and be grounded in the goal of eliminating a potentially confounding effect on the outcome of the study. For example, in a study of the impact of home visits by mental health nurses on postpartum depression in Japanese women, the researcher used the following criteria when selecting the sample:

Japanese women aged 18 years or older. Women were excluded if they lived outside the district, had delivered prematurely (before 36 weeks' gestation), if their infant had any congenital or serious disease, if they did not have a singleton birth, or if they had received any antidepressant or other specific treatments during the study period. (Tamaki, 2008, p. 420)

How to Sample?

There are two categories of sampling strategies—probability and nonprobability sampling. Probability sampling employs specific strategies designed to yield an unbiased (i.e., representative) sample by giving each element the possibility of being selected. The elements, which are each potential members of a sample, are chosen at random (by chance). Nonprobability sampling does not include random selection of elements and, therefore, has a higher possibility of yielding a biased (i.e., nonrepresentative) sample. In this case, researchers use elements that are accessible and available, and there is no way of estimating the probability that an element will be included in the sample.

? Think Outside the Box

Differentiate among the following terms: target population, accessible population, representative sample, population, and sample.

Whether to use a probability or nonprobability strategy is the choice of the researcher. This choice is based on the problem under investigation and the purpose of the study. Quantitative studies can use either probability or nonprobability sampling strategies. All decisions made about sampling in quantitative studies are based on maximizing the representativeness of the sample. Qualitative studies, because of their very nature, employ nonprobability sampling strategies. All decisions made about sampling in qualitative studies are based on maximizing the representativeness of the phenomenon of interest.

Probability Sampling Strategies

Probability sampling is the most well-respected type of sampling, because it is more likely to produce a representative sample. It is not the same thing as random assignment, however. Random assignment is the process of randomly placing subjects in an experimental study in different treatment groups. Random sampling involves processes in which each element of the population has an equal chance of being in the sample. Four probability sampling strategies are commonly used: (1) simple random, (2) stratified random, (3) cluster, and (4) systematic random.

Simple random sampling is a process in which the researcher defines the population, lists and consecutively numbers all elements of the population, and then randomly selects a sample from this list. The most simplistic method of simple random sampling is to put all of the numbers in a "hat" and draw out the desired number of elements. Obviously, this technique would work only for a study with a very small number of elements.

The random selection of the sample may also be accomplished by using a table of random numbers (Table 6-1). With this strategy, the researcher begins at any point on the list of numbers and reads consecutive numbers in any direction, choosing those numbers that correspond to the numbered elements in the population until the desired sample size is reached. For example, if you have a list of 50 elements from which to choose a random sample of 15, each element would be numbered from 01 to 50. If you closed your eyes and pointed at the data in Table 6-1 and your finger ended up on the numeral 91254, deciding to go across the rows to the right, the first two-digit number would be 91 (**91**254), which is not in your range of possibilities. The next two-digit number would be 25 (91**25**4); that element would be selected, as would 42 (19254 **24**090), and 40 (24**0**90). The next two-digit number would be 90 (240**90**), which is not in your range, followed by 25 (**25**752), which you have already selected, and 75 (25**75**2), which is not in your range. Thus the next elements selected would be 24 (25752 **24**831), 28 (42**83**1), and 31 (428**31**). This process would continue until 15 elements were

Table 6-1				
Excerpt from a Table of Random Numbers				
39634	62349	74088	65564	16379
14595	35050	40469	27478	44526
30734	71571	83722	79712	25775
64628	89126	91254	24090	25752
42831	95113	43511	42082	15140
80583	70361	41047	26792	78466

Excerpted from http://www.mrs.umn.edu/~sungurea/introstat/public/instruction/ranbox/randomnumbersII.html.

selected. Simple random selection is not widely used, because it is rather cumbersome and inefficient. Furthermore, it is rare to have the ability to list every element in the population.

Stratified random sampling is a variation on the simple random sampling technique. When the composition of a population with respect to some characteristic important to the study is known, the population is divided into two or more strata (groups) based on that characteristic. Simple random selection is then used to pick elements from each group. This selection strategy makes each group homogenous as far as the characteristic of interest is concerned. Examples of characteristics upon which stratification may be made include gender, age, ethnicity, occupation, education, and so forth. For example, if a researcher wanted a sample of 100 people to be stratified in terms of gender, the elements would be divided based on gender, and a random selection of 50 people from each list would be chosen for the sample.

If desired, the researcher may use proportional sampling to ensure that the sample accurately reflects the composition of the population on the characteristic by which the population was stratified. If, for example, 60% of the known population is male, the researcher might want to randomly select 60 males and 40 females for a total sample of 100. Proportional sampling is not generally a wise choice if the strata are of extremely disproportionate sizes.

To demonstrate how this technique works, consider a study of prevalence and family characteristics associated with incest in South Korea (Kim & Kim, 2005). In this study, proportional stratified random sampling was used to select 1,672 adolescents—1,053 middle and high school students and 619 adolescents from juvenile detention facilities. Stratification was based on where the participant lived (urban versus rural) and the type of institution (middle school versus high school versus detention center). In this way, the researchers ensured representation of adolescents from all four strata without underrepresenting or overrepresenting either urban or rural dwelling adolescents, or those from the school system or detention facility.

Cluster sampling, also called multistage sampling, is a probability sampling strategy in which not all of the elements of the population need to be known. This strategy employs random selection of first larger sampling units (clusters), then successively smaller clusters, either by simple or stratified random selection techniques. It is a particularly efficient strategy when the population is large and spread out over a large geographic area. For example, in a rapid assessment of the health impact and the needs of the citizens of two Florida counties after Hurricane Ivan struck in 2004, 30 clusters (neighborhoods) were identified and 7 households in each cluster were interviewed (Bayleyegn et al., 2006). Interviewing the entire target population (all households in the two counties) would have been an impossible task. By identifying and selecting neighborhoods and then households within neighborhoods, however, researchers could conduct an overall assessment in a short period of time.

? Think Outside the Box

Why is the use of a randomly selected population a stronger sampling method than the use of a nonrandomized sample? Discuss the value of having the strongest sampling method possible for the research to be conducted.

Systematic random sampling is a probability sampling technique in which elements are randomly selected from the population at predetermined, fixed intervals. The researcher first determines the desired sample size and then decides on the sampling interval. If the researcher has a list of the elements in the population, the sampling interval is determined by dividing the total population by the desired sample size. Suppose the population includes 750 individuals and the sample size is 50; in this case, the sampling interval would be 15. The researcher selects the first element randomly and then selects every fifteenth element thereafter to obtain the 50 elements for the sample. If the list is exhausted before the sample size is reached, counting resumes at the top of the list.

This technique produces a random sample in a more efficient manner than is possible with simple randomization. For example, in a study of the types of intravenous fluids used in oxytocin dilution, systematic random sampling was used to select 700 obstetric units from a list of eligible hospitals prepared by the American Hospital Association (Ruchala, Metheny, Essenpreis, & Borcherding, 2002). Questionnaires were then mailed to the nurse managers of each of the 700 obstetric units.

Nonprobability Sampling Strategies

The second broad category of sampling strategies is nonprobability sampling. These techniques are less likely to produce samples that are representative of the population. Nonetheless, they are more widely used in many disciplines, including nursing, because such samples are generally easier to obtain. Commonly used nonprobability sampling strategies include (1) convenience sampling, (2) quota sampling, (3) purposive sampling, (4) snowball sampling, and (5) theoretic sampling.

Convenience sampling is the process of selecting elements to be in the sample simply because they are readily available. Also called accidental sampling, it is the simplest and potentially least representative of all the sampling strategies. It is also currently the most frequently used sampling strategy in nursing research studies.

Quota sampling begins with the researcher identifying strata of the population and then determining the number of elements in each stratum necessary to proportionately represent the population. Actual selection of elements from each stratum is then accomplished in the same way as in convenience sampling. In an evaluation of an educational program for women receiving radiation therapy for breast cancer, quota sampling was used to make sure that equal numbers were recruited from specific age categories assumed to represent three menopausal states—premenopausal, perimenopausal, and postmenopausal (Jahraus, Sokolosky, Thurston, & Guo, 2002).

Purposive sampling, also called judgmental sampling, is a sampling strategy in which participants are handpicked by the researcher, either because they are typical of the phenomenon of interest or because they are knowledgeable about the issues under investigation. This strategy is often used when the researcher desires a sample consisting of experts. McMurry (2006) used this strategy to identify 10 patients who had participated in each of three smoking cessation programs in his evaluation of smoking relapse rates among military personnel.

Snowball sampling, also known as network sampling, is a sampling strategy in which participants already in the study are asked to provide referrals to potential study subjects. Doherty and Scanell-Desch (2008), for example, in describing the recruitment of the 10 women in their study of the lived experience of widowhood during pregnancy, stated:

> One investigator obtained the name of a September 11th widow from a nursing colleague. This woman was pregnant at the time of her husband's death, agreed to participate in the study, and referred the researchers to other potential participants. The investigator also obtained the names of several pregnant military widows from a retired military nurse. (p. 104)

Snowball sampling is a particularly good strategy to use when potential participants in the study are challenging to find, as might be the case with vegetarians, drug abusers, persons engaged in prostitution, people with a specific disability or rare condition, and homeless individuals.

Theoretical sampling is generally restricted to qualitative research methods, especially in conjunction with grounded theory. It is most analogous to the purposive sampling strategy. As the study unfolds and the interviews conducted with the first few participants are analyzed, conceptual categories and themes are identified. Subsequent decisions as to who will provide data and which data will be gathered are then based on who has already been sampled and which data have already been provided. Sampling and data collection continue until all of the categories and themes are "saturated"—that is, no additional categories or themes are emerging and no new facets of existing categories and themes are uncovered. Calvin (2004), for example, used theoretical sampling to select the 20 participants for a grounded theory explanation of how persons on hemodialysis make end-of-life decisions.

How Many to Sample?

Once the researcher has decided who to sample and how the sampling will be done, it is time to make the decision about how many elements need to be in the sample. The question of sample size is a crucial one when the objective is the ability to generalize the findings to a larger population. The generally accepted recommendation is to sample as many elements as possible. It is wise to remember, however, that the validity of a study begins with the design. Even the largest of samples cannot make up for faulty design.

? Think Outside the Box

Convenience sampling is the most commonly used sampling method. Which steps would you expect to see used within a study to strengthen the study in this type of sampling method?

Quantitative Studies

Several factors that are taken into consideration when decisions are made about desired sample size in quantitative studies, including factors related to (1) the population, (2) the study design, (3) measurement, and (4) practicability.

Population Factors

Population-related factors that influence required sample size include the homogeneity of the population as well as the expected rate of the phenomenon, event, or outcome being measured and the anticipated attrition rate. In a population that is fairly homogenous (i.e., in which sampling elements are very similar to one another), the required sample size is generally smaller than if the population were more heterogeneous. Similarly, if the phenomenon, event, or outcome occurs frequently, a smaller sample size is needed than if occurrences are infrequent.

In longitudinal studies, attrition may be a problem. When this phenomenon is anticipated to occur, researchers often "over-enroll" participants in the research. If, for example, a study were expected to have an attrition rate of 20% (i.e., if 100 subjects were to begin the study, only 80 would complete it), then the researcher would enroll 120 participants so as to have the desired 100 at completion.

Design Factors

Design factors influencing sample size include the type of study, the number of variables, and the sampling strategy. Quantitative studies, in general, require larger sample sizes than do qualitative studies. Some differences also occur in relation to the quantitative designs themselves. First, a study that is more complex requires a larger sample size. For example, a study employing a longitudinal data collection plan needs to enroll increased numbers of participants at the beginning because of the increased possibility of losing subjects over the course of the study (sample attrition). Second, as the number of variables being measured increases, so does the needed sample size. Third, the sampling strategy itself can affect the required sample size. Stratified random sampling and quota sampling techniques, for example, allow the researcher to use smaller sample sizes than would be needed in studies employing simple random or convenience sampling, because some of the representativeness is already built into the stratification procedure.

Measurement Factors

Measurement factors that influence sample size include the sensitivity of the research instruments and the effect that the process has on the outcome. Data collection instruments in which measurement error is minimal are said to be precise. The less precise the instrument, the larger the sample size might need to be. Because interval-level data are generally more precise, from a sample size perspective it is best to measure at that level if at all possible, because a smaller sample size may be used.

Practical Factors

Practical factors such as cost and convenience also influence sample size. Although population factors, design factors, and measurement factors certainly affect the ideal sample size, it is these practical factors that often prove most influential. When this is the case, adjustments in design and/or sampling strategies need to be made to strengthen the internal validity of the study.

Given these factors discussed, how do researchers determine the sample size needed for a particular study? Some use the "rule of 30": There should be 30 subjects for each group or 30 subjects for each variable. This notion is based on the central limit theorem, which asserts that, in a randomly generated sample of 30 or more subjects, the mean of a characteristic will approximate the population mean (Hinkle, Wiersma, & Jurs, 1988). It is essential to remember, however, that representativeness is more important than sample size. The "rule of 30" should, therefore, be considered the minimum acceptable sample size rather than the ideal.

The gold standard in determining sample size is power analysis, a statistical calculation of the number of subjects needed to accurately reject the null hypothesis (Cohen, 1989; Kraemer & Thiemann, 1987). The actual calculation of sample size is beyond the scope of this book. The most commonly used significance level is .05 and the standard power is .80. The effect size is estimated based on pilot studies undertaken by the researcher or on reports in the literature drawn from previous studies on the same or similar problems. Performing the power analysis prior to conducting a study strengthens the study's credibility concerning the size of the sample utilized. For example, here is the description of the power analysis for a study of the impact of a relative's clinic on next-of-kin satisfaction with care received by patients in critical care:

> The study was powered to detect a difference in mean satisfaction score of 0.5, assuming a 50% response rate, 150 participants in each group and a standard deviation of 1.0 using an unpaired two-tailed t-test. The alpha and beta levels selected were 0.05 and 0.2, respectively. (Steel, Underwood, Notley, & Blunt, 2008, p. 122)

Power analysis formulas are sometimes applied after the fact to determine the power of a test given the sample size and results obtained. Sometimes the formula is used on a post hoc basis to determine the optimal sample size. For example, in a study of interventions to assist smokers with smoking cessation in a sample of 42 patients randomly assigned to treatment and control groups, the required sample size to achieve an effect size of .25 was determined post hoc to be 140 (with 70 in each group) to reach a significance level of .05 with a power of .80 (Buchanan, El-Banna, White, Moses, Siedlik, & Wood, 2004).

Qualitative Studies

Qualitative studies generally employ relatively small, nonrandom samples. Because the aim of qualitative research is to describe and analyze the meanings and experiences of particular individuals or groups, large sample sizes are not generally appropriate or feasible in these scenarios. Instead, the sample size should be sufficient to provide enough information to answer the research question based on the notion of data saturation. Participants continue to be enrolled in a study until no new information is being uncovered; that is, redundancy occurs in all subsequent data collection encounters.

Redundancy may be achieved with a limited number of participants when the sample is homogenous. For this reason, it is not unusual to have very small sample sizes in phenomenologic studies. For example, Schneider and Mannell (2006) had 12 participants in their study of spirituality and faith in parents of children with cancer, and Barnett (2005) interviewed 10 participants for her study of the lived experience of patients with chronic obstructive pulmonary disease.

? Think Outside the Box

What would be the implications of the "rule of 30" applied to qualitative research?

In contrast, for ethnographic or grounded theory studies, in which the sample is usually more heterogeneous, larger sample sizes are generally the norm. For example, a focused ethnography approach was used with 61 nurses in an evaluation of the implementation of evidence-based nursing activities on two intrapartum units (Angus, Hodnett, & O'Brien-Pallas, 2003), and 21 participants supplied the data upon which a grounded theory of readjustment following myocardial infarction was developed (Brink, Karlson, & Hallberg, 2006).

Specific Evidence-Based Practice Considerations

Evidence-based clinical decisions are essential for the practice of nursing. Melnyk and Fineout-Overholt (2005) have rightly asserted, "The goal of EBP is to use the highest quality of knowledge in providing care to produce the greatest impact on patients' health status and healthcare" (p. 75). It is imperative, therefore, to have the ability to critically examine the available research and to determine the strength of the evidence. Several guiding questions can help direct reading about and critiquing sampling plans. While these questions are similar in some respects in both quantitative and qualitative research, they differ in many other respects (Table 6-2).

Table 6-2

Guidelines for Critiquing the Sample for Evidence-Based Practice
Quantitative Research Studies
1. How and when was the desired sample size determined?
2. Was the sample size adequate to answer the research question?
3. What were the inclusion and exclusion criteria?
4. Was the sampling strategy one of probability or nonprobability? Was this strategy appropriate to the research question?
5. Is the sample for the study clearly described?
6. Are there potential biases in the sample selection or the sample itself that could have an effect on the outcome of the study?
7. Is the sample representative of the target population? Is it representative of your own patients?
Qualitative Research Studies
1. Which sampling strategy was used to choose the participants?
2. Was the sample size adequate to answer the research question?
3. Is the sample for the study clearly described?
4. Is the sample representative of the phenomenon of interest?

Quantitative Evidence Critique

A well-written quantitative research report contains a detailed explanation of the sampling strategy (including sample size determination) and the inclusion and exclusion criteria together with the rationale for their use. Lee and Laffrey (2006), for example, provided the following description of the sampling plan in their examination of the predictors of physical activity in older adults with borderline hypertension:

> Sample size for this cross-sectional explanatory study was determined according to Bentler's (1995) criterion of five participants per free model parameter. The proposed model, with 48 free parameters, required 265 participants. A nonprobability sample of 316 men and women was recruited from 16 senior centers with nutrition programs in four cities in central Texas. The BP [blood pressure] range for participants was between 130 and 160 mm Hg systolic or 85 and 100 mm Hg diastolic. This BP range was selected because lifestyle modification, such as regular PA [physical activity], has been recommended for preventing hypertension in persons with a high normal BP as well as for initial treatment of persons with mild to moderate hypertension (NHLBI, 1997, 2003). Participants were (a) aged 60–75 years, (b) able to read and write English, and (c) able to walk without assistance. Persons with cognitive impairment were excluded. (p. 112)

The well-written quantitative research report also thoroughly describes the demographic characteristics of the sample that actually participated in the study:

> Of the 316 participants, 267 (84%) completed the study. The average age of the participants was 69 years. . . . 183 (68.5%) were women, and 172 (64.4%) were Caucasian. The participants were well educated. . . . forty percent lived alone and 44% reported family incomes over $30,000. (Lee & Laffrey, 2006, p. 112)

Descriptions such as these allow the reader to determine the representativeness of the sample for their own population and establish the strength of the evidence for implementing the findings.

Qualitative Evidence Critique

A well-written qualitative research report also contains a detailed explanation of the sampling strategy as well as a description of the sample obtained. Sullivan-Bolyai, Knafl, Tamborlane, and Grey (2004), for example, described the plan they used to recruit participants in their study of parents whose children were using insulin pumps as follows:

> A list of patients less than 12 years old was obtained from the pediatric diabetes clinic staff at the hospital. The principal investigator contacted the parents of each of these children regarding participation in the study. . . . Fourteen mothers and seven fathers (six couples and nine single parents) of 16 children (including a set of twins) with type 1 diabetes were identified. All agreed to participate except two mothers. . . . All participating parents (n = 21) were Caucasian and well educated . . . with a mean age of 38 ± 3 years. All were married, except one divorced mother. (p. 317)

Evaluating the Evidence for Implementation

Once the sample characteristics and size have been critically analyzed, the next step in determining appropriateness for consideration for EBP is to establish whether this evidence, however good, is applicable in the local situation. For example, in the study of a smoking cessation intervention, "the typical participant was married or partnered, Caucasian, and employed, had a high school education and mean annual income of $19,800 (±$9,876)" (Buchanan et al., 2004,

p. 327). A nurse working with a predominately Hispanic population of migrant workers who wanted to implement a smoking cessation program with proven success would need to carefully consider whether the strategy designed by these researchers could be applied in the local setting. An alternative in this situation would be to examine the smoking cessation strategies employed in the study conducted by Malchodi et al. (2003), whose sample was predominately Hispanic, single, and unemployed, with more than 50% having less than a high school education. Although Malchodi et al. conducted their study in a sample of pregnant women, their strategies may well be more appropriate for the local situation because of the sociocultural similarities of the populations.

? Think Outside the Box

Specific evidence-based practice considerations: Identify the demographic characteristics of a sample that would be representative of the population with whom you are currently working in a clinical course.

Sampling Decisions for an Evidence-Based Project

After identifying the clinical question or problem on which to build an evidence-based project and deciding, based on the strength of the evidence, on an appropriate intervention or change in practice, a sampling decision must be made. Based on the information contained in this chapter, it should be clear that the best (i.e., the strongest) sampling technique would be a random assignment of patients to either the nursing intervention or the standard of care. If it were not possible to randomize the participants, then a nonrandom sampling plan would be appropriate if efforts to build in representativeness through matching or purposive sampling procedures were used.

Final Comments on Sampling

Although they are only one component in the overall research process, sampling decisions affect both the internal validity and the external validity of a study. As such, critical analysis of the sampling strategy, the sample size, and the quality of the sample are essential in determining the relevance of the results of one study, or a group of studies, to EBP for nurses.

Summary Points

1. Sampling allows a researcher to draw conclusions about the research problem under investigation based on information from a portion of the population, rather than the whole population.

2. The researcher selects a sample from an accessible population that is representative of the target population to whom the findings may be generalized.

3. Probability sampling strategies employ random selection of elements of the population. Probability strategies include simple random, systematic random, stratified random, and cluster sampling.

4. Nonprobability sampling strategies employ nonrandom selection of elements of the population. Nonprobability strategies include convenience, quota, purposive, snowball, and theoretical sampling.

5. Sampling decisions in quantitative research are made based on the desire to have a representative sample. Sampling strategies include both probability and nonprobability strategies.

6. Sampling decisions in qualitative research are made based on the desire to obtain data that are representative of the phenomenon of interest. Sampling strategies are almost always nonprobability strategies.

7. Critiquing studies to determine their relevance for evidence-based practice (EBP) involves evaluation of the sampling plan, sampling strategies, and sample size for their appropriateness to the research question and the research design.

RED FLAGS

- Randomization of a sample group strengthens a study. Bias within the sampling process is decreased by randomization.
- The appropriate sample size for a quantitative study is best established by performing a power analysis before the study gets under way.
- Convenience and snowball sampling methodologies are weak sampling methods owing to their higher potential for lack of generalizability and potential for bias.
- At the least, inclusion criterion should be documented for review within the research report. Both inclusion and exclusion criteria should be provided.
- Failure to utilize the "rule of 30" can weaken a study.
- Inadequate or unclear description of the sampling strategy results in confusion when others attempt to understand the study's conclusions.
- Failure to use a sampling strategy that would produce a sample size appropriate for the particular research method leads to a limitation for the study.
- Attempts to generalize findings past the representativeness of the sample are inappropriate.
- Failure to acknowledge limitations resulting from sample size or sample selection decisions is problematic.

Multiple Choice Questions

1. Sampling criteria may be defined as

   A. The identification of eligibility or ineligibility to participate in a study.
   B. The population in which the investigator is interested.
   C. The selection of a subset of a population to represent the whole population.
   D. A technique used to ensure that each person has a chance of being included in a study.

2. Another term for cluster sampling is

   A. Systematic sampling.
   B. Quota sampling.
   C. Multistage sampling.
   D. Network sampling.

3. You are to select a set of five subjects using systematic random sampling and a random numbers table. The total population includes 50 subjects. Your pencil was initially placed on the fifth column from the left and the third row down. The decision is to move across the columns to the right.

   13 25 31 40 23 29 10 17 12 32
   49 42 21 48 38 14 35 34 07 02
   45 15 26 11 06 24 04 44 40 50
   08 22 20 35 01 43 09 33 28 16
   03 37 19 54 47 18 43 27 46 05

   What will the subject numbers be?

   A. 06, 01, 47, 29, and 14
   B. 06, 11, 26, 15, and 45
   C. 06, 38, 23, 29, and 10
   D. 06, 24, 04, 44, and 40

4. Which of the following types of studies would require the largest sample size?

   A. Correlational
   B. Ethnography
   C. Grounded theory
   D. Phenomenologic

5. A researcher has decided to conduct a satisfaction survey among all of the patients who presented to the emergency department over a two-month period of time. This is an example of

   A. Stratified random sampling.
   B. Cluster sampling.
   C. Convenience sampling.
   D. Purposive sampling.

6. A total of 20 nursing students are randomly selected from a random sample of five nursing programs in one state. This is an example of

    A. Simple random sampling.
    B. Cluster sampling.
    C. Convenience sampling.
    D. Purposive sampling.

7. Power analysis is conducted to

    A. Determine a large effect size.
    B. Estimate sample size.
    C. Test for internal validity.
    D. Set the level of significance.

8. Determination of the appropriate sample size in qualitative research is based on the principle(s) of

    A. Power analysis.
    B. The "rule of 30."
    C. Saturation and redundancy.
    D. Convenience.

9. Which of the following samples is least likely to be representative of the overall population?

    A. Convenience
    B. Quota
    C. Random
    D. Stratified random

10. In interpreting quantitative research results, the representativeness of the sample is most closely tied to

    A. Internal validity.
    B. External validity.
    C. Sample validity.
    D. Research validity.

Discussion Questions

1. You are a nurse working in the labor and delivery suite in an academic medical center. You are interested in nonpharmacologic pain management for your patients and would like to implement an evidence-based change project on your unit. Which particular sampling concerns will you examine in the research studies about nonpharmacologic pain management for the laboring patients?

2. You are a BSN student enrolled in a research course. The instructor has given you the following problem statement: "Does music affect the perception of pain in patients who have undergone hip replacement?" Describe one probability sampling plan and one nonprobability sampling plan for answering this question.

3. Read the excerpt below from an article describing an intervention to increase mothers' knowledge regarding infant immunization and answer the following questions:
   1. What is the sampling strategy used?
   2. What were the inclusion and exclusion criteria?
   3. What are the sample characteristics?
   4. Is this sample representative?
   5. How could the sampling strategy be improved?

   Fifty-four mothers were recruited and randomized to either a control or an experimental group. Women who had low income, received immunization and well-baby care at the study sites, and had children younger than 2 years were eligible to participate in the study. Eligible participants were identified by the health center staff during well-baby visits and approached by a member of the research team. . . . The mean age of the participants was 26 years (SD = 7.8 years), ranging between 18 and 52 years. The average income was between $10,000 and $15,000, and nearly half of the mothers were unemployed (47%). Seventy-eight percent of the mothers were head-of-household single parents with an average of two children in each family. All the participants were African Americans (Wilson, Brown, & Stephens-Ferris, 2006, p. 8).

Suggested Readings

Claudio, L., & Stingone, J. A. (2008). Improving sampling and response rates in children's health research through participatory methods. *Journal of School Health, 78*(8), 445–451.

Hedges, C., & Bliss-Holtz, J. (2006). Not too big, not too small, but just right: The dilemma of sample size estimation. *AACN Advanced Critical Care, 17*(3), 341–344.

Higginbottom, G. M. (2004). Sampling issues in qualitative research. *Nurse Researcher, 12*(1), 7–19.

Jackson, R. (2005). Sampling errors. *Health Care Food & Nutrition Focus, 22*(1), 2.

Trochim, W. (2006). *Research Methods Knowledge Base: Sampling.* Retrieved September 17, 2009, from http://www.socialresearchmethods.net/kb/sampling.php

Yoon, S. L., & Horne, C. H. (2004). Accruing the sample in survey research. *Southern Online Journal of Nursing Research, 2*(5), 1–17.

References

Angus, J., Hodnett, E., & O'Brien-Pallus, L. (2003). Implementing evidence-based nursing practice: A tale of two intrapartum nursing units. *Nursing Inquiry, 10*(4), 218–228.

Barnett, M. (2005). Chronic obstructive pulmonary disease: A phenomenological study of patients' experiences. *Journal of Clinical Nursing, 14*(7), 805–812.

Bayleyegn, T., Wolkin, A., Oberst, K., Young, S., Sanchez, C., Phelps, A., et al. (2006). Rapid assessment of the needs and health status in Santa Rosa and Escambia counties, Florida, after Hurricane Ivan, September 2004. *Disaster Management Response, 4*(1), 12–18.

Beauchesne, M. A., Kelley, B. R., Patsdaughter, C. A., & Pickard, J. (2002). Attack on America: Children's reactions and parents' responses. *Journal of Pediatric Health Care, 16*(5), 213–221.

Brink, E., Karlson, B. W., & Hallberg, L. R. (2006). Readjustment 5 months after a first-time myocardial infarction: Reorienting the active self. *Journal of Advanced Nursing, 53*(4), 403–411.

Buchanan, L. M., El-Banna, M., White, A., Moses, S., Siedlik, C., & Wood, M. (2004). An exploratory study of multicomponent treatment intervention for tobacco dependency. *Journal of Nursing Scholarship, 36*(4), 324–330.

Calvin, A. O. (2004). Haemodialysis patients and end-of-life decisions: A theory of personal preservation. *Journal of Advanced Nursing, 46*(5), 558–566.

Cohen, J. (1989). *Statistical power analysis for the behavioral sciences* (2nd ed.). Hillsdale, NJ: Lawrence Erlbaum Associates.

Doherty, M. E., & Scannell-Desch, E. (2008). The lived experience of widowhood during pregnancy. *Journal of Midwifery & Women's Health, 53*(2), 103–109.

Hinkle, D., Wiersma, W., & Jurs, S. (1988). *Applied statistics for the behavioral sciences* (2nd ed.). Boston: Houghton-Mifflin.

Jahraus, D., Sokolosky, S. Thurston, N., & Guo, D. (2002). Evaluation of an education program for patients with breast cancer receiving radiation therapy. *Cancer Nursing, 25*(4), 266–275.

Kim, H. S., & Kim, H. S. (2005). Incestuous experience among Korean adolescents: Prevalence, family problems, perceived family dynamics, and psychological characteristics. *Public Health Nursing, 22*(6), 472–482.

Kraemer, H. C., & Thiemann, S. (1987). *How many subjects? Statistical power analysis in research.* Newbury Park, CA: Sage.

Lee, Y. S., & Laffrey, S. C. (2006). Predictors of physical activity in older adults with borderline hypertension. *Nursing Research, 55*(2), 110–120.

Malchodi, C. S., Oncken, C., Dornelas, E. A., Caramanica, L., Gregonia, E., & Curry, S. L. (2003). The effects of peer counseling on smoking cessation and reduction. *Obstetrics and Gynecology, 101*(3), 504–510.

Malloch, K., & Porter-O'Grady, T. (2006). *Introduction to evidence-based practice in nursing and health care.* Sudbury, MA: Jones and Bartlett.

McMurry, T. B. (2006). A comparison of pharmacologic tobacco cessation relapse rates. *Journal of Community Health Nursing, 23*(1), 15–28.

Melnyk, B. M., & Fineout-Overholt, E. (2005). *Evidence-based practice in nursing and health-care: A guide to best practice.* Philadelphia: Lippincott Williams & Wilkins.

Ruchala, P. L., Metheny, N., Essenpreis, H., & Borcherding, K. (2002). Current practice in oxytocin dilution and fluid administration for induction of labor. *Journal of Obstetric, Gynecologic, and Neonatal Nursing, 31*(5), 545–550.

Schneider, M. A., & Mannell, R. C. (2006). Beacon in the storm: An exploration of the spirituality and faith of parents whose children have cancer. *Issues in Comprehensive Pediatric Nursing, 29*(1), 3–24.

Steel, A., Underwood, C., Notley, C., & Blunt M. (2008). The impact of offering a relatives' clinic on the satisfaction of the next-of-kin of critical care patients: A prospective time-interrupted trial. *Intensive Critical Care Nursing, 24*(2), 122–129.

Sullivan-Bolyai, S., Knafl, K., Tamborlane, W., & Grey, M. (2004). Parents' reflections on managing their children's diabetes with insulin pumps. *Journal of Nursing Scholarship, 36*(4), 316–323.

Tamaki, A. (2008). Effectiveness of home visits by mental health nurses for Japanese women with post-partum depression. *International Journal of Mental Health Nursing, 17*(6), 419–427.

Wilson, F. L., Brown, D. L., & Stephens-Ferris, M. (2006). Can easy-to-read immunization information increase knowledge in urban low-income mothers? *Journal of Pediatric Nursing, 21*(1), 4–12.

Chapter 7

Quantitative Research Design

Sharon Cannon

Chapter Objectives

At the conclusion of this chapter, the learner will be able to

1. List characteristics of quantitative designs
2. Discuss descriptive designs
3. Identify control for quantitative designs
4. Compare experimental, nonexperimental, time-dimensional, and quasi-experimental designs
5. Examine research design and quality improvement programs
6. Select a quantitative design for research utilization in an evidence-based practice clinical situation

Key Terms

➤ Comparative design

➤ Control

➤ Correlational design

➤ Dependent variable

➤ Descriptive design

➤ Experimental design

➤ Independent variable

➤ Manipulation

➤ Meta-analysis

➤ Nonequivalent control group

➤ Nonexperimental design

➤ Quantitative design

➤ Quasi-experimental design

➤ Randomization

➤ Research design and quality
   improvement project

➤ Secondary analysis

➤ Time-dimensional design

Introduction

The most commonly used research design is a quantitative design. But precisely what is a quantitative design? This question, as well as the characteristics and types of designs for use in evidence-based practice (EBP) clinical situations, are discussed in this chapter.

Before exploring the characteristics of a study design, it is necessary to define quantitative research. Quantitative research is often identified with the traditional scientific method that gathers data objectively in an organized, systematic, controlled manner so that the findings can be generalized to other situations/populations (Brockopp & Hastings-Tolsma, 2003; Burns & Grove, 2009; Fain, 2009; Polit & Beck, 2008). A design is a plan on how to proceed; thus a quantitative research design can be defined as an objective, systematic plan to gather data that has application to other situations/ populations. Quantitative design may be (1) experimental, (2) non-experimental, or (3) quasi-experimental. Studies utilizing an experimental design use treatment and control groups; those with a nonexperimental design generate questions for experimental design; and studies having a quasi-experimental design lack randomization or may not include a control group.

Characteristics of Quantitative Research Design

The characteristics of quantitative design center on the why, where, who, what, when, and how questions. The quantitative researcher must state why (purpose) the study is being done, where (setting) the study is being conducted (i.e., laboratory, hospital, or clinic), who (subjects) is being studied (i.e., animals or humans), what type of data is being collected, when the data are to be collected, and how (design) the data are to be collected.

Within the framework of these questions, quantitative research looks for cause and effect in an experiment. When considering potential causes and effects, different groups participating in the study are viewed in terms of being either treatment or control groups. Control is one of the most common and important characteristics of quantitative design. To understand the concept of control, it is necessary to understand variables. A variable can be a quality, characteristic, attribute, or property of a person, thing, or situation (Burns & Grove, 2009; Polit & Beck, 2008). The two types of variables found in quantitative research are dependent and independent variables. The dependent variable is the outcome caused by the independent variable; the independent variable is a treatment, intervention, or experiment. Consider the situation in which a nurse researcher studies the effect of patient teaching (independent variable) about wound care in an attempt to reduce the likelihood of wound infection (dependent variable) when the surgical patient is discharged from the hospital. In this example, the teaching is what affects the rate of wound infection.

? **Think Outside the Box**

Considering these two examples, which type of research design could be used to provide the strongest methodology possible:
- What information has been used to determine the method of catheterizing for a laboring mother?
- What information serves as the basis for the range of blood sugars used within elderly persons who are newly diagnosed with diabetes?

Closely connected to the issue of control is manipulation of the independent variable. The researcher wants to make sure that the treatment is the only explanation for the outcome. In the example given previously, the nurse researcher wants to ensure that the patient education on wound care delivered prior to discharge is the reason why the rate of wound infections in discharged surgical patients decreases. Control or manipulation in this situation would involve providing patient education to surgical patients who are not taking antibiotics when discharged from the hospital. Obviously, because patients who are taking antibiotics would be least likely to develop a wound infection, the use of antibiotics would be a variable that might skew the results.

Another important characteristic of quantitative research is randomization. Randomization is the assignment of subjects to a group in such a manner that each subject has an equal opportunity of being selected to participate in the study. In the example previously given about wound care, the researcher might have two groups: The control group would include those subjects who did not receive any wound care education, whereas the experimental group would include those subjects who did receive the patient education. Randomization would occur when the patients were assigned to either group in a way that each patient had an equal opportunity for inclusion in either group. This could be done by selecting every third patient discharged to be a member of a group. Another way to randomize the sample might be to give each patient a number, draw the numbers out of a hat, and alternate assignment to the groups. Randomization helps to eliminate bias. For example, the nurse who thinks that only her patients should be in the treatment group would be biased; randomization of subjects would eliminate that possibility. Although randomization strengthens a study, be aware that not all studies can be randomized. Randomization can be costly and time-consuming, and there may not be enough participants to randomize them effectively. Thus not all study samples can be randomized.

In any quantitative research study, it is important to control the influence of extraneous variables, such as gender, age, and ethnicity. Randomization provides for internal validity of a study because the groups are equal at the beginning of the study. External validity is achieved when the outcome can be applied (generalized) to the target population; generalization helps strengthen the study results. Using the wound care example, control of the extraneous variable could involve not providing patient education to pediatric patients, but rather providing it only to the adult patients.

Manipulation, control, and randomization are three essential characteristics of quantitative research design. These characteristics enable the researcher to be confident that the outcome is caused by the intervention and not by other variables, and that it can be generalized to a target population.

Descriptive Design

Descriptive design examines the characteristics of just one sample population. According to Burns and Grove (2009), this type of research design may be used for theory development, practice problems, rationale for current practice, generating hypotheses, or clinical decision making based on what others are doing. Examples of descriptive design include comparative (looks at differences in two or more groups), time-dimensional (occurring over an extended period of time), cross-sectional (stages of development simultaneously), trends and events, and correlational (relationships) designs. A descriptive design describes or explains the variables being studied and provides flexibility in examining a problem from many different angles. The two most commonly used types of descriptive designs are comparative and correlational.

The comparative design involves no manipulation or control of the independent variable, with the dependent variable being the only variable measured in two or more groups (Brink & Wood, 2001). This type of design can also be retrospective in nature. Using the wound care example, a comparative design would assign patients with wounds to a group of surgical patients or to a group of patients with wounds resulting from trauma to compare the rates of post-discharge infections. The research question might be, "Is the rate of infection higher in trauma patients than in surgical patients?" The patients' past histories would then be examined for prior surgeries or trauma wounds. Cause and effect remain the focus of this design, in that the two groups being compared for infection rates are identified according to the type of wound.

? Think Outside the Box

Explore the idea of control within a quantitative design methodology. Which aspects of the study design are important to consider and why?

Perhaps the most widely used type of descriptive design is the correlational study. Simply stated, a correlational design examines the relationships between two or more variables within a situation without knowing the reason for the relationship. The researcher may use this design when there is uncertainty about whether the variables are related and, if so, how they are related. However, the researcher assumes that the variables *are* related and seeks to discover and explain that relationship. Correlational designs do not conclude that only one variable causes another because the independent variable cannot always be controlled (Polit & Beck, 2008).

Another aspect of a correlational design is that it is "ex post facto," meaning "from after the fact" (Polit & Beck, 2006). For example, a study that compares a variable occurring in the past with a variable occurring currently would be characterized as using a retrospective correlational design. In other words, a study that looks at a variable after the fact is a retrospective study. For instance, the nurse researcher might conduct a chart review on all discharged surgical patients to determine if any patient education on wound care occurred prior to discharge from the hospital and then to check whether any of those patients were readmitted for a wound infection.

Prospective correlational designs are usually considered stronger than retrospective designs, because the researcher may be able to control or rule out explanations for some outcomes (Polit & Beck, 2008). These designs require the researcher to assume cause and effect and to implement the study under those assumptions.

Correlational designs may also be predictive in nature. In this type of study, one variable occurs prior to another variable—that is, the independent variable occurs prior to the dependent variable. Again using the wound care example, a predictive correlational study research statement might be, "The rate of wound infection will decrease 1 week post discharge after receiving the wound care educational program in the outpatient clinic."

Experimental Design

Experimental design looks for cause and effect (outcome). Obviously, there must be a preceding cause and a relationship between the cause and the outcome without any influencing variables to warrant the conclusion that a cause-and-effect relationship exists.

Several issues related to experimental design should be addressed before discussing the designs themselves. The first issue is that not all variables can be manipulated. In the prior wound care example, not every patient has a wound. As such, the researcher cannot inflict a wound on all individuals so as to obtain a large random sample.

Another issue is that of ethics. Consider the famous Tuskegee Syphilis Study, an experiment that was conducted over 40 years to examine the progress of syphilis in adult black males. Many of the subjects in this study were not even aware that they were participants. Also, even though an effective treatment for syphilis (penicillin) was available, not all subjects with syphilis in this study were given penicillin. To satisfy ethical concerns, some variables should not be manipulated.

Feasibility is another issue in experimental design. Some experiments may be too expensive, require cooperation from individuals from multiple key areas, require too much time, or not have enough subjects for participation.

In experimental design, another significant issue is that of the Hawthorne effect. Simply stated, the Hawthorne effect arises when the subjects know that they are part of the study and change their behavior accordingly; that is, the act of observing changes the observed's behavior.

Keeping in mind these issues, we now move on to an examination of experimental design. The most classic experimental design is a pre-test/post-test design. With this approach, subjects are assigned to one of two groups: a control (comparative) group that does not receive the treatment (intervention) or an experimental group that does receive the treatment. In the wound care example, patients would be assigned to a group that receives no specific wound care

Figure 7-1

Experimental design examples.

Pre-test/Post-test

$$R \quad O_1 \quad X_1 \quad O_2$$

$$R \quad O_1 \quad X_2 \quad O_2$$

Two-Group Post-test Only

$$R \quad X_1 \quad O_1$$

$$R \quad X_2 \quad O_1$$

Three Groups

$$R \quad X_1 \quad O_1$$

$$R \quad X_2 \quad O_1$$

$$R \quad O_1$$

Four Groups

$$R \quad O_1 \quad X_1 \quad O_2$$

$$R \quad X_1 \quad O_2$$

$$R \quad O_1 \quad X_2 \quad O_2$$

$$R \quad X_2 \quad O_2$$

Note: O = Outcome/measurement; R = Random assignment; X = Treatment/intervention.

instructions (control group) or to the group that receives patient education regarding wound care (experimental group).

Another experimental design of considerable importance in the healthcare arena is the randomized controlled trial (RCT). The RCT is considered the true experiment. This design may involve two, three, or four groups. The tests used may involve both a pre-test and post-test, a post-test only, or repeated measures (Figure 7-1).

Nonexperimental Design

Some studies do not lend themselves to an experimental design; that is, manipulation of variables is not possible, nor is randomization controlled. Studies with this kind of nonexperimental design occur in the here and now and are observational rather than interventional in nature. Two types of nonexperimental designs used in EBP are secondary analysis and meta-analysis.

Secondary analysis follows the course implied by its name: It examines data obtained in another study and allows researchers to examine large and small data sets collected via different approaches. A secondary analysis asks new questions about data previously collected for another purpose. For example, a nurse researcher interested in the effects of patient education on decreased wound infection rates might examine one or several previously conducted studies. By analyzing a variable that had not been studied previously, such as the age of the patient, a secondary analysis might show a relationship to wound healing, especially for geriatric patients.

Meta-analysis also looks at previous studies. Brockopp and Hastings-Tolsma (2003) indicate that meta-analysis, through calculation of statistics, can help researchers establish the existence of bias and confounding variables in the cause-and-effect relationship identified in multiple studies. Polit and Beck (2006) suggest that a data set is "the total collection of data for all sample members for analysis" (p. 642). The data set analysis carried out as part of a meta-analysis is similar to that performed for individual studies through statistical tests. The key to understanding meta-analysis is the application of statistics to multiple studies looking at the same phenomenon (Burns & Grove, 2009).

❓ Think Outside the Box

If you have elected to use a nonexperimental design, how can you strengthen the confidence in the research project's findings?

Although secondary and meta-analyses are of particular importance for research utilization in EBP, caution should be taken when considering their findings. Not all studies focus on the same subject, and information may even be missing from some studies. Care should be taken before leaping to conclusions or making generalizations in applying findings to specific populations because bias can result, especially in other studies with small sample sizes. The researcher should keep in mind the adage that "one size does not fit all."

Time-Dimensional Design

When establishing a research project, attention must always be given to the dimension of time. The determination of when and how long data are to be collected is an essential component to any research design. If data have already been collected, then the study is considered to utilize a retrospective design. An example of a retrospective design would be that of a chart review. Perhaps a new procedure has been implemented to decrease length of stay (LOS). The nurse might go to the Medical Records department and conduct a chart review for the average LOS for patients who did not receive the new procedure versus those who did receive it.

A second type of time-dimensional design comprises a cross-sectional design. The cross-sectional design measures only what is currently in existence; it does not examine anything that happened in the past or future. An example of this design world could be a retrospective chart review of lung cancer patients for the past five years to discover how long they had smoked cigarettes. Many cross-sectional studies are retrospective in nature, but they all collect data at a specific point in time.

The third type of time-dimensional design is the longitudinal study. As is implied by the name, a study with a longitudinal design relies on data that are collected at various intervals over time. The times for data collection may be short or long depending on the rate of change. This design is useful to examine changes that occur over time and assist in determining causality (Polit & Beck, 2008). Longitudinal designs are considered stronger than cross-sectional study designs because longitudinal designs allow for the possibility that changes and trends might emerge. However, longitudinal studies also face the extra danger of having subjects drop out over time, and they are generally more expensive to manage.

Each of the time-dimensional designs has its own set of advantages and disadvantages that must be considered by the researcher. In addition, the strengths and weaknesses of each study design must be considered before the results of the studies are applied to practice.

Quasi-Experimental Design

Given that randomization is often not possible in research studies, quasi-experimental design is the most frequently used quantitative research design. With this approach, the independent variable is still manipulated, but there is no randomization or control group. The purpose of quasi-experimental design is to examine causality, though it is acknowledged that this design is not as strong as the experimental design, which has a control group and randomization. Nevertheless, quasi-experimental design is considered stronger than descriptive design, and it is more practical when true experimental design is not possible.

Types of quasi-experimental design include (1) post-test only with nonequivalent groups, (2) one-group pre-test/post-test, (3) untreated control group with pre-test/post-test, (4) removal treatment and reversal treatment, (5) nonequivalent control group, and (6) time series. The two most commonly used designs—nonequivalent control group and time series—are discussed here.

The nonequivalent control group design (sometimes called a comparison group) compares two groups that are not randomized. The initial baseline measurement (O_1) is used to determine if the subjects assigned to groups are similar. A treatment/intervention (X) is applied, and then a second measurement (O_2) is performed to see if the outcome is a result of the treatment/intervention (Figure 7-2).

Using the prior example of wound care, all patients would be assigned to group 1 or group 2. A pre-test assessment would be conducted. The intervention (patient education program) would then be implemented. Each group would then be tested to see if its members experienced a decreased infection rate (outcome). When using this type of study design, the nurse researcher should keep in mind potential confounding factors such as the Hawthorne effect as well as the threat of history. History, in this instance, refers to some other variable that might have occurred. In the wound care experiment, an

---

Figure 7-2

Quasi-experimental design examples.

Nonequivalent Control Group

O_1 X O_2

O_1 O_2

Note: O_1 = Baseline measurement; X = Treatment/intervention; O_2 = Outcome

measurement.

Time Series (Simple)

O_1 O_2 O_3 X O_4 O_5 O_6

Note: O_1, O_2, O_3 = Baseline measurements at various levels; X = Treatment/intervention;

O_4, O_5, O_6 = Outcome measures at various intervals.

example of the history variable might be the patients who received additional instruction by the doctor's office staff prior to undergoing surgery or again after the educational program was administered.

The second quasi-experimental design to be discussed is the time-series design. This type of study may be conducted over a long period, in which case it is also called a longitudinal study. With a time series design, participants are not randomized, nor is a control group used. Data are collected at various intervals prior to the treatment as well as after the treatment (see Figure 7-2). Returning to the wound care example, in a time-series design, the first observation might be on days 2 and 3 postoperatively, with a subsequent observation being recorded on the day of discharge. The educational program would then be conducted. The next three measurements might be on days 5, 7, and 9 postoperatively.

A variable that should be considered as an alternative explanation for the outcome measurement within time-series studies is maturation. Maturation refers to change that occurs throughout the entire span of time that the experiment is conducted. It might be a result of the repetition of testing, which might influence the scores that follow. For instance, if the patients were tested about wound care knowledge prior to receiving the educational program, they might become aware of what was needed for wound care to prevent infection just because of the questions used to test their baseline knowledge.

? Think Outside the Box

Discuss how you would use the ranking of research designs' strength in evidence-based practice.

Another area of concern with the time-series design is the potential for attrition of subjects. Because the study occurs over time, subjects may drop out of the study for various reasons. As a result, the sample size may be too small when the study ends, causing the study's findings to not be generalizable to other situations or populations.

The two quasi-experimental designs discussed here offer a practical approach when an experimental design is not possible. Nurse researchers should be alert to the possible threats of the quasi-experimental design that can lead to other reasons for the study's outcomes.

Control

As indicated earlier in this chapter, control of variables is critical when the researcher is seeking to determine the extent of a cause-and-effect relationship for the treatment/intervention applied as part of a study. Randomization helps control extraneous variables, both internal and external, to a research project, especially when the study employs an experimental design.

In studies using nonexperimental and quasi-experimental designs, which do not have randomization or control groups, using subjects who are similar helps control extraneous variables that can influence the outcome. As a result, history, maturation, and attrition threats must be considered when designing the research project so as to maintain control. Variables can be controlled through the establishment of specific inclusion/exclusion criteria for selection of subjects, timing of test intervals, use of scripts for data collectors, and the setting in which the study is conducted.

Research Design and Quality Improvement Projects

Care must be given when designing quantitative research. Even though research and quality improvement (QI) activities are focused on patient outcomes, they are different processes (Kring, 2008). QI results can provide direction for improving practice but are not necessarily considered true "scientific inquiry." For example, chart reviews may reveal a trend but do not inspire the same level of confidence as results produced from a quantitative retrospective research design. QI projects can and often do contribute additional evidence, and it may even give significance to previous findings. Nevertheless, research designs take a more rigorous approach toward producing results and have more significant implications for practice. Both research design and QI projects may have implications for evidence-based practice, however, and their relationship should be considered within the totality of quantitative research design.

Evidence-Based Considerations

Utilization of quantitative research design in EBP requires the nurse to be able to comprehend the various designs and understand both their benefits and their shortcomings. Whether the nurse is participating in research or is applying research findings in practice, the type of design is essential to guide clinical decision making. The concepts of randomization and control in quantitative research provide information about generalization of outcomes in experimental, nonexperimental, and quasi-experimental studies to current practice.

If a nurse wants to look at the relationship between an educational program and the rate of wound infections, a correlational design would be appropriate. In contrast, if a nurse wants to examine the effect of a wound care educational program in producing a decreased rate of wound infections, the appropriate quantitative design would be experimental or quasi-experimental. Use of a secondary analysis or meta-analysis is another way a nurse might use quantitative research to validate existing practice or the need to change practice.

Manipulation, control of variables, and randomization are essential components of quantitative research. Extraneous variables in the practice setting must be examined carefully so that the evidence obtained will be applicable to nursing practice. Thus knowing whether the research design is experimental, quasi-experimental, or nonexperimental influences the strength and generalizability of a study's findings to the current practice being considered. This point is of particular significance when conducting a secondary analysis or meta-analysis of research for the purpose of making clinical decisions.

Quantitative research design and QI projects are important when examining evidence to improve practice. Nurses need to make sure they fully understand the distinctions between QI and quantitative research designs, as well as how both are relevant in EBP.

Summary Points

1. Quantitative research is often identified as corresponding with the traditional scientific method, which gathers data objectively in an organized method to allow findings to be generalized to other situations/populations.
2. A quantitative research design is an objective, systematic plan to gather data.
3. Characteristics of quantitative designs center on why, where, who, what, when, and how questions.
4. Quantitative research examines relationships for cause and effect in an experiment.
5. Manipulation of the independent variable, control of extraneous variables, and randomization are essential to quantitative research.
6. In comparative designs, there is no manipulation or control of the independent variable.
7. The most commonly used descriptive design is the correlational design, which examines relationships between two or more variables within a situation without knowing the reason why the relationship exists.
8. Correlational designs may be ex post facto, prospective, or predictive.
9. Experimental designs look for cause and effect (outcome).

10. Issues such as ethics, inability to manipulate all variables, feasibility, and the Hawthorne effect must be addressed when considering studies with experimental designs.
11. The most classic experimental design is the pre-test/post-test design.
12. The randomized controlled trial (RCT) is considered to be a true experimental design.
13. Two types of nonexperimental designs are used in evidence-based practice (EBP): secondary analysis and meta-analysis. Both look at previously completed studies and create data sets from those earlier studies to be analyzed in a different approach.
14. Quasi-experimental designs are used most frequently because the independent variable can still be manipulated even when no randomization or control group is possible.
15. The two most commonly used quasi-experimental designs are the nonequivalent control group and time-series designs.
16. The nonequivalent control group design compares two groups whose members are not randomized.
17. The time-series design is not randomized, and there is no control group. Data are gathered at various intervals.
18. Control of threats such as history, maturation, and attrition is of prime importance in quantitative designs and is of significance when making clinical decisions based on outcomes from quantitative research.
19. Understanding the implications for utilization of quantitative research in EBP requires a working knowledge of quantitative design.
20. Quality improvement projects and quantitative research are important in confirming evidence for EBP.

RED FLAGS

- For a study to be classified as an experimental (quantitative) design, the design must incorporate control, randomization, and an intervention.

- Experimental (quantitative) design is considered to be the strongest research design. Quasi-experimental (quantitative) design has less strength, and non-experimental (quantitative) design has the least strength.

- When a small sample size is used for a quantitative study, the results of the study need to be examined closely for their generalizability to other populations.

- Prospective designs are stronger than retrospective design formats.

- Control of variables is critical when results are related to cause and effect.

- A comparative design does not involve any manipulation or control of the independent variable.

Multiple Choice Questions

1. Which of the following characteristics is *not* part of a quantitative research design?
   A. Randomization
   B. Manipulation
   C. Saturation
   D. Control

2. Which of the following is *not* an independent variable?
   A. Outcome
   B. Treatment
   C. Intervention
   D. Experiment

3. Quantitative research is often identified with which method of gathering data?
   A. Triangulation
   B. Saturation
   C. Ethnography
   D. Scientific

4. Nonexperimental designs generate _____ for _____ designs.
   A. answers; quasi-experimental
   B. questions; experimental
   C. solutions; quantitative
   D. problems; experimental

5. One of the most common and important characteristics of a quantitative design is
   A. The dependent variable.
   B. The independent variable.
   C. Control.
   D. The relationship.

6. Manipulation of which variable is connected to control?
   A. Independent
   B. Dependent
   C. Extraneous
   D. Attribute

7. Randomization helps to eliminate
   A. Confounding data.
   B. Ethics.
   C. Subjects.
   D. Bias.

8. Generalization can _____ a study.

    A.   weaken
    B.   strengthen
    C.   shorten
    D.   lengthen

9. A comparative design has

    A.   No manipulation and control of the dependent variable.
    B.   Only measurement of the dependent variable.
    C.   No manipulation and control of the independent variable.
    D.   Both B and C.

10. A correlational study looks at the

    A.   Cause of two or more variables.
    B.   Relationship of two or more variables.
    C.   Effect of two or more variables.
    D.   Both A and D.

11. Issues related to experimental design include

    A.   Manipulation of all variables, ethics, and feasibility.
    B.   The Hawthorne effect, ethics, and sample size.
    C.   Treatments, interventions, and no manipulation of variables.
    D.   Feasibility, the Hawthorne effect, and research questions.

12. An example of a randomized controlled trial (RCT) design is as follows (where R = randomization, O = measurement, and X = treatment):

    A.   R O X O
    B.   O X O
    C.   O O X O O
    D.   O O O X O O O

13. Meta-analysis is the examination of multiple studies through statistical analysis to establish

    A.   The nonexistence of bias.
    B.   New data sets for analysis.
    C.   The nonexistence of confounding variables.
    D.   Correlation of the variables.

14. A quasi-experimental design is one in which

    A.   The dependent variable is manipulated with randomization and a control group.
    B.   The independent variable is manipulated with randomization and a control group.
    C.   The independent variable is manipulated with no randomization and no control group.
    D.   The dependent variable is manipulated with no randomization and no control group.

15. The initial baseline measurement in a nonequivalent control group is used to determine if the subjects assigned to the group are

    A. Different.
    B. Equal.
    C. Bonded.
    D. Similar.

16. The research design that collects data at various intervals is called a(n)

    A. Long study.
    B. Time-series study.
    C. Experimental study.
    D. Nonexperimental study.

17. An area of concern in a time-series design is

    A. Randomization.
    B. Control.
    C. Manipulation.
    D. Maturation.

18. Some ways of controlling variables for nonexperimental or quasi-experimental designs are

    A. Timing of test intervals and the setting.
    B. Randomization of subjects and control groups.
    C. Flexible inclusion and exclusion criteria.
    D. Control of history and maturation.

19. In evidence-based practice, a nurse using quantitative research for clinical decision making must be most knowledgeable about how

    A. To calculate statistics.
    B. To write research reports.
    C. The study design applies to practice.
    D. To design a research study.

20. Using research in practice requires the nurse to be most aware of

    A. Limited funding.
    B. Generalizability of the results to current practice.
    C. Exclusion of subjects.
    D. The credentials of the researcher.

21. Quality improvement (QI) projects are considered

    A. The same as scientific inquiry.
    B. Different from scientific inquiry.
    C. To focus on only patient satisfaction.
    D. A rigorous approach for research.

Discussion Questions

1. You are a nurse in a pre-op holding area in which all patients are classi-fied as "nothing by mouth" (NPO) after midnight to prevent possible aspiration. You wonder why that policy is necessary, and you and a surgical team want to design a research project to investigate the potential for providing at least some liquid nourishment to pre-op patients. The team decides to do a two-group post-test only design.

2. Using the same example as in Question 1 (all surgical patients being NPO after midnight), how would you and the surgical team conduct a meta-analysis?

3. Using a nonequivalent control group design in the NPO scenario, explain how this design would be constructed.

Suggested Readings

Bott, M., & Endacott, R. (2005). Clinical research: Quantitative data collection and analysis. *Intensive & Critical Care Nursing, 21*(3), 187–193.

Chulay, M. (2006). Good research ideas for clinicians. *AACN Advanced Critical Care, 17*(3), 253–265.

Freshwater, D. (2005). Integrating qualitative and quantitative research methods: Trend or foe? *Journal of Research in Nursing, 10*(3), 337–338.

Kinn, S., & Curzio, J. (2005). Integrating qualitative and quantitative research methods. *Journal of Research in Nursing, 10*(3), 317–336.

O'Neill, R. (2006). *The advantages and disadvantages of qualitative and quantitative research methods.* Available at: http://www.roboneill.co.uk/papers/research_methods.htm

Onwuegbuzie, A., & Leech, N. (2005). Taking the "Q" out of research: Teaching research methodology courses without the divide between quantitative and qualitative paradigms. *Quality & Quantity, 39*(3), 267–295.

Walker, W. (2005). The strengths and weaknesses of research designs involving quantitative measures. *Journal of Research in Nursing, 10*(5), 571–573.

Yoder, L. (2005). Evidence-based practice: The time is now! *MedSurg Nursing, 14*(2), 91–92.

References

Brink, P. J., & Wood, M. J. (2001). *Basic steps in planning nursing research from question to proposal* (5th ed.). Sudbury, MA: Jones and Bartlett.

Brockopp, D. Y., & Hastings-Tolsma, M. T. (2003). *Fundamentals of nursing research* (3rd ed.). Sudbury, MA: Jones and Bartlett.

Burns, N., & Grove, S. K. (2009). *The practice of nursing research: Appraisal, synthesis, and generation of evidence* (6th ed.). St. Louis, MO: Saunders Elsevier.

Fain, J. A. (2009). *Reading, understanding, and applying nursing research* (3rd ed.). Philadelphia: F. A. Davis.

Kring, D. L. (2008). Research and quality improvement: Different processes, different evidence. *MedSurg Nursing, 17*(3), 162–169.

Polit, D. F., & Beck, C. T. (2006). *Essentials of nursing research methods, appraisal and utilization* (6th ed.). Philadelphia: Lippincott Williams & Wilkins.

Polit, D. F., & Beck, C. T. (2008). *Nursing research: Generating and assessing evidence for nursing practice* (8th ed.). Philadelphia: Wolters Kluwer/Lippincott Williams & Wilkins.

Chapter 8

Qualitative Research Methods

Donna Scott Tilley

Chapter Objectives

At the conclusion of this chapter, the learner will be able to

1. Define qualitative research
2. Compare qualitative and quantitative research
3. Describe the various types of qualitative research methodology
4. Discuss reliability and validity issues in relation to qualitative research
5. Discuss analysis of qualitative data
6. Determine the benefits of using qualitative methods in nursing research

Key Terms

➤ Adequacy

➤ Appropriateness

➤ Case study

➤ Confirmability

➤ Content analysis

➤ Credibility

➤ Dependability

➤ Ethnography

➤ Grounded theory

➤ Phenomenology

➤ Qualitative research

➤ Saturation

➤ Transferability

➤ Triangulation

Introduction

Human beings are complex, multidimensional systems. Much of what drives humans is difficult to understand or measure. Perhaps not surprisingly, then, understanding such complex systems is a challenging task. Qualitative research methods, based on the assumption that truth is dynamic, offer an avenue for the exploration and understanding of elements of humanity that are not possible through quantitative research methods.

Qualitative research is not easily defined. The objectives of qualitative research vary according to the discipline involved. For example, the marketing researcher who uses qualitative methods to determine why an advertising technique is effective with adolescents has a very different goal in mind for the research than the nurse scientist who seeks to understand the experience of the transition from middle school to high school.

In addition, many types of qualitative research are possible, including case studies, ethnography, grounded theory, and phenomenology, to name but a few. These specific types are discussed in detail later in this chapter.

The word *qualitative* means that one is examining the quality of something rather than its quantity, amount, intensity, or frequency. Examining the quality of something implies a level of subjectivity. Denzin and Lincoln (1998) state that the qualitative researcher stresses the socially constructed nature of reality, the intimate relationship between the research and the subject of the research, and the situational factors that shape inquiry. Thus the social experience shapes the meaning of reality.

Prior to the 1970s, qualitative research methods were used primarily in the fields of anthropology and sociology. During the 1970s and 1980s, however, use of qualitative research methods expanded, as they were effectively applied in the disciplines of education, social work, management, nursing, and women's studies.

Nursing has traditionally focused on the person as a whole. This holistic approach to the person lends itself well to examination by qualitative methods. As a result, qualitative methods have become increasingly common in nursing research. Qualitative methods continue to gain recognition as having value for the science of nursing, as studies based on this approach contribute to areas in which little research has been done or variables for quantitative research have yet to be defined. With the increased use of qualitative methods, efforts to design such methodologies that offer holistic understanding of persons while still offering reliability and validity are also improving.

A Comparison of Quantitative and Qualitative Methods

It is not uncommon for both researchers and consumers of research to have strong opinions about the value of quantitative or qualitative methods. Those who favor quantitative methods may dismiss qualitative studies as lacking reliability and validity or structure. Those who favor qualitative methods may claim that quantitative studies are shallow or do not paint a complete and accurate picture of a phenomenon. In truth, both types of research have great scientific merit. One experienced researcher likened her preference for quantitative methods to handedness: While she is predominantly right-handed (a quantitative researcher) and finds that quantitative methods come more easily to her, she occasionally needs to use her left hand (qualitative methods) and certainly is a stronger researcher for being able to use both methods (Stiles, 2009).

Morse (1991) has identified three features that distinguish the qualitative research approach from the quantitative approach. First, qualitative research approaches phenomena from the "emic" perspective. That is, the perspective of the participant provides the source of meaning rather than the perspective of the researcher. Second, qualitative research utilizes a holistic approach to the participant. The participant brings values and life experiences that affect his or her perspective on the phenomena of interest. Whereas quantitative methods often seek to minimize the effects associated with these values and experiences, qualitative methods embrace these individual differences. Finally, qualitative methods are inductive and interactive rather than deductive. In other words, qualitative methods reach conclusions about larger groups based on observed instances.

Notably, quantitative methods require strict control to assure that the research findings actually result from the intervention being studied; thus they require that the researcher not deviate in the data collection process from one subject to another. In contrast, qualitative methods embrace the data that heterogeneous samples provide and allow the researcher to adapt his or her inquiry as understanding of the phenomena grows.

The consumer of research may also note that research participants are described differently in these two types of studies. Quantitative

Table 8-1			
Differences Between Quantitative and Qualitative Research Methods			
Point of View	**Attachment to the Participant**	**Process of Inquiry**	**Sample**
Quantitative Etic—analyzed without considering their role as a unit within a system	Seeks to minimize the differences among subjects	Deductive	Larger sample sizes required
Qualitative Emic—analyzed with consideration of their role as a unit within the system	Embraces the different perspectives of each participant	Inductive	Individuals; a small sample size is typical

researchers typically refer to the individual of interest in a study as a "subject." Qualitative researchers may refer to the individual of interest in a study as an "informant" or a "participant."

Qualitative and quantitative methods differ significantly in acceptable sample size as well. Sample sizes in qualitative studies are generally smaller than the sample sizes in quantitative studies. Because the focus of the qualitative data is on the quality of the data collected, each participant is a source of a large volume of data. Thus a smaller sample size is reasonable and common in qualitative research (Table 8-1).

The differences between qualitative and quantitative methods are clearly significant, but, in many cases, combining both methods is a viable option for researchers. A researcher might choose to combine methods in an effort to supplement the data, validate the data, or determine via pilot studies the best approach to data collection with a larger group. Combining qualitative and quantitative methods may be referred to as triangulation or as a mixed methods study.

Mixed Method Studies

Mixed method studies combine and apply one or more research methodologies in the study of a phenomenon. Mixed methods can be used in studies that are primarily either quantitative or qualitative. The benefits of convergence of qualitative and quantitative methods can include increased confidence in study data, expanded understanding of a phenomenon, the revelation of unique data, and integration of theories. Although the use of mixed methods is very effective in providing a clearer understanding of a phenomenon, mixing methods will not strengthen a flawed study (Thurmond, 2001).

Mixed methods (i.e., triangulation) might be used in four basic ways in a study: (1) data triangulation, (2) researcher triangulation, (3) theory triangulation, and (4) methodologic triangulation. Triangulation is a process where the research process along with the data is analyzed from several different directions. This process is employed to decrease the potential for biases within the research process and the analysis of the day while validating the results obtained.

? Think Outside the Box

Look at Table 8-1, which compares quantitative and qualitative research designs. Which other aspects can you identify that might be added to this table to further delineate the differences and similarities between these two research design methods?

Data triangulation involves the use of multiple data sources to validate conclusions (Polit & Beck, 2004). It includes at least three types—time, space, and person triangulation. In time triangulation, the researcher collects data on the same phenomenon or about the same informant at different times. Intervals between data collection points may be hours or months. The goal of time triangulation is to observe how the informant or phenomenon changes over time. In space triangulation, the researcher collects data on the same phenomena at different sites, which allows for assessment of consistency of data across sites. Finally, person triangulation involves data collection from different types of people or informants. Nurses are very familiar with the concept of the family as the "unit of care"; person triangulation is a similar concept. The patient experiencing a phenomenon might have a very different perspective on that phenomenon than his or her spouse, which may be different from the perspectives of siblings, parents, caregivers, or friends. Collecting data from many of the parties, therefore, widens the perspective on the phenomenon of interest.

In researcher triangulation, several observers are used rather than a single observer. More than one researcher may collect data or to analyze and interpret data as part of the same study. This technique is often used in qualitative studies as a way to ensure the validity of the research. The goal of researcher triangulation is to minimize the occurrence of researcher bias and to enhance the depth and breadth of the data analysis.

In theory triangulation, the researcher uses more than one theory or hypothesis as data are analyzed and interpreted. This strategy allows for flexibility in analysis and interpretation. Theory triangulation also helps the researcher avoid allowing preconceived ideas to guide data analysis and interpretation, and the resulting conceptualization of the phenomenon. In quantitative research, the corollary to theory triangulation is construct validation.

Methodological triangulation is the combination of qualitative and quantitative data collection techniques, which allows the researcher to more fully understand a phenomenon and link dimensions of the phenomenon. It also allows the researcher to sort through competing ideas about factors that might explain the phenomenon of interest. For example, a researcher interested in alcoholism and violence towards partners among college-age males might conduct individual interviews with young men who have been charged with battering an intimate partner while intoxicated or public intoxication. In these interviews, the subject's perspective on the degree to which alcohol is a problem for him might be discussed. The researcher might also ask the subject to complete a quantitative instrument such as the Short Michigan Alcohol Screening Test (SMAST), a ten-item questionnaire designed to objectively rate the likelihood that a person has the disease of alcoholism. Another tool, a measure that uses a Center for Epidemiologic Studies Depression Scale, would provide a different view of the mental states of the individual. Combining the interview data with the quantitative tool data paints a far more complete picture of the phenomenon of alcohol use than either the interview alone or the SMAST alone could provide (Table 8-2).

Table 8-2

An Example of Methodological Triangulation

Research Area

The development of violence in men who batter their intimate partners

Quantitative Questions

What is the prevalence of alcohol/drug use among men who batter intimate partners? (measure using a Short Michigan Alcohol Screening Test)

What is the prevalence of depression among men who batter intimate partners? (measure using a Center for Epidemiologic Studies Depression Scale)

What is the average age of onset of violence among men who batter intimate partners? (collect along with other basic demographic data)

Qualitative Questions

Which processes contributed to the violence in your relationship with your intimate partner?

What were your experiences with violence as a perpetrator, victim, or witness throughout your life?

Which life events do you identify as significant in your becoming violent?

Qualitative Research Methods

Although all qualitative research methods have the overall goal of describing complex human experiences, they may differ in the ways in which they collect, analyze, present, and use data. Of the many qualitative inquiry methods of merit, this chapter discusses four: case studies, ethnography, grounded theory, and phenomenology.

Case Studies

Case study research is often used when the selected case might offer insight into a unique situation or when researchers want to know more about a particular phenomenon within a real-life context (Rosenburg & Yates, 2007). Using case study methodology, researchers are able to maintain the richness and complexity of the concept of interest, while simultaneously highlighting specific details (Hentz, 2007; Stake, 1995).

The three major types of case studies—descriptive, exploratory, and explanatory—have different purposes. Descriptive case studies allow researchers to describe characteristic features or qualities of a yet unstudied person, institution or situation. Exploratory case studies offer an opportunity to clarify key concepts, ask more relevant questions, and better understand a concept of interest, often as a prelude to undertaking a larger study of the issue (Yin, 2002). Explanatory case studies can be used as pilot studies in the development of a conceptual framework, which can serve to organize the data collected in a larger study (Gerring, 2006). Explanatory case studies give new or refined meanings to previously explored concepts while the researchers hold extant theories and prior assumptions in abeyance (Tilley, Rugari, & Walker, 2008). Each type of case study uses multiple data sources and data collection methods to obtain a broad view of the phenomenon (Gerring, 2006). For example, a researcher interested in end-of-life issues could conduct a case study of a person recently diagnosed with terminal cancer. The investigator might choose to conduct a case study of nurses at a hospice agency.

The researcher engaging in a case study is typically seeking to understand which common features characterize a case as well as what is unique about a case (Stake, 1998). Stake has stated that to fully understand commonalities and unique features of a case, the researcher is likely to explore case features such as the following:

- The nature of the case
- The historical background of the case

■ The physical setting
■ Other contexts, including economic, political, legal, and aesthetic
■ Other cases through which this case is recognized
■ Those informants through whom the case is known

Data collected and examined within a case study might be both qualitative and quantitative. For instance, a case study might collect data such as temperatures or pain ratings (quantitative), along with data about the person's experience of pain and discomfort (qualitative). Together, such data paint a more complete picture of the disease experience.

Data analysis in case studies involves content analysis—that is, the researcher looks for patterns and themes. For example, the researcher might identify the themes of "feeling powerless" and "wishing I could take this away from my child" in a case study of parents of a child with cystic fibrosis (CF).

The readers or consumers of a case study should expect to be able to apply the findings from a case to their practice when the researcher has clearly bounded the case or defined the object of the study, identified patterns of data, and developed generalizations or assertions about the case. They should avoid applying findings from a case to their practice when the case is a single, unique instance or is a poor representation of a population, or when a single case as a negative example is applied to general populations. For example, findings from a single case about intractable pain that is poorly managed should not be used to guide policy. Conversely, analysis of several cases illustrating effective management of pain through the application of guided imagery might well be used to guide policy about the use of guided imagery in a hospice agency.

Ethnography

Ethnography involves collection and analysis of data about groups. The ethnographer seeks to understand the culture of the group or to gain an understanding of the values, norms, and rules that characterize the group. Groups of interest may include organizational, experiential, ethnic, and geographic entities.

Data collection for ethnography is usually accomplished through reading documents that were created within the culture, conducting interviews, observation, or a combination of these methods. Key informants or people who are most knowledgeable about the culture are usually primary sources of interview data.

Data analysis in ethnography occurs simultaneously with data collection. As the data evolve, new questions emerge. Data analysis requires bracketing by the researcher—that is, a process in which the researcher identifies his or her own personal biases and beliefs and purposefully sets them aside so as to fully understand the culture of the informants. Bracketing allows for a more open interpretation of the evolving data.

The reader or consumer of studies based on this method might find practice applications if the ethnography informs one how to do the following:

- Behave when with a certain group
- Approach a person within the group
- Recognize and respond to needs of a person within the group

For example, a nurse might find ethnographic data about the experiences of a group of parents of children with CF helpful in the provision of care to a child with the disease. Such an ethnographic study might provide the nurse with insight about the needs of the parents, the ways in which the parents can access assistance within the community of parents of children with CF, and the experiences and feelings that are commonly experienced by the parents of children with CF.

Grounded Theory

Grounded theory is a general methodology for developing new theory that is rooted in data that have been systematically gathered and analyzed (Denzin & Lincoln, 1998). There is an explicit expectation that theory development and theory verification will occur in conjunction with this method.

With this technique, data are drawn from interviews and observation. Data collection in grounded theory involves purposive sampling, theoretic sampling, and data collection to saturation. Purposive sampling entails deliberately choosing subjects who are most able to shed light on the phenomena of interest (Strauss & Corbin, 1998). Rather than seeking subjects with similar perspectives on the phenomena, the researcher seeks out subjects with diverse perspectives. Theoretical sampling is the process of choosing new research sites or cases to compare with a site or case that has already been studied, with the goal of producing a deeper understanding of the data. Data collection to saturation implies that a degree of data analysis is undertaken as data collection occurs. Saturation occurs when the researcher begins to hear repetition or redundancy in the themes or patterns in the data; no new information is obtained with new informants. Depending on the phenomena of interest, saturation may occur with a very small number of informants or may require a large number of subjects.

? **Think Outside the Box**

Carefully consider the idea of saturation. Discuss how you can determine that saturation has occurred within a research project.

Data analysis in grounded theory is systematic and deliberate. The process begins with open coding, which involves categorizing the information and examining properties and dimensions of the data (Strauss & Corbin, 1998). The next step is axial coding, in which the researcher identifies relationships between categories and subcategories. Selective coding, the final step in data analysis, is the integration of concepts around a core category and the filling in of categories in need of further development and refinement (Strauss & Corbin, 1998). Saturation is a relevant concept in data analysis as well as data collection, in that the researcher continues data analysis until no new codes or categories emerge.

The final product of the grounded theory method is a theory that is rooted in the data collected and analyzed for the phenomenon of interest. The consumer of grounded theory research could expect to apply the model while developing interventions for a population. For example, reading a grounded theory about the attachment patterns of elderly adults might guide the nurse who is assisting a family in relocating their aging parent from a home environment to an assisted-living environment.

Phenomenology

As the name implies, phenomenology is the study of phenomena from a human perspective. This type of research seeks to develop an understanding of lived experience. The first-hand report or description of one's experience of the phenomenon is central to understanding the phenomenon. The meaning one creates in the world is socially constructed and is rooted in the experiences of the person; in other words, meaning occurs through ongoing social processes.

Data collection in phenomenology is done through unstructured interviews and inductive analysis. The guiding question in a phenomenological study typically centers on the essence, structure, or lived experience of a phenomenon. Data analysis occurs simultaneously with data collection; with this technique, the researcher identifies patterns and themes and develops new questions as new data emerge.

To understand phenomenology as a research method, an understanding of the concepts of bracketing and hermeneutics is also necessary. As with ethnography, the researcher identifies his or her own personal biases and beliefs about the phenomenon and sets them aside (bracketing) in an effort to fully understand the lived experience of the informants. Depending on the specific phenomenology framework, the author may or may not identify deliberate bracketing as part of the research report. Some phenomenologic researchers, for example, choose to acknowledge their own personal biases in the data analysis process.

Hermeneutics is the orderly interpretation and understanding of data through a structured framework. With this perspective, data are considered part of a whole that cannot be considered in isolation. When data are analyzed with the guidance of a nursing framework, the researcher is conducting hermeneutical analysis (Norwood, 2000).

The reader or consumer of a phenomenological study can use the findings to understand the experiences of clients who are experiencing a similar event. For example, reading a phenomenological study about the lived experience of a victim of sexual assault might assist the emergency department nurse in communicating more effectively and providing meaningful education to a client who has been sexually assaulted (Table 8-3).

Both qualitative and quantitative research methods require the researcher to strive for rigor, or the criteria for trustworthiness of data and interpretation of data. The major methods for ensuring rigor in qualitative studies are intricately linked with reliability and validity checks. The four criteria for rigor as presented by Lincoln and Guba (1985) include (1) credibility, (2) transferability, (3) dependability, and (4) confirmability. The following discussion considers how each criterion can be achieved to establish the trustworthiness of a study.

Credibility, or the truth value of data and data analysis, can be achieved in conjunction with a proposed study through several

Table 8-3			
Qualitative Research Methods			
	Data Collection	**Data Source**	**Data Analysis**
Case Study	Questionnaires; interviews; observation; participant journals	Individuals or groups	Patterns and themes in the data
Ethnography	Documents; interviews; observation	Individuals within a culture	Ongoing throughout the data collection process
Grounded Theory	Interviews; observation	Individuals	Systematic coding (open, axial, and selective)
Phenomenology	Unstructured interviews; new questions emerge as the data evolves	Individuals	Inductive analysis; data collection and analysis occur simultaneously

methods. First, when possible, the data should be taken back to the subjects to ensure accuracy. Upon coding of data, the coded data can be checked with available participants. Additionally, coded data can be reviewed by experts both in the area of research and in the method used for the study. These checks usually consist of validation of data, validation of findings, and checking of interpretations.

Transferability refers to the applicability of findings to other populations in different contexts. Often, this goal is accomplished by providing a thorough description of the sample, setting, and data in the report on the research to allow the reader to determine the transferability of the study's findings.

Dependability in qualitative research can also be described as auditability. If other researchers can follow the investigator's decisions throughout the study and come to similar conclusions, then the study is considered auditable (Lincoln & Guba, 1985). Thus an audit trail also provides an element of rigor to any study. The audit trail documents the development of the project and provides an adequate amount of evidence for interested parties to reconstruct the process by which the investigators reached their conclusions (Morse, 1998).

Confirmability represents freedom from bias, or neutrality (Lincoln & Guba, 1985). It is important to analyze data in a way that keeps researcher biases, assumptions, and perspectives separate from the analysis. These elements should be clearly identified early in the proposal process. Reviewing the analyzed data with informants or study participants and review by experts also serves to mitigate the effects of researcher bias.

? Think Outside the Box

Judiciously ponder the idea of mixed method studies. Which elements would need to be present to reflect effective use of quantitative methods in a qualitative research project? Explain your answer.

In addition to the criteria for rigor established by Lincoln and Guba (1985), two other criteria set forth by Morse (1991) include the concepts of adequacy of data and appropriateness of data. Adequacy of data, or the amount of data collected (rather than the number of subjects interviewed), is an important measure of rigor; it is attained when variations in data are accounted for and understood. Appropriateness of data refers to the selection of information according to the theoretic needs of the study. Purposive sampling provides concurring and confirming data, and ensures saturation (Morse, 1998). The researcher can ensure adequacy of data by collecting data until saturation occurs and ensure appropriateness by using selective sampling.

The consumer of research should consider whether the qualitative study under consideration has adequately addressed the majority of the criteria for reliability and validity—credibility, transferability, dependability, conformability, adequacy of data, and appropriateness of data. Although there are many ways to establish the quality of qualitative data, researchers can select the appropriate criteria for the topic under investigation. It is not necessary for all of these criteria to be incorporated into each study project. Application of any research results to practice, whether qualitative or quantitative, must be considered in light of the study's reliability, validity, and generalizability.

Qualitative Data Analysis

From the brief descriptions of data analysis in the methods introduced earlier in this chapter, one can see that qualitative data analysis can be quite complex. Whereas quantitative data analysis usually involves numbers and statistics, qualitative data analysis focuses on deep examination of large volumes of written or other forms of data.

The qualitative research methods of grounded theory, phenomenology, and ethnography require specific steps in data analysis. In contrast, other qualitative methods have no specific "rules" for the analysis of data. In such cases, a researcher might simply state that content analysis was conducted. "Content analysis" is a generic term for the process of data being analyzed and categories of data being created by experts.

Many researchers prefer to analyze their qualitative data by hand. This often involves reviewing the data many times to create categories in which to organize the data and to code data. The researcher may also choose to use data analysis software to sort and categorize data. Many software packages are available for qualitative data analysis, most of which offer the ability to store, edit, and assemble data according to category or code (Table 8-4).

Contributions of Qualitative Research Methods to Nursing and Evidence-Based Practice

Qualitative research has made and continues to make many contributions to the practice of nursing. Reflecting the value of these potential contributions, the development of qualitative research in nursing is accelerating in both quality and quantity (Morse, 1991). Additionally,

Table 8-4		
Qualitative Data Analysis Software		
Software	**Uses**	**Vendor**
NVivo	Analysis of small or large bodies of text; focus group summaries; open-ended answers in surveys	QSR International
Ethnograph	Project data files; documents in interview transcript form; field notes; open-ended survey responses; other text-based documents	QualisResearch Associates
ATLAS.ti	Large bodies of text; graphic data; audio data; video data	Scolari Sage Publications Software
N VIVO	Action research; grounded theory; ethnography; literature reviews; phenomenology	QSR

the scope of qualitative research is broad: There is virtually no area within nursing that does not lend itself to qualitative study.

Nursing practice should be guided by nursing theory that is solidly grounded in research data. Qualitative studies are often the first step in the development of a theoretical framework for a phenomenon that has not been fully explored. For example, Andrews and Waterman (2005) collected interview and observation data using the grounded theory approach in their study about how hospital-based staff use vital signs and the Early Warning Score to predict physiologic deterioration in clients. These authors reported that quantifiable evidence is the most effective means of referring patients to doctors and improving communication between professionals. Furthermore, they concluded that the Early Warning Score leads to successful referral of patients by providing an agreed-upon framework for assessment, increasing confidence in the use of medical language, and empowering nurses.

? Think Outside the Box

Discuss how sample sizes for qualitative versus quantitative research projects differ. How do researchers determine optimal sample size for qualitative studies as opposed to quantitative studies?

Qualitative research affords opportunities to explore human issues that have previously been understood only by way of assumption or simply not understood at all. For example, the high turnover and burnout rate among nursing staff has historically been assumed to be a function of long hours, physically strenuous work, and lack of power. The studies using combined qualitative and quantitative methods that were undertaken by Cohen-Katz and colleagues (2004) have illuminated the issue of nursing burnout and led to system-wide changes to help nurses manage stress and burnout.

The results of qualitative studies often have immediate clinical applicability. These studies are a source of rich descriptions of a wide range of physical and psychosocial experiences of healthcare consumers. By gaining a deeper understanding of those experiences, nurses can provide counseling, plan interventions, and develop programs to meet the needs of clients in similar conditions. A study that described the experience of managing lymphedema in breast cancer survivors provides an example (Fu, 2005). In this study, a descriptive phenomenologic method was used to explore how 12 breast cancer survivors managed lymphedema in their daily lives. Findings of the study provided an insightful alternative to the compliance approach to lymphedema management. Instead of merely evaluating breast cancer survivors' degree of compliance with treatment, the author suggested that researchers and practitioners should also assess the impact of the presence or absence of the women's intentions on lymphedema management.

Conclusion

Qualitative research lends itself well to the study of complex human issues. It focuses on the study of the quality of something rather than the quantity, amount, or frequency of something. Subjectivity is an expected trait of a qualitative study.

Qualitative and quantitative research methods differ in many ways. Qualitative studies approach phenomena from the emic perspective—the perspective of the participant provides the meaning rather than the perspective of the researcher. Quantitative studies, by contrast, approach phenomena from the perspective of the researcher—that is, from the etic perspective. Qualitative methods are inductive, as opposed to the deductive approach that characterizes quantitative methods. Although quantitative methods seek to minimize differences among subjects, qualitative methods embrace differences among participants. Sample size in qualitative research is often small compared with the requisite larger sample sizes in quantitative research.

Mixed method studies, also called triangulation, are commonly used by researchers in health care. Mixed method studies allow researchers to fully understand a phenomenon of interest through convergence of qualitative and quantitative data.

Case studies can be used with individuals or groups to identify both commonalities and unique features of cases. Ethnography focuses on the culture of a group of people in an attempt to understand the views and rules of the group. Grounded theory is a deliberate approach to qualitative data collection that aims to develop theory about the phenomena. Phenomenology is a method of inquiry that focuses on the lived experiences of humans.

Saturation is a concept that is important to both data collection and data analysis. In data collection, saturation occurs when no new data or theme emerges. In data analysis, saturation occurs when no new codes emerge or the data analysis becomes redundant.

Reliability and validity are important to the consumer of qualitative research. The reliability and validity of qualitative research can be ensured by verifying credibility, transferability, dependability, conformability, adequacy of data, and appropriateness of data.

Qualitative data analysis is often a tedious and time-consuming process. Although many qualitative researchers prefer to analyze data by hand, software programs are available to assist in the organization and coding of data.

Qualitative research brings offers of increased knowledge to the evidence-based practice of nursing. These research methods are often used to develop theories needed to guide future quantitative studies. Qualitative studies can illuminate issues that are poorly or inaccurately understood. Finally, qualitative studies often yield results with immediate clinical applicability and can guide teaching and practice.

Summary Points

1. Qualitative research is the study of the quality of something rather than the quantity, amount, or frequency of something. Subjectivity is an expected trait of a qualitative study.
2. Qualitative research is conducted from the emic perspective.
3. Sample size in qualitative research is often small compared with the requisite larger sample sizes in quantitative research.
4. The criteria for reliability and validity of a qualitative study include credibility, transferability, dependability, conformability, adequacy of data, and appropriateness of data.
5. Mixed research methods—that is, combinations of qualitative and quantitative methods—are used to supplement or validate data.
6. Saturation occurs in data collection or analysis when there is repetition or redundancy in the themes or patterns in the data.

RED FLAGS

- Attention must be given to the auditability of the data collected via a qualitative methodology.
- Within a qualitative research report, the reader should be able to pick out aspects that demonstrate credibility, transferability, dependability, and confirmability of the research.
- Qualitative research designs use an inductive reasoning process.
- Patterns and/or themes coming from the data should be documented and supported by the discussion.
- Given that qualitative research deals with volumes of written data, the documentation of statistic results would cause concern when evaluating a project.

Multiple Choice Questions

1. Qualitative research examines which of the following characteristics of a phenomenon?

   A. Frequency
   B. Quantity
   C. Quality
   D. Intensity

2. Which of the following best illustrates the emic perspective in research?

   A. Finding a quality of a phenomenon and looking for examples of the quality
   B. Taking an outsider's view of a phenomenon
   C. Exploring the way members of a group view themselves
   D. Validating perspectives about a group through interviews

3. Which of the following types of studies is considered qualitative research?

   A. Delphi technique
   B. Cross-sectional design
   C. Ethnography
   D. Survey

4. Combining qualitative and quantitative methods in a single study is known as

   A. Systematic analysis.
   B. Transferability.
   C. Prospective design.
   D. Triangulation.

5. A researcher explores the phenomenon of how nurses make decisions about when to discuss end-of-life issues with clients. From this research, a model is developed to explain the decision-making process. Which type of research does this represent?

   A. Grounded theory
   B. Ethnography
   C. Phenomenology
   D. Case study

6. A researcher examines the norms, rules, and values of the staff of a large long-term care facility. Which type of research does this represent?

   A. Grounded theory
   B. Ethnography
   C. Phenomenology
   D. Case study

7. A researcher conducts a study in which participants are asked to describe the lived experience of being a caregiver of a parent with Alzheimer's disease. Which type of qualitative study does this represent?

    A. Grounded theory
    B. Ethnography
    C. Phenomenology
    D. Case study

8. Which of the following statements is true with regard to comparing qualitative and quantitative research methods?

    A. Qualitative studies often require a larger sample size than quantitative studies.
    B. Qualitative studies don't require evidence of reliability and validity.
    C. Qualitative studies don't allow for the use of computerized data analysis.
    D. Qualitative research is often inductive in nature, whereas quantitative research is deductive in nature.

9. When writing up a research project, the researcher describes in detail the audit trail used as conclusions about data were drawn. Which criterion for reliability and validity was met?

    A. Credibility
    B. Transferability
    C. Dependability
    D. Confirmability

10. When writing up a research project, the researcher describes in detail the sample, setting, and data. Which criterion for reliability and validity was met?

    A. Credibility
    B. Transferability
    C. Dependability
    D. Confirmability

11. When writing up a research project, the researcher describes in detail how biases, assumptions, and personal perspectives were identified and set aside, or bracketed. Which criterion for reliability and validity was met?

    A. Credibility
    B. Transferability
    C. Dependability
    D. Confirmability

12. The researcher collecting data notices that she is beginning to hear the same things repeatedly and that no new themes are emerging. The researcher recognizes that what has occurred?

    A. Triangulation
    B. Saturation
    C. Quantizing
    D. Redundancy

Discussion Questions

1. You are the nurse manager of a perinatal care unit. You have read a phenomenology research report on the positive effects of music on the labor and delivery process for mothers. Consider the following: The study is one of many of this type with similar findings, there were five informants in the study, and the researcher did not provide a discussion of reliability and validity in the write-up. Will you use this study to support the practice of ensuring that all labor and delivery rooms are equipped to play music throughout the labor and delivery process? Support your answer.

2. You are the charge nurse on a medical–surgical floor. After reading several qualitative research reports on pet therapy, you approach your nurse manager about the possibility of implementing a pet therapy program on your floor. Your nurse manager states that no changes should be made based on qualitative research, because the sample sizes are always too small. What is your best response?

3. You are reading a research report about a long-term care facility. The researcher describes in detail the demographics of administration, staff, and clients. There is a lengthy discussion about how problems are solved in the facility, how various departments communicate, and how the facility values family involvement in client care. Which type of qualitative study does this represent? Support your answer.

Suggested Readings

Freshwater, D. (2005). Integrating qualitative and quantitative research methods: Trend or foe? *Journal of Research in Nursing, 10*(3), 337–338.

Freshwater, D., Walsh, L., & Storey, L. (2002, February). Prison health care part 2: Developing leadership through clinical supervision. *Nursing Management, 8*(9), 16–20.

Grassley, J., & Nelms, T. (2008). The breast feeding conversation: A philosophic exploration of support. *Advances in Nursing Science, 31*(4), E55–E66.

Halcomb, E., & Andrews, S. (2005). Triangulation as a method for contemporary nursing research. *Nurse Researcher, 13*(2), 71–82.

Kinn, S., & Curzio, J. (2005), Integrating qualitative and quantitative research methods. *Journal of Research in Nursing, 10*(3), 317–336.

Law, M., Stewart, D., Letts, L., Pollock, N., Bosch, J., & Westmoreland, M. (1998). *Guidelines for critical review of qualitative studies.* Retrieved July 11, 2009, from http://www.usc.edu/hsc/ebnet/res/Guidelines.pdf

O'Neill, R. (2006). *The advantages and disadvantages of qualitative and quantitative research methods.* Retrieved December 31, 2006, from http://www.robneill.com.uk/papers/research_methods.htm

Onwuegbuzie, A., & Leech, N. (2005). Taking the "Q" out of research: Teaching research methodology courses without the divide between quantitative and qualitative paradigms. *Quality & Quantity, 39*(3), 267–295.

Paton, B., Martin, S., McClunie-Trust, P., & Weir, N. (2004, July/August). Doing phenomenological research collaboratively. *Journal of Continuing Education in Nursing, 35*(4), 176–181.

Priest, H., Roberts, P., & Woods, L. (2002). An overview of three different approaches to the interpretation of qualitative data. Part 1: Theoretical issues. *Nurse Researcher, 10*(1), 30–42.

Rapport, F., & Wainwright, P. (2006). Phenomenology as a paradigm of movement. *Nursing Inquiry, 13*(3), 228–236.

Shih, J. (1998). Triangulation in nursing research: Issues of conceptual clarity and purpose. *Journal of Advanced Nursing, 28*(3), 631–641.

Silverstein, L., Auerbach, C., & Levant, R. (2006). Using qualitative research to strengthen clinical practice. *Professional Psychology: Research & Practice, 37*(4), 351–358.

Vishnevsky, T., & Beanlands, H. (2004, March/April). Qualitative research. *Nephrology Nursing Journal, 31*(2), 234–238.

References

Andrews, T., & Waterman, H. (2005). Packaging: A grounded theory of how to report physiological deterioration effectively. *Journal of Advanced Nursing, 52*(5), 473–481.

Cohen-Katz, J., Wiley, S., Capuano, T., Baker, D., & Shapiro, S. (2004). The effects of mindfulness-based stress reduction on nurse stress and burnout: A quantitative and qualitative study. *Holistic Nursing Practice, 18*(6), 302–308.

Denzin, N., & Lincoln, Y. (1998). *The landscape of qualitative research: Theories and issues.* Thousand Oaks, CA: Sage.

Fu, M. (2005). Breast cancer survivors' intentions of managing lymphedema. *Cancer Nursing, 28*(6), 446–457.

Gerring, J. (2006). *Case study research: Principles and practice.* Cambridge, UK: Cambridge University Press.

Hentz, P. B. (2007). Case study: The method. In P. I. Mulhall (Ed.), *Nursing research: A qualitative perspective* (3rd ed., pp. 359–384). Sudbury, MA: Jones and Bartlett.

Lincoln, Y., & Guba, E. (1985). *Naturalistic inquiry.* Beverly Hills, CA: Sage.

Morse, J. (1991). *Qualitative nursing research: A contemporary dialogue.* London: Sage.

Morse, J. (1998). Designing funded qualitative research. In N. Denzin & Y. Lincoln (Eds.), *Strategies of qualitative inquiry* (2nd ed., pp. 56–85). Thousand Oaks, CA: Sage.

Norwood, S. (2000). *Research strategies for advanced practice nurses.* Upper Saddle River, NJ: Prentice Hall.

Polit, D., & Beck, C. (2004). *Nursing research: Principles and methods* (7th ed.). New York: Lippincott Williams & Wilkins.

Rosenberg, J. P., & Yates, P. M. (2007). Schematic representation of case study research designs. *Journal of Advanced Nursing, 60*(4), 447–452.

Stake, R. E. (1995). *The art of case study research: Perspectives on practice.* Thousand Oaks, CA: Sage.

Stake, R. (1998). Qualitative case studies. In N. Denzin & Y. Lincoln (Eds.), *Strategies of qualitative inquiry* (pp. 119–150). Thousand Oaks, CA: Sage.

Stiles, A. (2009). Personal communication, Texas Woman's University, Denton, Texas.

Strauss, A., & Corbin, J. (1998). *Basics of qualitative research: Techniques and procedures for developing grounded theory* (2nd ed.). Thousand Oaks, CA: Sage.

Thurmond, V. (2001). The point of triangulation. *Journal of Nursing Scholarship, 33*(3), 253–259.

Tilley, D. S., Rugari, S. M., & Walker, C. A. (2008). Development of violence in men who batter intimate partners: A case study. *Journal of Theory Construction and Testing, 12*(1), 28–32.

Yin, R. K. (2002). *Applications of case study research.* Thousand Oaks, CA: Sage.

Chapter 9

Data Collection

Carol Boswell

Chapter Objectives

At the conclusion of this chapter, the learner will be able to

1. Compare a researcher's decision to use accessible data versus new data
2. Contrast different forms of data collection methods

Key Terms

➤ Accessible data

➤ Biophysiological data

➤ Closed-ended questions

➤ Data collection

➤ Focus group

➤ Interview

➤ In vitro

➤ In vivo

➤ Meta-analysis

➤ Novel data

➤ Observation

➤ Open-ended questions

➤ Primary data

➤ Questionnaire

➤ Secondary data

➤ Test

Overview of Data Collection Methods and Sources

Data come in many forms and are obtained through multiple methodologies. Data collection is the foundational piece within the monitoring and evaluation required for the research process (Asia-initiative, n.d.). As a result, the process of collecting data essentially establishes boundaries for a project. As a researcher begins to conceptualize the implementation of a research project, the question of the appropriate facts required to address the PICOT question(s), research question(s), research purpose(s), and/or hypothesis(es) become critical. According to LoBiondo-Wood and Haber (1998), "The major difference between the data collected when performing patient care and the data collected for the purpose of research is that the data collection method employed by researchers needs to be objective and systematic" (p. 308). Although many methods of data gathering are available, all of them are implemented in the same manner no matter what the anticipated project. The objectivity and organization of the data collection process provide for generalizability of a research project's resulting outcomes to a broader population.

The specification of the outcome for each phase of the data collection plan is mandatory. When all aspects of the data required for the study are established prior to the initiation of the study, the selection of the appropriate data collection method can be effectively addressed as part of this specification. Thus this process decreases the potential for unintentionally omitting a key component of the data. Because data collection is fundamental to the entire process, careful consideration for the use of a mixture of types can prove to be a valuable option as the decisions about data collection methods are confirmed.

Before delving into a discussion of the functions of data collection source and data collection tools/instruments, it is helpful to have an understanding of the definitions of selected concepts. "Data collection 'source' means the mechanism or method for collecting data—for example, surveys, focus group discussions, observations, project progress reports, routine project statistics, etc." (Asia-initiative, n.d., p. 72). The sources for data collection can be varied but require a somewhat direct connection with the participants. Data collection "tools/instruments" comprise the actual physical devices employed to collect the information that is under investigation. The use of a tool/instrument does not mandate a direct connection with the participants, as these tools could be delivered by mail or through the Internet.

There are seven major methods of data collection:

- Tests
- Questionnaires

- Interviews
- Focus groups
- Observations
- Biophysiological data
- Existing or secondary data

The data set identified by the researcher for any selected study can usually be accessed by several of these methods.

According to Polit and Beck (2008), the researcher must try to determine which data will effectively address the question under investigation, describe the sample characteristics, establish methods for controlling extraneous variables, analyze impending biases, recognize subgroup effects, and check for manipulation of the data. Creswell (2003) reinforces this notion by identifying the data collection steps to include (1) establishing the boundaries for the study, (2) accumulating the data through the appropriate methodologies, and (3) clarifying the process for recording and managing the data collected. As a result, the researcher has the responsibility to understand the different formats of data collections, the strengths and weaknesses of the different methods, and the specific needs recognized for the topic under evaluation.

Accessible Data Versus Novel Data

As the researcher begins the process of clarifying the data collection process, a key question arises concerning the type of information that will be used to satisfy the question being investigated. Two types of data can be identified—accessible (existing) or new (novel). The aspects of each of these data types need to be conscientiously considered as the researcher distinguishes the data collection process.

Accessible data may also be called existing data; as such, it provides an essential source for use in research endeavors. This information may be located in preexisting reports (e.g., hospital records, databases, historic documents), and it can be used as the basis for a secondary analysis of the data gathered in a previous study or of records developed for some other reason, such as hospital patient records. The use of preexisting records, often called a retrospective chart review, is common in nursing research because these documents are an economical and convenient source of information. Questions do arise with this form of data, however, as the records' biases and incompleteness cannot be thoroughly established. Secondary analysis of data allows for the use of data collected for a prior project to test one or more different hypotheses and illuminate fresh relationships evident within the data. When preexisting data can be used, this practice does eliminate the time-consuming and costly process subsumed within the practice of research. The use of accessible (existing) data serves as the foundation for evidence-based practice. Meta-analyses and meta-syntheses, which use obtainable research reports as their underlying database, integrate the material to provide the foundation for evidence-based protocol guidelines.

New or novel data comprise original information collected for a specific study. This type of data is unique to the question or questions under investigation, and the researcher needs to judiciously determine each component of data needed for the particular question(s). Within the time sequence allocated for the research project, all of the various pieces of data must be collected. The data collection plan should address each aspect of the needed information so that at some point during the process, it is all collected for use during the analysis process.

Another way to look at data is to classify it as either primary data or secondary data. Primary (novel) data are considered to be data generated through the actual conducting of an original study. In contrast, secondary (accessible) data are pulled from existing data and documents (Watershed Planning, n.d.). This process of using accessible or secondary data is termed "data mining."

Key Categories of Data for Nursing Studies

Within any research design, the data collection process must be matched to the stated study aims and/or purpose and reflect the particular strategies implemented during the study. Many data sources are available for use. They include secondary data from national surveys and other secondary data sources such as Medicaid, demographic indicators, nonclinical program data, clinical program data, public comments, informant groups, questionnaire/interview surveys, screenings, and epidemiology surveys. Researchers must carefully and thoroughly contemplate the various methods of data collection and the various sources of data, thereby ensuring they select the most appropriate options.

Orcher (2005) identified two feasible incentives for using established instruments. Established tools are identified as validated tools based on the number of times that the tool has been successfully used while fostering a reliable body of research. Each of the two incentives can have a profound impact on the quality of the research study outcomes:

■ Initially, time and energy should be expended to ensure that the data collected are appropriate for the study question(s) and the methodology is effective in capturing the total picture needed to address the research problem.

▓ Care should be given to identifying any confounded variables that could adversely affect the research outcomes.

? **Think Outside the Box**

Using the provided examples, select a data collection method and justify your selection. Examples to use include the following:
- Which information has been used to determine the method of catheterizing a laboring mother?
- Which information serves as the basis for the range of blood sugars used within newly diagnosed elderly diabetics?

Significant Facets of Data Collection Schemes

As the investigator establishes the data collection methodology for a study, questions concerning the consistency of the data collected from each participant become of paramount importance. The basic idea is that the data should be collected in the same manner for each of the participants so that unique environmental, societal, and physical effects are diminished. Concerns related to the Hawthorne effect, for example, must be carefully thought about to minimize the potential for participants to modify their behaviors because they are affected—either positively or negatively—by being included in a study. As studies of the Hawthorne effect have shown, the simple act of being selected to participate in a project can result in the modification of the behavior being evaluated. Because this effect is real, researchers must carefully consider all aspects of the data collection process to diminish the likelihood that the resulting modifications will be so pronounced that the data collected are of little value.

Another important aspect within the data collection process is the idea of inter-rater reliability. In those studies that employ more than one data collector, the goal is to ensure accuracy, such that each of the data collectors accumulates the information in the exact same way. According to Melnyk and Fineout-Overholt (2005), "It is important to train observers on the instrument that will be used in a study so that there is an inter-rater reliability or agreement on the construct that is being observed at least 90% of the time" (p. 277). If the 90% rate cannot be accomplished, the researcher and data collectors must establish a level of agreement for the specific project that considers the element of chance.

Within the data collection process, one method utilized within evidence-based practice is meta-analysis. According to materials developed by Northern Arizona University (2001), a meta-analysis is a process of merging the outcomes from multiple studies related to one primary topic. The strength of each set of conclusions is determined to provide an overall view of the evidence available on the identified topic. The methods used within the various studies, along with the quantification of the findings from the studies, are condensed into a summary document related to the topic under investigation. The effect size within a meta-analysis seeks to establish the relevance of the tests, treatments, and methods used in the research studies under consideration. These documents are then used to provide the context for the next steps in the research process and the determination of the reliability of the evidence related to that topic.

Now let's turn the attention to the different data collection methods. In the remainder of this chapter, for each method, an overview of the method expectations, strengths of the method, and limitations resulting from its use are discussed.

Test Methods

Overview

The use of tests within the research process is a fairly common methodology used to ascertain the explicit intelligence, talents, behaviors, or cognitive endeavor that is under investigation. Frequently, the terms "tool," "instrument," and "standardized test" are used interchangeably to describe this research method. These devices are used within research to appraise characteristics, aptitude, accomplishments, and performance. The use of self-reporting strategies when the goal is collection of vast amounts of research information appears to be an effective process. Directness and versatility are two key benefits associated with the use of tests (especially standardized tests) to discover the information that is sought within a research project.

The Educational Testing Service's ETS Test Collection Database (2006) contains descriptions of more than 25,000 instruments, including research and unpublished instruments. Another resource for locating possible tools is a review of literature on a topic. Other research reports may also provide insight concerning tools that have been used in other research projects about an identified topic.

When a tool cannot be located to address a particular topic, the eight steps identified by Orcher (2005, p. 121) for building an appropriate instrument can be used:

1. Develop a plan.
2. Have the plan reviewed.
3. Revise the plan in light of the review.
4. Write items based on the plan.

5. Have the items reviewed.
6. Revise the items in light of the review.
7. Pilot test the instrument.
8. Revise the instrument in light of the pilot test.

Because an instrument is essential in addressing a topic, the development of a unique instrument can be a suitable alternative when the researcher cannot locate an appropriate one for data collection.

Strengths

Because tests are structured, a comparable motivation encouraging completion of the tool is presented for each participant, thus allowing for consistency during the data collection process. Each potential participant is offered the same benefits for agreeing to participate in the study. The equivalency of the measurement across research populations is another benefit from using this form of data collection. According to the Harvard Family Research Project (2004), tests and assessments provide additional valid and reliable data, as they tend to reduce the identification of perceptions and opinions. Because the functionality of a test is established through its validity and reliability, the usability of the tool within multiple population samples certifies the effectiveness of that tool. As tools are used repeatedly, the availability of reference group data grows, providing additional support for the tool and the data collected via use of that tool.

Another advantage to using tests relates to the administration process for the tool. Frequently, tests can be dispensed within a group setting, which saves time, expense, and energy. When the data can be collected in a group setting, the response rate is higher owing to the greater control exerted with this type of administration.

An additional reward for using tests within the data collection process is the accessibility of an extensive assortment of tests. The wide variety of tests available for use in research projects reflects the many content areas that might be investigated. For this reason, the identification of a functional tool that is appropriate for use within a research project requires a persistent quest for the most applicable instrument. Because the same instrument/tool can be used both prior to and after an intervention has been delivered, changes in the results from both phases of the study can be compared.

The final advantage of tests within the research process derives from the practicality of undertaking data analysis because of the quantitative features of the data accumulated through use of this methodology. Because quantitative data are numerical in nature, those data can be easily used within the calculations used for statistical testing.

? **Think Outside the Box**

Discuss the ethical aspects of using covert data collection methods.

Limitations

Although tests have multiple strengths related to their use in research, several limitations must also be considered with this methodology. If a test requires that a fee be paid for each individual taking the test, the expense can be excessive when a large sample is required. Standardized tests must be evaluated for the presence of biases within the construction of the tool. These biases may be directed toward a certain group of individuals or a unique population. Because most tests are structured, this data collection method does not lend itself to open-ended and probing-type questions as easily as other methods do.

Another area the researcher must consider is the management of incomplete test documents. Will these incomplete forms be omitted from the data analyzed, or will the answered questions still be included? Does the inclusion of incomplete forms skew the results? When no responses are provided for selected aspects within any research instrument/tool, the appropriate management of the potential distortion of the results should be considered.

A final area of potential weakness or limitation with the use of tests relates to the problems encountered when an instrument/tool lacks psychometric data. In such cases, the project does not guarantee the validity or reliability for the device. When a tool lacks the foundational psychometric data, the use of the tool in other projects can provide validity and reliability of the tool, but it cannot certify the appropriateness of the tool for all uses.

Questionnaire Methods

Overview

When a questionnaire is the tool used for data collection, the data collection method is a survey process. A survey necessitates the querying of individuals through the use of some device that contains questions to be answered. A questionnaire is a data collection tool completed by a participant, where the researcher has the intent to discover what the individual thinks about a specific item. Questionnaires can be employed to gather information concerning knowledge, attitudes, beliefs, and feelings. Because it is a self-reporting device, a questionnaire can be provided as a paper-and-pencil device, a telephone survey, or a structured document uploaded onto the Internet, such as those called "Monkey Surveys." As a result, the device can be administered in person, by mail, by telephone, or through an Internet delivery method.

According to Brink and Wood (2001), questionnaires limit the replies possible, because they involve directed answers to prearranged questions. Several types of questions can be incorporated into the questionnaire format, including dichotomous (yes/no), multiple choice, cafeteria, rank order, forced-choice ratings, checklists, calendar, and visual analogue (Polit & Beck, 2008). The researcher should consider the question format while assessing the applicability of different tools.

Should a researcher elect to develop a tool specific for the topic under investigation, several facets of the instrument ought to be vigilantly contemplated in designing the questionnaire (**Table 9-1**). Of course, the entire tool must address the research focus as well as be appropriate for the target population. These two items are fundamental to the process of developing the different questions and the format for the tool. The language employed within the instrument must be free of jargon, use familiar words, and be easily understood by the potential participants. Each statement should be short and

---

Table 9-1

Design Tenets for Questionnaires

- Ensure that the tool addresses the research purpose, objectives, goals, and questions.
- Carefully consider the target population who will use the questionnaire so that the tool is easy to use.
- Use simple, familiar language without jargon and with correct grammar.
- Compose each question to be understandable, concise, and reasonably brief.
- Consider sequencing the questions from impersonal to personal, less sensitive to more sensitive, and broad to specific.
- Avoid using questions that hint at or direct responses, use double negatives, or embarrass the participant.
- Verify that each question addresses only a single topic.
- Structure the tool by beginning with questions that stimulate interest and group questions by topics.
- Cautiously word questions dealing with painful situations.
- Incorporate into the question all information necessary to address the issue under investigation.
- Construct the tool with the questions in the same order for each testing session to provide consistency in delivery and data collection.
- Ascertain the necessary format to accumulate the appropriate information: open-ended questions, closed-ended questions, mutually exclusive and exhaustive response categories, response categories for closed-ended questions (rating scales, ranking, semantic differential, checklists).
- Use various items and approaches to appraise conceptual ideas.
- Carefully consider the use of reverse wording on some of the questions to eliminate the possibility of a "response set."
- Determine the coding and/or weighting of the responses prior to the administration of the tool.
- Conduct a pilot test of the tool with a select group of the target population to confirm the applicability of the tool.

specific, while addressing only one concept. Care must be given to the wording to prevent any leading of the participants toward a specific response.

According to Boswell, "Good questions endeavor to scrutinize, evaluate, translate, illuminate, and reflect relationships about the multiple fragments of data assembled on any given topic" (in press, paragraph 1). While neutral wording for each statement should be the goal, the use of active verbs in the statement is conducive to analysis, synthesis, and evaluation of the situation, thus resulting in an optimal response (Boswell, in press).

The type of questions (open-ended versus closed-ended) is one of the initial concerns to be addressed in terms of the format of the instrument. Open-ended questions leave the direction of the answer up to the individual participant. This type of questioning is more frequently used to assess qualitative types of issues and exploratory research. In contrast, closed-ended questions force a response, because the researcher provides the answers. Closed-ended questions lend themselves to the collection of quantitative data and quantitative (confirmatory) research.

When developing closed-ended questions, the tool developer must ensure that the categories used for the answers are mutually exclusive and exhaustive. An example of a mutually exclusive category is the classification of years of service to an organization. The potential choices must not overlap, because overlapping of categories would cause confusion. Therefore, the ranges would need to be stated as follows:

Years of service: Less than 3, 4–6, 7–9, 10–12

For categories to be exhaustive, every possible option must be presented as a potential selection piece. In the ranges provided in the preceding example, individuals who had worked 13 or more years would not be provided with an option that they could select. However, keep in mind that the researcher may not want a certain range. In such a case, the researcher will need to provide a rationale for the exclusion. An example of when a lack of a specific range might be appropriate is when the researcher opens the year range to include every year possible.

The tool developer needs to carefully consider the information that is being sought through the use of the questionnaire. As that decision is confirmed, the tool then ought to address each and every potential aspect of the information being collected. For example, the type of response categories is an important consideration with closed-ended questionnaires. The instrument developer should consider several types of responses, including rating scales, ranking, semantic differential, and checklists (**Table 9-2**). Ultimately, the type of infor-

Table 9-2

Different Types of Questionnaire Responses

Type of response	Example of response
Rating scales	On a scale of from 0 to 10, with 10 being the most severe pain you can imagine and 0 being no pain at all, where does your current pain level fall? 0 1 2 3 4 5 6 7 8 9 10 No pain Most severe pain
Ranking	Nurses rank different things at different levels. Below is a list of items that many nurses value in the workplace. Please designate their order of significance to you by placing "1" beside the most significant, "2" beside the next most significant, and so on. _4_ Salary _2_ Competent peers _1_ Effective workplace _3_ Management workload _5_ Opportunities to advance
Semantic differential	On each of the combinations provided, place an "X" to reflect how you see yourself function related to the two associated terms. Competent !__!__!__!__!__!__! Incompetent Pleasant !__!__!__!__!__!__! Unpleasant Responsible !__!__!__!__!__!__! Irresponsible Successful !__!__!__!__!__!__! Unsuccessful
Checklists	Please check all of the applicable characteristics you think a nurse should have in order to participate in evidence-based practice (EBP). Critical thinking abilities ✓ Energy ✓ Knowledge about searching ✓ Years of nursing experience Desire for EBP ✓

mation that is being collected should drive the choice of response categories used for the tool.

Strengths

The use of questionnaires for data collection has several advantages. A primary reason for using this methodology is the ability to access a larger sample in a group setting at a minimum expense. Participants also seem to favor the use of questionnaires because this method of data collection provides a greater sense of anonymity. Another advantage identified by Brink and Wood (2001) is the potential to collect an enhanced quantity of data with an extensive variety of topics using a standard format. A final advantage to the use of this data compilation method is the opportunity to determine the validity and reliability of the tool, thereby strengthening the overall design of the research project.

Limitations

The use of questionnaires as a data collection method does present some notable problems, however. To ensure adequate sampling, the tool must be short and to the point. Long, cumbersome questionnaires result in individuals electing to not complete the tool, which in turn requires enrollment of additional sample participants to complete the research project and can delay the project.

Another limitation resulting from the use of questionnaires in data collection is the potential for participants to be nonresponsive to selected items within the tool. This nonresponsiveness to items results in a dilemma for the researcher, as the inclusion of an incomplete questionnaire becomes an important question to address prior to the actual use of the tool within a study.

A final limitation resulting from the use of this method is the time-consuming nature of the data collection process. For open-ended questions, the differences within the verbal responses must be carefully considered and correlated. This process is time-consuming because the verbal responses are not preselected responses. Determinations concerning the comparability between terms must be made carefully, and supported by documentation to reflect the thought processes used. For closed-ended questions, the establishment of the data set, the process of data input, and the actual inputting of the quantitative data must be considered and planned, because it requires focused time by someone to manually enter each piece of data.

Interview Methods

Overview

Brink and Wood (2001) identified the key variation between questionnaires and interviews as the presence of an individual to conduct the interview; this "personal touch" is the basic difference between the two data collection methods. Otherwise, the expectations and concerns about interview questions are the same as arise in the development of a questionnaire or survey.

Within this compilation design, the use of an interviewer to direct the questioning process requires that trust and rapport be developed between interviewer and interviewee. The interviewer has to present a positive, supportive manner to engage the individual being queried. If the individual does not perceive the environment to be appropriate, the data collected will be skewed accordingly. Thus the environment selected for the session is of paramount importance. Because the questions are presented by the interviewer, the ordering of the questions and the environment wherein the questions are presented should allow for openness from the interviewee and the increased depth of the resulting responses. If a room is too hot, too cold, too noisy, or too open, the participant may elect not to continue the interview or may be less open to engaging in dialogue. According to the Harvard Family Research Project (2004), "Questions [in an interview] are generally open-ended and responses are documented in thorough, detailed notes or transcription" (p. 3).

Interview data collection can pull together information from both the quantitative and qualitative realms. When quantitative information is sought from the interview process, the questions are completed through the use of a structured format. Frequently, closed-ended questions are administered by means of a standardized test. Each question is asked in the same pattern or flow. The environment of the interview is controlled in an attempt to reduce the effect of confounding environmental variables.

If the purpose of the planned data collection is to seek qualitative information, the entire process can be managed in a less structured manner. Often, the questions used for this type of interview are geared more toward the open-ended type. When an informal conversational interview format is used, the process is impulsive and freely structured. According to Asia-initiative (n.d.), the interviewer functions "as a moderator, guiding the respondent from one topic to another. It is best to start with a topic that is important to the respondent and not sensitive" (p. 81).

The flexibility of the interview process is perceived as both an advantage and a disadvantage for this data collection method. Because of the openness of the data collection process, the interviewer collects not only verbal data, but also nonverbal data. By juxtaposing the nonverbal communication with the verbal statements, clarification related to the meanings of the comments and data is improved and facilitated. The disadvantage is related to the wealth of data that can be collected and then must be utilized or analyzed to determine the appropriateness of the material. The volumes of data collected can make the data analysis process seem very overwhelming and cumbersome.

Strengths

One of the initial strengths noted with the interview data collection design is the resulting powerful and abundant information accumulated, which paints an extensive portrait of the issue at hand and may have far-reaching implications. Another benefit gained from using this design is the ability, through the use of communication, to highlight issues that may present themselves only during the course of discussion as the interview progresses. The ability to measure attitudes, probe feelings, pose follow-up questions, gather internal meanings and ways of thinking, and control the depth of information amassed are other advantages associated with the use of the interview data collection method. An extra advantage is that interviews allow for the collection of data without the requirement that the participant be able to read or write.

Limitations

The interview data collection process does present some limitations that must be considered as a researcher decides which method to use. This methodology for gathering information can be both expensive and time-consuming. Conducting individual interviews requires time-intensive interactions and close observation of the nonverbal communication that helps to clarify the verbal communication. The interviewer must be able to elicit the information expected for the research project. Another weakness to consider is the potential for the participants to say what they perceive is appropriate or socially desirable, instead of what they actually believe. In addition, the sample size is often small when the interview methodology is used, which in turn makes generalizations to a larger population more difficult. Finally, analysis of the open-ended, subjective data collected via interviews requires time and thought to ensure that the results are valid and supported by the information.

Focus Group Methods

Overview

Although focus groups share many of the characteristics discussed in relation to interviews, a focus group entails a type of "coordinated interview," in which 6 to 12 homogeneous individuals are led in the discussion of a selected topic at the same time. Each focus session tends to last approximately one to three hours. To facilitate the data collection process, the sessions typically are audiotaped or videotaped for analysis at a later time.

The focus group leader should understand where the session should come together in regard to the data to be collected. This leader must ensure that the research topic is adequately covered during the discussion. According to Asia-initiative (n.d.), "The moderator's role is to encourage all to participate in the discussion, stimulate discussion between participants, guide the group from one discussion topic to another, remain neutral and refrain from expressing a personal opinion on a subject, and retain control over the discussion, but not act as an expert" (p. 83).

Many different features within the process need to be controlled and manipulated. The participants must understand that their opinions and experiences are important, such that no answers are inappropriate within the context of the subject under investigation. Care concerning the setting for the focus group should address comfort, privacy, and convenience. Although the session is recorded in some manner, the moderator and researcher must ensure that the participants feel secure in the knowledge that the recording will be used only to pull out the information provided.

The researcher should also give thought and consideration to the membership of the group. A homogeneous grouping with regard to gender, age, and socioeconomic status enhances the generalizability of the resulting data. Putting thought into the size and composition of each focus group is essential to maximize the effectiveness of the data collection process.

Strengths

Many of the same advantages listed previously for interviews also hold true for the focus group data collection method. Because the collection of data is done in an open and revealing manner, exploration of ideas and concepts can grow and develop as the session progresses. As members of the focus group discuss the different aspects presented through the process, the moderator can probe the in-depth information for additional understanding of the phenomenon. Each individual is allowed to react to other participants without having to carry the entire data collection process by himself or herself.

Limitations

Limitations of this design process relate to the sizing and management of the focus groups. The moderator must be adept at conducting the process. Getting the right moderator, organizing the appropriate focus group members, conducting the session, and completing the management of the data can also be quite expensive. Within each group, extrovert personalities must be controlled, while involvement of introvert personalities is encouraged.

Observation Methods

Overview

According to Wood and Ross-Kerr (2006), "Observation is a method of collecting descriptive, behavioral data and is extremely useful in nursing studies because one can observe behavior as it occurs"

(p. 171). The entire process of observing individuals results in an interactive engagement. Frequently, what a person says and what a person does can be two different pieces of information. Observation allows for the confirmation of what is said by the viewing of specific behaviors and activities. It is an articulation of individualism, character preconceptions, and beliefs. Each individual assesses a situation based on his or her unique background and philosophy of life. As a result, the selectivity of this type of data collection must be highly patterned by the expectations of the study. Clarity related to the behavioral information under investigation is imperative.

LoBiondo-Wood and Haber (1998) specified four conditions needed for the use of observation as a data collection method:

■ "Observations undertaken are consistent with the study's specific objectives,

■ Standardized and systematic plan for the observation and the recording of data,

■ All of the observations are checked and controlled, and

■ Observations are related to scientific concepts and theories" (p. 312).

The complexity of the process requires attention to be given to the operationalization of the variables. The variables are frequently the behaviors being observed. Consequently, the individual characteristics and conditions (traits, symptoms, verbal communications, nonverbal conditions, activities, skills, or environmental aspects) should be clearly and distinctly documented for the integrity of the data collection process. Another issue that arises with this type of data collection process is whether the observer will be directed to try to provoke some behavior/action within the individuals being observed.

? Think Outside the Box

Select an evidence-based topic, and then develop open-ended and closed-ended questions that could be used to address the topic. Debate the benefits of using open-ended versus closed-ended question formats.

Both quantitative and qualitative observations can be used within this research effort. Because generalizability of the results is desired, a checklist of the behaviors/observations is frequently used to provide a structure for the analysis phase of the process. Put simply, quantitative observations require the standardization of those items to be counted or not counted. Likewise, clear directions related to the operational definitions of the selected behaviors must be given. When these behaviors are unmistakably defined, the observational sessions produce the quantitative data expected from the research process. The definition should include the "who, what, when, where, why, and how" for the behavior on which data are to be collected within the study. As an example, if one piece of data that a researcher wants to collect is the number of times a person made eye contact during a lecture presentation, clarification is needed as to what duration of eye contact would be counted. In this case, the researcher might establish that each time the lecturer made eye contact with a student for at least 45 seconds, the contact would be counted.

In contrast to quantitative observation, qualitative observation is investigative and open-ended. The resulting information provides massive amounts of field notes to analyze.

Four diverse observer roles create a continuum of data collection with the observation methodology:

- *Complete participant*. The observer takes the role of member within the sample; the data is collected via a covert (hidden) process; the members of the group are not informed about the data collection process.
- *Participant-as-observer*. The observer continues to work from within the group but collects the data through an overt (informed) process; the members of the group are aware that the observer is taking on the dual roles of member of the group and spectator.
- *Observer-as-participant*. The observer does work from within the group but spends more time in the role of spectator, instead of member of the group; data are collected in an overt manner.
- *Complete observer*. The observer is totally in the role of watcher; covert observations are used to collect the data.

? Think Outside the Box

Using a PICOT question format, describe how you would collect data.

For each data collection session, the researcher would take time to conscientiously consider which of these depths of observation was appropriate for the study population. Because some of the methods require covert (undercover) data collection, the researcher must also justify why this clandestine method for accessing the data is needed. In these situations, the question is raised as to the necessity of collecting information without the individual's knowledge and the ethics of that undisclosed process. The researcher must diligently document the manner in which the individuals would be protected from harm.

On the other side of the picture, when the participants know they are being watched, the researcher has to work to ensure that behaviors are not modified due to this knowledge (the Hawthorne effect). Frequently, the course of action used to ensure that individuals are behaving naturally is related to the length of time the observations are occurring. The researcher/observer may have to be immersed in this situation of being observed for a long period of time so that the participants become comfortable with him or her being there. As their comfort with the researcher's presence increases, the individuals return to their normal behaviors, allowing the observer to then see the normalcy of the situation.

Strengths

According to the Harvard Family Research Project (2004), the observation method provides "highly detailed information from an external perspective on what actually occurs in programs" (p. 3). The depth of the information obtained is the primary benefit from collecting data in this manner. Having someone watch the activity under investigation allows events that might otherwise be detected in everyday life to be identified and discussed. Observation as a data collection process is seen as an effective method for understanding important related items of a designated setting. Another advantage of this method is that it can be used with any individual regardless of educational preparation. Thus the behaviors, attitudes, and involvement of individuals who may have weaker verbal skills can be evaluated and researched.

Limitations

The limitations of this data collection practice flow from the time-consuming, labor-intensive, and expensive nature of completing the observation process. Inter-rater reliability for the observers and the training of these individuals have equally important implications for the quality of the resulting data. Without the assurance that the observers are knowledgeable about the entire process, the excellence of the data may be questioned.

Bias is a major problem that must be addressed throughout the observation time period. Researchers and observers should be upfront about the presence of any biases that might potentially compromise the integrity of the study results. It becomes imperative that all biases are identified and reported. Because biases cannot be completely removed, the acknowledgment of the existence of the predispositions provides validation of the results. Consumers of the research results can then be aware that these preconceptions were recognized.

Secondary (Existing) Data Methods

Overview

The data collection process using secondary (existing) data builds on the information collected from another study. Because it takes the data compiled for another reason and applies it in a different manner, this method of reevaluating should be carefully considered and contemplated. The researcher must explain which pieces of the primary data will be used in reassessment of the information. Within this process, the researcher reconsiders a part of the information accumulated through some other manner in an attempt to address a follow-up type of question.

The data used for these secondary assessment projects might include documents, physical data, and/or archived research data, for example. When documents are used, they could include personal documents, such as letters, diaries, or family pictures, as well as official documents, such as attendance records, budgets, annual reports, newspapers, yearbooks, minutes, or client records.

Strengths

The advantages of using this method to assess existing records result from the availability of the records. A data collection process that relies on secondary data can be completed without any intrusion into the lives of people. The extra time gained by using the sources already assembled can be devoted to collecting key pieces of information that previously were overlooked or not valued.

In addition, the reevaluation of documents allows for exploration of alternative conclusions. The environmental aspects and historic perceptions can augment the interpretation of the data. A fuller evaluation of the information can be completed, thereby providing a more comprehensive understanding of the phenomena under investigation. By using previously collected records, researchers can identify trends, because the entirety of the incident can be manipulated. For the most part, the use of secondary (existing) data is also less expensive than collection of primary data.

Limitations

Some of the weaknesses of this data collection method revolve around the restrictiveness of the data sources. The only data that can be collected and analyzed are the data that were initially amassed. The researcher cannot add questions and can access only the information that has been compiled. Among the other barriers presented by the use of secondary data is the potential for the data to be out-of-date.

Another obstacle a researcher may encounter related to this type of data collection results from the restriction on accessing certain documents. If the documents are controlled to protect individual privacy, access to the information could be problematic.

An additional hindrance ensuing from this method is the limitation resulting from the sample used for the initial data collection. Specifically, the original sampling inclusion and exclusion criteria could negatively affect the secondary assessment of archived research data.

A final problem with the use of secondary (existing) data is the lack of open-ended or qualitative data related to the question. The researcher would need to acknowledge the unavailability of this type of data, which might or might not affect the quality of the project. If the project did not require the inclusion of qualitative data, then a secondary assessment of data would be appropriate. If qualitative data were desired to paint the total picture of the occurrence under investigation, the likelihood of accessing the original sample to gain further data would be highly problematic, if not impossible. Thus the reevaluation of secondary sources for additional results can pose difficulties because of the lack of initially collected information relating to the topic under current discussion.

Biophysiological Methods

Overview

The final type of data collection method is the use of biological indicators to organize the data being sought for the research activity. The research community views biophysiological measures as objective data. Researchers may use the biophysiological data collection process either alone or in combination with other methods.

This method of data collection necessitates the use of specialized equipment to establish the physical and/or biological condition of the subjects. Two types of biophysiological methods are possible:

■ In vivo: Requires the use of some apparatus to evaluate one or more elements of a participant. Examples of the types of items evaluated include blood pressure measurements, electrocardiograms, temperatures, muscular activity, and respiratory rates and rhythms.

■ In vitro: Requires the extraction of physiological materials from the participants, frequently via a laboratory analysis. Examples of the types of items within this realm include bacterial counts and identifications, tissue biopsies, glucose levels, and cholesterol levels.

This type of data collection process is frequently used with experimental and quasi-experimental research designs. Typically, the data are used to advance the implementation of specific nursing actions. Because of the type of information collected through this method, the research projects gathering biophysiological data tend to be more structured and controlled.

? Think Outside the Box

Discuss the challenges involved in using in vitro and in vivo data collection methods.

Strengths

The advantages of using this kind of data collection are the objectivity, precision, and sensitivity of the information compiled. The facts acquired from the use of specialized equipment have the tendency to be viewed as having increased independence from bias and subjectivity. As a result, the research community views this level of data with enhanced respect.

Limitations

The disadvantages related to the use of the specialized apparatus include the cost of obtaining the measurements and calibrating the instruments, which can be enormous with some data collection processes. Also, the acquisition of data by instrumentation requires specialized knowledge and training to be able to accurately gather the data. Additional research assistants may be required to perform the testing processes, leading to escalating costs, greater time commitments, and concerns related to inter-rater reliability.

A final problem resulting from this type of data collection is the potential reluctance of the accessible population to participate in such a study. Some members of the accessible population may decline to allow the physiological and biological measurements. The researcher must obtain informed consent from each individual prior to the collection of data.

Achievement of the Data Collection Strategy

Each of the data collection strategies profiled in this chapter has both benefits and limitations. The researcher must carefully consider the PICOT question, research purpose, research question/hypothesis, research design, sampling method, cost considerations, and time restrictions as he or she tries to identify the appropriate data collection plan. According to the Harvard Family Research Project (2004), "Using multiple methods to assess the same outcomes [e.g., using surveys and document review to assess program management] provides a richer, more detailed picture" (p. 5). Although it certainly adds to the richness of the results, the use of multiple methods of data collection also increases the resources (cost, personnel, and tools) required to carry out the project.

Each researcher must carefully consider the many different strategies available for accessing the information needed to address the identified research problem. In singling out the appropriate data collection process, justification for those choices needs to be documented. Because each method does have its own set of strengths and limitations, the primary objective for the researcher is to substantiate the rationale for the choices made to dispatch the research challenge.

In determining the strategy, the objectives of the project, along with the type of data required, should be taken into account during the decision-making process. Once the strategy for a research or evidence-based project has been determined to be the use of a tool, several aspects must be considered. The selection of a tool, the questions that need to be developed, and the method for implementing the tool/questions must all be contemplated. In addition, the environment of the data collection process is just as important as the individual questions to be addressed. Within the environment, the participants must be made to feel secure with the process, or the resulting data could be gibberish.

Evidence-Based Practice Considerations

Within the realm of evidence-based practice (EBP), the focus is more on the idea of outcome measures. According to Melnyk and Fineout-Overholt (2005), "The effectiveness and usefulness of outcomes measurement is affected by: the quality of the data, the consistency and accuracy of the data collection process, the commitment and ability of those collecting the data and making decisions based on findings, and the timing of data collection" (p. 306). The principal issues for data collection, as viewed from the EBP perspective, are the quality of the process and the content of the data collected. Each choice made by a researcher concerning the data to be collected, the method or methods to be used, and the environment used to collect the data must be founded on reliable, sensible judgments. The rationales for these decisions can make or break the study by determining the validity and reliability of the results produced by the study. If the decisions are not supported by appropriate thought processes and planning, then the entire inquiry is in jeopardy.

A principal investigator need not select the strongest data collection methods possible, but researchers must select the optimal strategies for getting the data needed to answer the questions asked and provide an appropriate justification for each of those decisions. The key idea is to make a decision and justify the selection with sound reasoning and a sound decision-making process. The entire research or evidence-based process rests on the quality of the data. The data form the foundation on which the results, recommendations, and outcomes of a study are based; the merit of the data becomes the underpinning for the research or evidence-based conclusions. The researcher must provide a sound rationale and strong support for the decisions made concerning the data collection process.

Summary Points

1. Data come in many varieties, and data collection is achieved through numerous methodologies.
2. Data collection sources are items or strategies for accumulating the information desired.
3. Data collection tools are the tangible devices used to complete the collection of the data.
4. The major methods of data collection are tests, questionnaires, interviews, focus groups, observations, secondary (existing) data, and biophysiological data.
5. Attention must be given to the information that actually exists and the information that is accessible. These two types of data may not be the same.
6. The basic objective in research is to collect the data in the same manner for each of the participants so that unique environmental, societal, and physical dimensions are diminished.
7. Another key aspect of the data collection process is the idea of establishing inter-rater reliability when more than one data collector is used to gather evidence.
8. Tests are used to ascertain the specific knowledge, talents, behaviors, and cognitive endeavor that are being investigated.

9. A questionnaire/survey is a data collection tool that is completed by a participant and allows the researcher to discover what the individual thinks about a specific item.
10. When interviews are used as the data collection process, establishing trust and rapport between interviewer and interviewee is essential.
11. Environmental aspects of the study setting must be taken into account when the plan is to conduct interviews and focus groups.
12. Observation allows for the confirmation of what is said by viewing the participant's specific behaviors and activities.
13. Several ethical issues need to be carefully considered as the method for the process of observation is determined.
14. A data collection process that uses secondary (existing) data builds on the information collected from another study or document.

RED FLAGS

- Tools used for quantitative data collection should have documentation of their validity and reliability indices.
- If desired, effective discussion of the entire data collection process should be provided in the report of the study results to allow for replication of the study.
- The use of appropriate tools to collect the information being sought must be addressed.
- The type of information needed to satisfy the research question must be reflected in the study design.
- The potential for a Hawthorne effect must be evaluated.
- If two or more data collectors are used within a study, inter-rater reliability must be established.

Multiple Choice Questions

1. Which of the following examples is not a data collection source used as a mechanism for amassing the information?

    A. Focus group discussions
    B. Observations
    C. Work excitement instrument
    D. Project progress reports

2. Which of the following processes is not a major method of data collection?

    A. Observations
    B. Open-ended questions
    C. Secondary (existing) data
    D. Tests

3. When considering the different data collection schemes, researchers must be careful to contemplate the presence of the Hawthorne effect. The Hawthorne effect is defined as

    A. A process in which the participant does not modify his or her behavior to meet the expectations of the study.
    B. A process in which the researcher modifies his or her behavior because of conducting the study.
    C. A process in which the researcher modifies the participants' behavior based on the data collected.
    D. A process in which the participant modifies his or her behavior as a result of engagement in the study.

4. As a researcher, you are attempting to gather data about the effects of a drug on individuals between the ages of 20 and 40 years. On the developed tool, the age ranges are provided as follows: 20–25; 25–30; 30–35; 35–40. Which problem is evident in this set of responses related to the question seeking to know a person's current age?

    A. The categories are not mutually exclusive.
    B. The categories are not exhaustive.
    C. The categories are written in a closed-ended format.
    D. There is no problem with this set of response categories.

5. Which of the following are tenets for use when designing a questionnaire?

    A. Use a variety of items and approaches to appraise conceptual ideas.
    B. Ensure that the tool addresses the research purpose.
    C. Use simple but appropriate jargon for the designated topics.
    D. Both A and B.

6. Which of the following is a method of data collection?

  A. Experimental
  B. Grounded theory
  C. Observation
  D. Cross-sectional

7. When developing questions for an instrument, a researcher should be careful in the wording to

  A. Provide hints toward the response.
  B. Use jargon as needed.
  C. Use single-topic questions.
  D. Use cultural aspects to provide context.

8. Both open-ended and closed-ended questions are used to collect data for research endeavors. Which of the following statements is true?

  A. Open-ended questions are used to collect primarily quantitative data.
  B. Closed-ended questions are used to collect quantitative data information, because the researcher provides the answers for selection.
  C. Open-ended questions provide confirmatory information, because the data are focused by the question.
  D. Closed-ended questions are used to collect exploratory data, because the information is left up to the individual.

9. Open-ended questions provide primarily _____ data.

  A. confirmatory
  B. exhaustive
  C. qualitative
  D. quantitative

10. Which of the following statements is true concerning observation?

  A. Clear directions related to the operational definitions of the selected behavior must be determined.
  B. Ethical considerations are a minor concern within this method of data collection.
  C. Observation data collection strategies result in manageable amounts of field notes to analyze.
  D. Within observational sessions, the observer is always known to the participant.

11. When creating a questionnaire, it is essential to do each of the following except

  A. Be concise and reasonably brief.
  B. Code and weight the responses prior to the administration of the tool.
  C. Conduct a pilot testing of the tool with a select group of the target population.
  D. Use double-negative questions regularly within the tool.

12. A researcher decides to use observation as the data collection method for a study. To effectively collect the needed data from college-age students, the researcher enrolls in a selected college course to be able to observe and collect data about the behaviors of the students. The researcher is using which observation role?

    A. Complete participant
    B. Participant-as-observer
    C. Observer-as-participant
    D. Complete observer

13. A class of preschool children is observed via a one-way mirror for a research project designed to determine the aggressive behaviors of boys and girls. The parents of the students are not informed about the research project, as no intervention is planned. Which type of data is being collected?

    A. Quantitative
    B. Covert
    C. Overt
    D. Time sequence

14. Which of the following terms best describes data compiled for another reason and applied in a different manner?

    A. Primary data
    B. Secondary data
    C. Novice data
    D. Experimental data

15. Which of the following biophysiological tests is an example of in vivo data?

    A. Complete blood count
    B. Urinalysis
    C. Respiratory rate
    D. Bacterial count

Discussion Questions

1. A researcher begins to develop the demographic section for use within a project. The three questions developed are the following:
   1. How many years have you been practicing professional nursing?
      - 0–5 years
      - 5–10 years
      - 10–15 years
      - More than 15 years
   2. What is your highest nursing degree?
      - ADN
      - BSN
      - MSN
      - Doctorate
   3. I have never been identified in a legal case.
      - Yes
      - No

   Which problems are present within these three questions that need to be corrected?

2. A researcher initially planned to use covert data collection techniques (observing a class of preschool children via a one-way mirror) for a research project designed to determine the aggressive behaviors of boys and girls. The parents of the students were not to be informed about the research project, as no intervention was planned. Which other observational role might the researcher use to make the data collection process an overt one?

3. A researcher has decided to conduct a structured interview with nursing students concerning their perceptions of what makes a good clinical instructor. Write three open-ended questions and three closed-ended questions related to this idea.

Suggested Readings

Ahern, N. R. (2005). Using the Internet to conduct research. *Nurse Researcher, 13*(2), 55–70.

Colling, J. (2004, June). Coding, analysis, and dissemination of study results. *Urology Nursing, 24*(3), 215–216.

Halcomb, E., & Andrews, S. (2005). Triangulation as a method for contemporary nursing research. *Nurse Researcher, 13*(2), 71–82.

Happ, M. B., Dabbs, A. D., Tate, J., Hricik, A., & Erlen, J. (2006, March/April). Exemplars of mixed methods data combination and analysis. *Nursing Research, 55*(2), S43–S49.

Priest, H., Roberts, P., & Woods, L. (2002). An overview of three different approaches to the interpretation of qualitative data. Part 1: Theoretical issues. *Nurse Researcher, 10*(1), 30–42.

Vishnevsky, T., & Beanlands, H. (2004, March/April). Qualitative research. *Nephrology Nursing Journal, 31*(2), 234–238.

References

Asia-initiative (n.d.). *Methods of data collection. Chapter 7.* Retrieved March 15, 2009, from http://www.asia-initiative.org/pdfs/chapter7.pdf

Boswell, C. (in press). Questioning students to develop critical thinking. In L. Caputi (Ed.), *Teaching nursing: The art and science* (2nd ed.). Glen Ellyn, IL: College of DuPage Press.

Brink, P. J., & Wood, M. J. (2001). *Basic steps in planning nursing research: From question to proposal.* Sudbury, MA: Jones and Bartlett.

Creswell, J. W. (2003). *Research design: Qualitative, quantitative, and mixed method approaches* (2nd ed.). Thousand Oaks, CA: Sage.

Educational Testing Services. (2006). *ETS test collection database.* Retrieved March 15, 2009, from http://www.ets.org/testcoll

Harvard Family Research Project. (2004, August). Detangling data collection: Methods for gathering data. *Out-of-School Time Evaluation Snapshot, 5,* 1–6. Retrieved March 15, 2008, from http://www.hfrp.org/publications-resources/browse-our-publications/detangling-data-collection-methods-for-gathering-data

LoBiondo-Wood, G., & Haber, J. (1998). *Nursing research: Methods, critical appraisal, and utilization* (4th ed.). St. Louis, MO: Mosby.

Melnyk, B. M., & Fineout-Overholt, E. (2005). *Evidence-based practice in nursing and healthcare: A guide to best practice.* Philadelphia: Lippincott Williams & Wilkins.

Northern Arizona University. (2001). *Module 2: Methods of data collection: Chapter 2 on-line lesson.* Retrieved December 16, 2008, from http://www.prm/mau.edu/prm447/methods_of_data _collection_lesson.htm

Orcher, L. T. (2005). *Conducting research: Social and behavioral science methods.* Glendale, CA: Pyrczak.

Polit, D. F., & Beck, C. T. (2008). *Nursing research: Generating and assessing evidence for nursing practice* (8th ed.). Philadelphia: Lippincott Williams & Wilkins.

Watershed Planning. (n.d.). *Conducting a social profile: Selecting data collection methods.* Retrieved December 16, 2008, from http://www.watershedplanning.uiuc.edu/profile_steps/step3.cfm

Wood, M. J., & Ross-Kerr, J. C. (2006). *Basic steps in planning nursing research: From question to proposal* (6th ed.). Sudbury, MA: Jones and Bartlett.

Chapter 10

Mixed Method Research

JoAnn Long and Carol Boswell

Chapter Objectives

At the conclusion of this chapter, the learner will be able to

1. Discuss the components involved in utilizing mixed method (multimethod) studies
2. Contrast the goals and distinctive features of mixed method research
3. Characterize the advantages of mixed method (multimethod) research

Key Terms

➤ Action research

➤ Concurrent research

➤ Convergent validity

➤ Mixed method research

➤ Multimethod research

➤ Sequential research

➤ Triangulation

Introduction

Mixed method research, broadly defined, is a combination of quantitative and qualitative research methods and techniques for collecting and analyzing data (Bliss, 2001; Creswell, Fetters, & Ivankova, 2004). This form of research is also referred to in the literature by several other names—multimethod, triangulated, and integrated designs.

Mixed method research is often possible within the clinical arena. For example, nurses often believe that the dryness of quantitative research needs to be tempered with the "touchy-feely" aspects of qualitative data. Within the realm of evidence-based nursing practice, a nurse might realize that the time spent in the surgical holding area causes increased stress to the patients. A study could collect physiologic data related to stress, such as blood pressures and time in the surgical holding area, as well as observed signs of stress and emotional data (e.g., verbal comments about the experience while in the surgical holding area awaiting the surgical procedure). The conclusions resulting from the collection of both types of data would reveal each aspect of the individual's experiences while in the surgical holding area. This example of a mixed method study would provide needed data to facilitate the provision of evidence-based nursing practice within the institution.

? Think Outside the Box

Debate the benefits and restrictions involved in using a mixed methodology for a research project.

Quantitative research, which is considered the foundational method, permits the researcher to make inferences only about the data that are being examined. The strengths of this method are the generalizability of study findings and the ability to control for individual variables. These studies, however, are not designed to detect contextual nuances, which may produce a biased understanding of the variables being studied. By comparison, qualitative research spreads a much broader net, allowing for in-depth examination of elements of a phenomenon not considered when research is conducted using quantitative methods. Qualitative studies have their own drawbacks. However, they almost always use small sample sizes and often lack quantitative controls; therefore, they do not produce findings that can be applied to the larger population (Borkan, 2004; Polit & Beck, 2008).

Because both quantitative and qualitative methods have strengths and weaknesses, neither can perfectly establish the full truth about phenomena of interest to nursing (Polit & Beck, 2008). Joining methods is done to reduce the biases associated with one design alone, provide insight into the complexity of the problem under study, and introduce rigor into the study design (Elliott, 2004). This form of research entails more than just the combination of two or more methods in a single study. Multimethod (mixed method) research implies the integration of both numbers and narrative, while offering the potential of producing enhanced results in terms of quality and span (Borkan, 2004). An example of what is meant by multimethod research can be seen when a questionnaire includes both closed-ended questions (numbers) to provide quantitative data and open-ended questions (narrative) that require qualitative analysis.

Simply stated, mixed method design views both quantitative and qualitative research as useful and important, while avoiding the constraints that might hamper a study carried out using a single research methodology (Johnson & Onwuegbuzie, 2004). Each method brings both strengths and weaknesses to the research process. Researchers must carefully consider each of the different pieces to determine the optimal method for addressing the research problem identified.

As the field of research has advanced, the use of mixed methods has sometimes been referred to as "action research." According to Dodd (2008), "Action research promotes change as well as describing, understanding, and explaining the focus of the research" (p. 13). Within action research, the process can take the direction of being cyclical (recurring steps in similar sequence), participative (all individuals working as partners within the process), qualitative (dealing with language, not numbers), or reflective (critically reflecting on the process and outcomes) (Dodd, 2008). The idea behind action research (mixed methods) is to reduce the "'inappropriate uncertainty,' where one 'right answer' derived from a certain method is cross-checked by employing the second method" (Dodd, 2008, p. 13). The best aspects of both kinds of research are pulled together to strengthen and offset problems in an endeavor to find the best evidence for the problem under investigation. Action research (also called design-based research) is frequently used in educational research (Barab, 2006). Action research methods may be employed to facilitate a change in strategy based on feedback about what is being observed in real time (Goodnough, 2008; Kwok, 2009).

Components of Mixed Method Procedures

In using mixed method procedures, the researcher attempts to blend a combination of methods (qualitative and quantitative) that have complementary strong points, while defusing the non-overlapping weaknesses. Bliss (2001) has stated, "A common misconception about mixed method research is that it requires a blending of contradictory or competing research paradigms" (p. 331). This view is also supported by Johnson and Onwuegbuzie (2004): "Mixed methods research is an attempt to legitimate the use of multiple approaches in answering research questions, rather than restricting or constraining researchers' choices (i.e., it rejects dogmatism)" (p. 17).

Although quantitative and qualitative methods each have an established focus, the two are neither contradictory nor competing. Within the delivery of the methodology, the two research designs are frequently meshed within the sampling, data collection, and analysis aspects of the research project. Although these aspects are the current levels, the process does not restrict the versatility or variety of the potential combinations within the two methodologies. Bliss (2001) has noted that "mixed method research seems to offer an opportunity to deepen our insights, sharpen our thinking, develop sensitive methods, and accelerate our advances" (p. 331). By allowing the researcher to identify a combination of methods, this process merges the best of both worlds of research to address the identified healthcare problem in the optimal manner available to the profession. The primary restriction on the joining of the methodologies is the obstruction occurring through lack of vision and risk taking on the part of the researcher.

According to Creswell, Fetters, and Ivankova (2004), mixed method (multimethod) research possesses the potential for rigor, methodologic effectiveness, and investigation within the primary care setting. Even though rigidity is not a problem within this kind of research, the aspects of each methodology employed must still be carefully considered and weighted by the researcher. Within any of the research designs, each method has identified strengths and limitations. As a researcher tries to maximize the complementary points while modifying the limitations, certain concerns emerge to be considered.

? Think Outside the Box

How would you handle a PICOT question format when using a mixed methodology?

According to Patton (1990), one of the main advantages of using the mixed method approach to research is the idea of triangulation. This principle states that the validity of the results from the use of various research approaches determines the appropriateness of the resulting outcomes of the analysis. A mixed method design allows for the utilization of words, pictures, and narrative within the data collection process. Each of these qualitative aspects of the study augments the data provided via the statistical process. Numbers provide the precision, while the words, pictures, and narrative supply the textural aspects of the experience.

As a result of having this intensity of data available for data analysis of the event, an extensive and more comprehensive array of research questions and/or hypotheses can be answered. Put simply, the researcher is not limited regarding the breadth of the questions to be searched within the study. Because both quantitative and qualitative aspects of the issue are being addressed through the mixed methods, the research team draws from the different designs to develop the optimal research project to address the identified problem.

An example of how the use of mixed methodologies uncovers perceptions that might otherwise be missed is illustrated in the work published by Chen and Goodson (2009), who studied barriers to adopting genomics into public health education. On the one hand, qualitative data were collected from a small number (n = 24) of public health educators through personal interviews. Quantitative data, on the other hand, were collected using a large (n = 1,607), Web-based survey method. The combined data gathered via the two methods highlighted barriers that extended beyond a lack of knowledge to more nuanced and complex issues of incompatibility of the individual's personal ethics and beliefs about genomics as factors in the adoption of genomics into public health education.

An additional strength visualized by the use of a mixed methodology for a research project relates to the enthusiasm of the evidence. This resulting power from the in-depth evidence comes about from the triangulation (convergence and corroboration) of the results identified (Johnson, n.d.). Because the evidence is managed through several different processes, the truth of the results is strengthened.

A further strength associated with use of mixed method strategies can be seen when complementary insights and perceptions arise that might have been missed if only one research methodology were employed. The use of both quantitative and qualitative methodology allows the researcher to pull together a wider and deeper understanding about the identified research problem, as it is considered from multiple viewpoints.

Mixed method strategies are not without limitations, however. When both quantitative and qualitative methods are employed, the researcher must be well versed in both methodologies, especially if the two methods are managed concurrently. If the researcher does not feel competent to implement both methods, a research team may be required to complete the process effectively. The combination of the two methods should not be engaged in haphazardly. When this strategy is selected for operationalization, care must be given to learning about the various methods and tactics to allow for the successful incorporation of the necessary approaches. Mixed methodology research can also be especially expensive to complete owing to the use of teams, and it can result in additional time-consuming expectations.

As any investigator elects to use this methodology, rationales for the decisions made must be documented and supported. These rationales need to be based on a thorough understanding of the relevant characteristics of both the quantitative and qualitative methodologies. Clear justification for the selection of a mixed method approach to the research problem must be provided to ensure that the research community comprehends the reasons for the decisions undertaken. These rationales are most often cited in the introduction section of the study report, the study aims discussion, or the overview of the section on methods to be used. As a researcher initiates this discussion concerning the rationales, the priority of the data collection process must be one key aspect that is presented clearly and concisely. This dialogue addresses the question of whether the quantitative and qualitative data are both emphasized equally. In whichever direction a researcher elects to go with the prioritization of the data, understandable and succinct logic for the choice should be carefully and thoroughly documented within the project.

Creswell, Fetters, and Ivankova (2004) have elaborated on the labor-intensive process needed for the involvement of multiple points of data collection and analysis. This process should not be seen as an easier way of arriving at results but rather as a process for obtaining richer and more thorough information about the phenomenon under investigation. Johnson and Onwuegbuzie (2004) contend that the fundamental piece driving this process should be the research question or identified problem. From the identified research problem, a researcher ought to be free to select those research methods that best address the research questions, thereby taking the best opportunity to obtain meaningful answers. If a single research design is considered the best option, then a researcher should utilize that design methodology. When the research problem is viewed as progressively complex, however, all avenues of research methodology should be contemplated to identify the best manner to successfully gain a thorough understanding of the phenomenon.

Mixed method strategies use both deductive and inductive inquiry methods in attempting to corroborate and complement the findings gained. The resulting analysis of the data tends to be a balanced approach to the research process with a common-sense conclusion to the project.

Types of Mixed Method Strategies

As researchers conceptualize using both quantitative and qualitative methodologies, at least three aspects of this process need to be considered: implementation, prioritization, and integration (**Figure 10-1**). Each of these three aspects results in one of two subtypes of mixed method models—within-stage or across-stage methods. Within-stage methods reflect the use of quantitative and qualitative approaches within one or more stages of the research process. An example of this method would be the inclusion of both open-ended questions and closed-ended questions on the same tool for adminis-tration at the same time. Across-stage mixed method approaches are seen when the two research designs are mixed transversely between at least two of the stages within the research endeavor. Returning to the example given earlier concerning the surgical holding room, the use of physiologic data collected while the individual is in the holding area, followed by development of a narrative regarding how the experience was perceived after the surgical process, is an example of the use of across-stage mixed methods. With this approach, the data

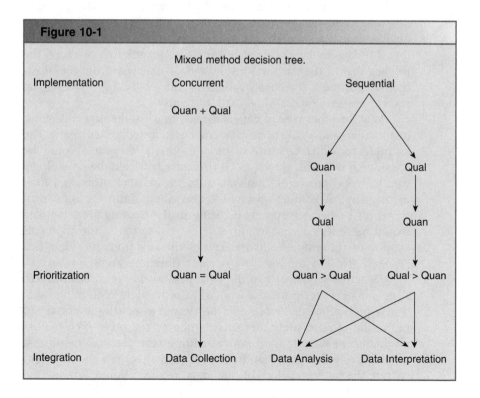

Figure 10-1

Mixed method decision tree.

are not collected at the same time but rather data collection at each stage builds on data collection from the other stages.

? Think Outside the Box

Discuss the risks and vision that may be needed by a researcher for joining quantitative and qualitative methodologies within a study.

In addressing the implementation question, the principal decision relates to whether the two methods—quantitative and qualitative —will be executed at the same time or sequentially. The research question aids in the determination of this aspect. At times, the information discovered within one of the methods is perceived as a valuable foundation for the gathering of the data within the following method. Consider the following example: To determine the extent of research use within an acute care facility, researchers could conduct focus groups with a select group of nurses to determine perceived barriers to the use of research. Based on the data collected via the focus groups, a questionnaire could be developed and given to all staff nurses to determine their level of agreement with the information identified by the focus group members. In this scenario, the qualitative data results and analysis are seen as critical forces determining the data to be collected within the quantitative piece of the project; that is, the statistical results and data analysis from the quantitative portion drive the qualitative data collection process. The reverse process could also be used, of course.

When neither type of data is needed to drive the data collection, quantitative and qualitative data can be collected concurrently. The example provided concerning the surgical holding area could be considered from this viewpoint. If the nurse collected the physiologic data of blood pressures, observation of stressed behaviors, and time in the surgical holding area while also questioning the individual about his or her perceptions of being in the holding area, the data would be collected concurrently. The determination of the appropriateness of this implementation comes directly from the identified research problem and resulting research questions and hypothesis.

Once the sequencing of the two methods has been determined, a researcher must resolve the issue of prioritization. Within this decision aspect, all of the data might be viewed as equally important to the resulting outcomes. Alternatively, one or the other type of data might also be viewed as of particular importance, so that the process would give either the quantitative or qualitative data more weight within the interpretation of the data results. Within any of the examples provided, a researcher would have to make the following decisions:

- Are the physiologic data or the verbal comments more important to the understanding of the stress?
- Is the focus group information concerning barriers to research utilization more appropriate than the results gained from the questionnaire?

The weighting of the data results is completely up to the researcher. Rationales for the weighting decisions must be provided in the report on the study so that the readers of the results can understand this process.

The third aspect to consider as the design is conceptualized concerns the integration of the data. The data can be merged at several different points within the process. Specifically, this merging of the methods could occur at the data collection, data analysis, and/or data interpretation stages. When the data are integrated at the data collection stage, the tool used for data collection would include both closed-ended questions (e.g., a Likert scale section) and several open-ended questions. If the decision were made to collapse the information during the data analysis and/or data interpretation phases, the researcher would be investigating all of the data to see where and how the data meshed into a defensible conclusion.

? Think Outside the Box

Consider a clinical situation that you have confronted. How could you address the clinical problem using both a quantitative method and a qualitative method?

As a researcher begins to consider the use of a mixed methodology with a study, these three aspects must be considered. The question concerning the sequencing of the two methodologies—quantitative and qualitative—provides the foundation for the investigation process. The investigator carefully considers whether both of the research designs will be conducted concurrently or consecutively.

If the decision is to conduct both the quantitative and qualitative data collection aspects at the same time, the process tends to be used to confirm, cross-validate, or corroborate findings within a single study (Creswell, 2003). Even when the two methods are conducted simultaneously, the question concerning how the information will be delivered must still be answered. If one method is embedded into the other method, then the process is termed "nesting." The idea is that the less predominant method is implanted into the other method.

An example of nesting would be the inclusion of open-ended questions at the conclusion of a previously validated quantitative tool. An advantage of using concurrent design for the mixed method process is the shortened data collection time period. Because all of the data are collected at one phase, the expense and time allocation can be reduced.

Within the concurrent implementation of the methodology, each piece of data is weighted equally within the data analysis phase. That is, for concurrent implementation, neither quantitative nor qualitative data are awarded a higher priority relative to the other; each aspect is judged on its own merits. Within this approach to mixed methods research, data integration begins during the data collection phase and continues through the data analysis phase and into the data interpretation phase. The data are interconnected for the initiation of the research process. When concurrent processing is selected for the research project, the investigator must be competent in both methodologies. This proficiency in both methods is imperative, because the researcher must ensure that the protocols for the quantitative and qualitative processes are appropriately carried out at each juncture of the research process.

When an investigator elects to use a sequential method for the mixed method process, several layers of decisions must be made. As the process begins, the researcher must establish which of the two methods will be the dominant method and which will be the lesser method. The principal rationale for considering a sequential format is to allow the results from the initial phase to guide the secondary data collection process. The secondary data results are then used to assist in the interpretation of the initial findings. As the plan is developed, the weighting of the different data formats must also be considered. Generally, within the sequential format, one data collection method is given more priority than the other format. Usually, the initial data collection method is the design that receives priority within the interpretation of the data. Justifications for the ordering and prioritization should be documented. Because the data are collected consecutively, it is integrated at either the data analysis or data interpretation segment. The sequential course of action tends to be easier to describe and to report. The data from the two types of methods are normally reported individually within the report. It is only in the data interpretation that the two groupings of data results may be integrated into a single synthesis of the material. This process allows the researcher to stay true to the quantitative and qualitative methodologies employed.

Data Collection Procedures

In research methods of all types, the collection of data refers to information collected and organized by the researcher. Research data are collected in an effort to measure specific variables that are relevant to the study (Macnee, 2004).

One often thinks first of data taking the form of numbers or statistics. Many preliminary steps must occur prior to the collection of such data in quantitative research. Polit and Beck (2008) describe the data collection plan in quantitative research as including the following steps:

1. Determining the data that need to be gathered
2. Considering the type of measurement to be used for each variable
3. Identifying the instruments available to capture each variable
4. Developing data collection forms/protocols
5. Collecting and managing the data

In mixed method research, data collection may also take nonquantitative forms. Narratives, verbal feedback from focus groups, transcripts, and videotapes are examples of sources of nonquantitative data (Vogt, 2005). The purpose of qualitative data collection in mixed record research may vary. For example, qualitative data may be collected for the purpose of developing questions in a quantitative survey or instrument. This step assists in developing a more comprehensive understanding of the dimensions of a construct under study or in generating hypotheses.

❓ Think Outside the Box

Debate which types of rationales are necessary when a mixed methods approach is used.

The rationale for the data collection process used in mixed method research studies should be stated clearly: Why and how did using one or more methods of collecting and integrating data contribute to the purpose of the study? The specific data that are collected by quantitative and qualitative methods, and the priority and emphasis given to each type of data, are determined by the researchers and driven by the research problem and goals of the study (Creswell et al., 2004). Johnson and Onwuegbuzie (2004, p. 21) describe their mixed method process as having eight distinct steps:

1. Determine the research question.
2. Determine whether a mixed design is appropriate.

3. Select the mixed method or mixed model research design.
4. Collect the data.
5. Analyze the data.
6. Interpret the data.
7. Legitimate the data.
8. Draw conclusions (if warranted) and write the final report.

Step 4 in Johnson and Onwuegbuzie's (2004) mixed method process focuses on data collection. Data collection in multimethod studies is frequently carried out such that quantitative and qualitative components of the study are kept separate during the actual conduct of the study and are combined only later in the interpretation and reporting of results (Creswell et al., 2004; Polit & Beck, 2008).

To illustrate this idea, consider the research reported by Long et al. (2006), in which quantitative methods were used to measure the differences among fruit, vegetable, and fat consumption before and after a Web-based intervention to prevent diabetes in adolescents. Qualitative methods were employed to understand adolescent perceptions and satisfaction with learning about healthy eating through a technology-based medium. In this pilot study, the researchers identified statistical analysis and significance testing of the effectiveness of the intervention as being research priorities. Structured interviews and checklists were used in combination with a computer-based self-report questionnaire to quantitatively measure fruit, vegetable, and fat intake in adolescents. The authors also used qualitative methods to collect data and analyze research questions of importance to the study. In particular, were adolescents satisfied—that is, how did they feel about learning how to prevent type 2 diabetes through the use of the World Wide Web? For the qualitative data collection, the researchers observed adolescent behavior during the study and held focus groups (unstructured group interviews) after the completion of the intervention (Long et al., 2006). They recorded data during the intervention by collecting field and interview notes to record the observations and the feedback obtained from the participants (Long et al., 2006).

Use of both quantitative and qualitative methods allowed these researchers to not only quantify and statistically analyze the effectiveness of the intervention, but also to seek to understand the perception of the adolescent subjects regarding this method of delivering health education and their satisfaction with the experience. Although the use of both research methods occurred concomitantly, data were collected and analyzed as separate "components" within the study and were brought together at the time of interpretation and reporting of study findings.

Data collection and analysis in mixed method research often treat quantitative and qualitative data as independent components in the research design. Creswell, Fetters, and Ivankova (2004), for example, analyzed five studies in which mixed methods had been used in primary care. The quantitative data collected in these five studies were obtained through the use of structured instruments, structured check-lists, and chart audits. The qualitative data were collected through interviews and field observations. Quantitative methods made use of a limited number of inferential analyses (correlation and regression). The authors' assessment of the five primary care studies using these methods suggests that their findings are typical of data collection and analysis processes in mixed method research (Creswell et al., 2004).

Data Analysis and Validation Procedures

How data are analyzed is inextricably tied to the type of information that has been collected. Quantitative data will, at minimum, be counted and described. Inferential statistical analysis will be applied depending on the type and level of data available to the researcher. Qualitative data analysis also takes multiple forms, but it generally involves the coding of narrative themes for depth of understanding. It is not surprising, therefore, that analysis of mixed method research mirrors the variety seen in analyses of both quantitative and qualitative methodologies.

The term "triangulation" is sometimes used when data analysis is performed for the purpose of corroborating data from multiple methods. Kirkman (2008) supports the idea of using triangulation to confirm and reflect the completeness of the confidence evident in the findings. An idea borrowed from the fields of aviation and mathematics, triangulation involves the use of more than one technique to understand or study the same thing. Two or more quantitative sources may be compared with one another, or a quantitative data source may be compared with qualitative findings. Triangulation is typically employed to resolve differences between two (or more) sources of data, with the ultimate goal being to enhance the validity of research findings (Ramprogus, 2005; Vogt, 2005). Triangulation used in this sense is also known as convergent validity and is employed by researchers to check the validity of one instrument or measurement against another.

To illuminate this point, consider the subset of data analysis in the study conducted by Long et al. (2006), which compared the results from two quantitative measurements of fruit, vegetable, and fat intake for convergent validity. Quantitative data from a computer-based self-report and from a structured interview were compared statistically (triangulated) and determined to have a small to medium correlation (Long et al., 2006). This form of mixed methodology is generative, and it assisted the researcher in determining the need for further development of the measurement methods used to determine fruit, vegetable, and fat consumption in an adolescent population. In the same study, the qualitative feedback obtained from observations of student enjoyment with using the Web-based educational intervention and verbal feedback from focus groups was analyzed and coded thematically to capture observed variances among learners, raising new questions about the population and about how to best provide meaningful health education to this group.

? Think Outside the Box

Think for a moment about your current workplace. Identify one problem, process, or policy in your work area whose improvement by the healthcare team would favorably affect patient outcomes. Once you have identified a problem, list ideas about which quantitative data would assist you and your colleagues in solving the problem. Further consider those aspects of the issue in which your understanding would be enhanced through collection of qualitative data. How could you apply best practices to solve the problem you identified using aspects of both research methods?

   Now consider an unmet educational need of new staff members on your unit. How might an "action research" mixed method approach assist you in understanding and meeting the changing educational needs of new staff members?

In summary, both quantitative and qualitative research designs can be complementarily combined through the use of a mixed method approach to data collection and analysis. The specific data collected by both methods and the emphasis given to each should be determined based on the research problem and the goals of the study. A research team whose members are experienced with use of both types of methods is important to the success of mixed method research. While each of the methods has its own strengths and weaknesses, mixed method research offers the opportunity for a more complete investigation into the problem being studied (Creswell et al., 2004; Elliott, 2004; Ramprogus, 2005). Given the complexities and the nature of the problems of interest to nursing, mixed method research holds promise for advancing evidence-based understanding that might lead to enhanced quality patient care.

Evidence-Based Practice Considerations and Mixed Method Research

Problems of interest to nursing are characteristically complex in nature. Nurses in clinical practice need to know how to find, evaluate, and use research so that they can implement best practices at the bedside (Lander, 2004). Understanding mixed method research is important, as it holds the potential for promoting methodologically sound studies that capture complexities which might otherwise be overlooked. According to Rolston-Blenman (2009), "Clinical stakeholders must participate in planning and championing the changes taking place. Staff must feel they have a voice in making decisions" (p. 21). Through the use of mixed methods (action research), the staff at the bedside can actively participate in different aspects of research, resulting in better management of the problems so identified. Action research is one means that nurses at the bedside can use to identify problems and be part of the solution given that multiple methods are employed in the research process.

According to Myers and Meccariello (2006), "It's critical to help nurses understand how crucial their role is in the research process and how they can improve patient care by validating their own trial and error experiences" (p. 24). Each day, individuals must realize the importance of connecting the research process to key activities that occur within the workplace—one patient at a time. This permeation of the workplace with a critical thinking mind frame allows for the deep consideration of multiple problems at the ground-zero level. The incorporation of the research thought process into the everyday workplace "forces us to move from our comfort zone of solely using tradition, intuition, trial and error, and past experiences to a new era in which we integrate all of these tools with what's substantiated through the literature" (p. 26). Taking advantage of the strengths of qualitative and quantitative research design methods, while planning for ways to overcome the limitations of the research designs, allows the discipline of nursing to advance the body of knowledge toward practice confirmed by evidence and practice.

Summary Points

1. Mixed method design (called multimethod, triangulated, and integrated design) is an amalgamation of quantitative and qualitative research methods and techniques used to collect and analyze data.
2. In mixed method studies, two research patterns are regularly interlocked within the sampling, data collection, or analysis aspects of the project.
3. The use of both methods permits the researcher to develop a wider and deeper understanding of the identified research problem as a result of the consideration of the problem from multiple viewpoints.
4. The fundamental force driving the use of mixed method research continues to be the clear and concise identification of the research problem.

5. The criteria used when choosing the combination of methods for inclusion in a mixed method study are related to implementation, prioritization, and integration needs.
6. The investigator must rigorously examine the issue of whether the two research designs should be conducted concurrently or sequentially.
7. Justification for the ordering and prioritization of the different methods must be documented, with rationales being presented for each of the decisions made concerning the research process.
8. During collection and analysis of data in mixed method research, quantitative and qualitative data are often treated as independent components in the research design.
9. The term "triangulation" is used to describe the situation in which data are analyzed for the purpose of corroborating data from multiple methods.

RED FLAGS

- Care must be given to explaining how different research methodologies are entwined as a single project.
- A lack of a rationale for using mixed methods is problematic.
- Any indication that quantitative and qualitative methods are competing with each other reflects lack of planning.
- When the rationale for weighting of the methods is not provided, then concerns must be raised about the results of the data analysis.
- The data collection process for each of the two research methodologies should be kept distinctive.
- If data collection methods are improperly conducted for the identified research methodology, then the validity of the results must be questioned.

Multiple Choice Questions

1. Another term used within the literature for mixed method design is
   A. Quantitative design.
   B. Qualitative design.
   C. Multimethod design.
   D. Experimental design.

2. When a researcher endeavors to use mixed method design to answer an identified research problem, the blending of the methods is based on
   A. Combining the methods to capitalize on their strong points while negating their flaws.
   B. Combining the methods to blend both their strengths and their weaknesses.
   C. Separating the strengths from the weaknesses within the different designs.
   D. Separating the weaker method from the stronger method.

3. The research designs are merged within which sections of the report on the research project?
   A. Introduction, sampling, and problem identification
   B. Problem identification, data collection, and analysis
   C. Sampling, data collection, and analysis
   D. Introduction, data collection, and analysis

4. The primary restrictions related to the researcher that prevent the use of mixed method research are
   A. Lack of understanding about the methods and the research community.
   B. Lack of willingness to engage in the use of, and lack of confidence in, one research method.
   C. Lack of vision and risk taking.
   D. Lack of willingness and overconfidence.

5. A nurse identifies individuals who seem to comply better with a treatment plan when several different teaching methods are used within the discharge planning process. In developing a mixed method design for researching which educational methods work best, a question concerning the type of data to be collected is confronted. Which of the following groups of data collection methods represents a mixed method format?
   A. Likert scale tool with a demographic component
   B. Observation of teaching sessions with videotaping
   C. Focus group discussion with audiotaping
   D. Likert scale tool with focus group discussion

6. The determination of the mixed method design approach must address the meshing of the qualitative and quantitative methodologies through the use of which of the following criteria?

   A. Implementation, prioritization, and integration
   B. Implementation, analysis, and investigation
   C. Analysis, prioritization, and integration
   D. Collection, prioritization, and analysis

7. A researcher has elected to conduct a mixed method research project. Within this project, the decision has been made to conduct the two types of data collection concurrently, with each type of data having equal weight within the analysis process. Based on these decisions, what must the researcher make sure is done for the reporting of the process?

   A. Establish a team to aid in the management of the study
   B. Reevaluate the decision, because quantitative research is the stronger method
   C. Ensure that confidentiality is maintained within the process
   D. Document the rationale for the decisions made within the process

8. Triangulation in mixed method research is utilized for the purposes of supporting _____ validity.

   A. criterion
   B. convergent
   C. construct
   D. variable

9. The data collected in mixed method research and the emphasis given to each type of data should be determined by the _____ and goals of the study.

   A. source of funding
   B. preference of the research team
   C. research problem
   D. literature

10. Qualitative data analysis seeks _____ in understanding of a phenomenon.

    A. rigor
    B. depth
    C. numbers
    D. statistics

11. A primary reason for using mixed research methodologies is the opportunity to _____ that might otherwise be overlooked.

    A. catch complexities
    B. define concepts
    C. describe problems
    D. uncover opportunities

12. In mixed method research, the collection of quantitative and qualitative data is often treated _____.
   A.   synchronously
   B.   stringently
   C.   independently
   D.   statistically

13. An advantage of using a mixed method design for a research study is to
   A.   Increase the biases associated with the use of two designs.
   B.   Provide insight into the complexity of the problem under study.
   C.   Impart rigor to the examination of the intricacies of the problem under study.
   D.   Decrease the impartiality associated with the use of one design.

14. Limitations related to the use of mixed method strategies include the
   A.   Cost and additional time required.
   B.   Extensive and comprehensive research questions involved.
   C.   Vivacity of the evidence provided.
   D.   Complementary insights and perceptions provided.

Discussion Questions

1. A nurse on the labor and delivery unit wants to study the effects of having small children participate with the family in the delivery process on the bonding process between mother and child. For this study, the nurse has determined that a questionnaire will be mailed out to families who elect to have their toddlers in the delivery room during the delivery of a sibling. The questionnaire will include both open-ended questions and closed-ended (Likert-type) questions. Which aspects of the study should be considered to provide a rationale for selecting this mixed method strategy?

2. A researcher working within a hospital striving to gain Magnet status wants to study the barriers to use of research at the bedside. For the design of this study, the individual is considering using a mixed method format. Which pieces of the design should be considered as the researcher prepares the study?

3. A group of researchers has developed a new instrument to assess the degree of destruction noted within decubitus ulcers (pressure ulcers). As part of their study, they are planning to compare the new instrument with instruments currently used within their acute care setting. Which components of the mixed method strategies need to be carefully considered as the researchers develop the study design?

Suggested Readings

Bader, M. K., Palmer, S., Stalcup, C., & Shaver, T. (2002). Using a FOCUS-PDCA quality improvement model for applying the severe traumatic brain injury guidelines to practice: Process and outcomes. *Online Journal of Knowledge Synthesis for Nursing, Clinical Column,* Document No. 4C.

Balas, E. A., & Boren, S. A. (2000). Managing clinical knowledge for healthcare improvements. In V. Schattauer (Ed.), *Yearbook of medical informatics* (pp. 65–70). Stuttgart, Germany: Schattauer.

Classen, S., & Lopez, E. (2006). Mixed methods approach explaining process of an older driver safety systematic literature review. *Topics in Geriatric Rehabilitation, 22*(2), 99–112.

Foss, C., & Ellefsen, B. (2002, October). The value of combining qualitative and quantitative approaches in nursing research by means of method triangulation. *Journal of Advanced Nursing, 40*(2), 242–248.

Hanson, W., Creswell, J., Clark, V., Petska, K., & Creswell, D. (2005). Mixed methods research designs in counseling psychology. *Journal of Counseling Psychology, 52*(2), 224–235.

Happ, M. B., Dabbs, A. D., Tate, J., Hricik, A., & Erlen, J. (2006, March/April). Exemplars of mixed methods data combination and analysis. *Nursing Research, 55*(2), S43–S49.

Melnyk, B. M., & Fineout-Overholt, E. (2006, Second Quarter). Advancing knowledge through collaboration. *Reflections on Nursing Leadership, 32*(2), 1–5.

Melnyk, B. M., Fineout-Overholt, E., Stetler, C., & Allen, J. (2005). Outcomes and implementation strategies from the first U.S. evidence-based leadership summit. *Worldviews on Evidence-Based Nursing, 2*(3), 113–121.

Miller, S., & Fredericks, M. (2006). Mixed methods and evaluation research: Trends and issues. *Qualitative Health Research, 16*(4), 567–597.

Sale, J., Lohfeld, L., & Brazil, K. (2002). Revisiting the quantitative–qualitative debate: Implications for mixed-methods research. *Quality & Quantity, 36*(1), 43–53.

Williamson, G. (2005). Illustrating triangulation in mixed-methods nursing research. *Nurse Researcher, 12*(1), 7–18.

References

Barab, S. (2006). Design-based research: A methodological toolkit for the learning scientist. In R. K. Sawyer (Ed.), *The Cambridge handbook of the learning sciences* (pp. 153–169). Cambridge, UK: Cambridge University Press.

Bliss, D. Z. (2001). Mixed or mixed up methods? *Nursing Research, 50*(6), 331.

Borkan, J. M. (2004). Mixed methods studies: A foundation for primary care research [Editorial]. *Annals of Family Medicine, 2*(1), 4–6.

Chen, L. S., & Goodson, P. (2009). Barriers to adopting genomics into public health education: A mixed methods study. *Genetics in Medicine, 11*(2), 104–110.

Creswell, J. W. (2003). *Research design: Qualitative, quantitative, and mixed methods approaches* (2nd ed.). Thousand Oaks, CA: Sage.

Creswell, J. W., Fetters, M. D., & Ivankova, N. V. (2004). Designing a mixed methods study in primary care. *Annals of Family Medicine, 2*(1), 7–12.

Dodd, T. (2008). Quantitative and qualitative research data and their relevance to policy and practice. *Nurse Researcher, 15*(4), 7–14.

Elliott, J. (2004). Multimethod approaches in educational research. *International Journal of Disability, Development and Education, 51*(2), 135–149.

Goodnough, K. (2008). Moving science off the "back burner": Meaning making within an action research community. *Journal of Science and Teacher Education, 19*(1), 15–39.

Johnson, B. (n.d.). *Chapter 14: Mixed research: Mixed method and mixed model research* [Online lecture]. Retrieved March 15, 2009, from http://www.southalabama.edu/coe/bset/johnson/dr_johnson/lectures/lec14.htm

Johnson, R. B., & Onwuegbuzie, A. J. (2004). Mixed methods research: A research paradigm whose time has come. *Educational Researcher, 33*(7), 14–26.

Kirkman, C. (2008). Establishing truthfulness, consistency, and transferability. *Nurse Researcher, 15*(4), 68–78.

Kwok, J. (2009). Boys and reading: An action research project. *Library Media Connection, 27*(4), 20–24.

Lander, J. A. (2004). Finding, evaluating, and using research for best practice. *Clinical Nursing Research, 14*(4), 299–302.

Long, J. D., Armstrong, M. L., Amos, E., Shriver, B., Roman-Shriver, C., Feng, D., et al. (2006). Pilot using World Wide Web to prevent diabetes in adolescents. *Clinical Nursing Research, 15*(1), 67–79.

Macnee, C. (2004). *Understanding nursing research.* Philadelphia: Lippincott Williams & Wilkins.

Myers, G., & Meccariello, M. (2006). From pet rock to rock-solid: Implementing unit-based research. *Nursing Management, 37*(1), 24–29.

Patton, M. Q. (1990). *Qualitative evaluation and research method* (2nd ed.) [Online]. Newbury Park, CA: Sage. Retrieved March 6, 2006, from http://www.ehr.nsf.gov/EHR/REC/pub/NSF97-153/CHAP_1.HTM

Polit, D. F., & Beck, C. T. (2008). *Nursing research: Generating and assessing evidence for nursing practice* (8th ed.). Philadelphia: Lippincott Williams & Wilkins.

Ramprogus, V. (2005). Triangulation. *Nurse Researcher, 12*(4), 4–6.

Rolston-Blenman, B. (2009). Nurses roll up their sleeves at the bedside to improve patient care. *Nurse Leader, 7*(1), 20–25.

Vogt, P. W. (2005). *Dictionary of statistics and methodology* (3rd ed.). Thousand Oaks, CA: Sage.

Chapter 11

Reliability, Validity, and Trustworthiness

James Eldridge

Chapter Objectives

At the conclusion of this chapter, the learner will be able to

1. Identify the need for reliability and validity of instruments used in evidence-based practice
2. Define reliability and validity
3. Discuss how reliability and validity affect outcome measures and conclusions of evidence-based research
4. Develop reliability and validity coefficients for appropriate data
5. Interpret reliability and validity coefficients of instruments used in evidence-based practice

Key Terms

➤ Accuracy

➤ Concurrent validity

➤ Consistency

➤ Construct validity

➤ Content-related validity

➤ Correlation coefficient

➤ Criterion-related validity

➤ Cross-validation

➤ Equivalency reliability

➤ Interclass reliability

➤ Intraclass reliability

➤ Objectivity

➤ Observed score

➤ Predictive validity

➤ Reliability

➤ Stability

➤ Standard error of measurement

➤ Trustworthiness

➤ Validity

Introduction

The foundation of good research and of good decision making in evidence-based practice (EBP) is the trustworthiness of the data used to make decisions. When data cannot be trusted, an informed decision cannot be made. Trustworthiness of the data can also be described as being only as good as the instruments or tests used to collect the data. Regardless of the specialization of the healthcare provider, nurses make daily decisions on the diagnosis and treatment of a patient based on the results from different tests to which the patient is subjected. To ensure that the individual makes the proper diagnosis and gives the proper treatment, the nurse must first be sure that the test results used to make the decisions are trustworthy or correct.

Working in an EBP setting requires the nurse to have the best data available to aid in the decision-making process. How can an individual make a decision if the results being used as the foundation of that process cannot be trusted? Put simply, a person cannot make a decision unless the results are trustworthy and correct.

This chapter presents three concepts to help the nurse determine whether the data upon which decisions are based are trustworthy: reliability, validity, and accuracy. Each defines a portion of the trustworthiness of the data collection instruments, which in turn defines the trustworthiness of the data, ensuring a proper diagnosis or treatment.

Reliability and validity are the most important concepts in the decision-making process. If either of these concepts is lacking in the data, the nurse cannot make an informed decision and, therefore, is more likely to make an incorrect decision. Because an incorrect decision in the medical field can have catastrophic consequences for the patient, one can see why reliability and validity are so important. But what do these concepts mean? What would happen if the same test were run on a person several times but the results were different each time? In the case of varying results, a decision becomes ambiguous because the results are unclear.

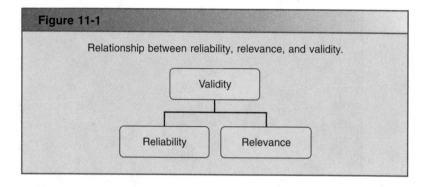

Figure 11-1

Relationship between reliability, relevance, and validity.

Validity

Reliability   Relevance

- Reliability = the instrument consistently measures the same thing.
- Validity = the instrument measures what it is supposed to measure.

Reliability is defined as the consistency or repeatability of test results. Other descriptors used to indicate reliability include "consistency," "repeatability," "objectivity," "dependability," and "precision." Accuracy is a function of reliability: The better the reliability, the more accurate the results. Conversely, the poorer the reliability, the more inaccurate the results and the greater the chance an incorrect decision could be made.

Validity is defined as the degree to which the results are truthful. It depends on the reliability and relevance of the test in question (**Figure 11-1**). Relevance is simply the degree of the relationship between the test and its objective, meaning that the test reflects what was reported to be tested.

An example of relevance is the measurement of the height of a patient. A nurse uses a stadiometer (a ruler used to measure vertical distance) to establish a patient's height. Is the stadiometer a relevant height measurement device? Height is the vertical distance from the floor to the top of the head, and a stadiometer measures vertical distance from the floor to any point above the floor; thus the stadiometer is a relevant measure of height.

Validity cannot exist without reliability and relevance, but reliability and relevance can exist independently of validity. **Figure 11-2a** depicts the case in which there is a high degree of reliability and a low degree of relevance. In this representation, even when reliability is high, validity is low owing to the lack of relevance. This figure shows that under the most reliable test, a low degree of relevance decreases the validity of the test.

Figure **11-2b** depicts the situation in which there is a high degree of relevance and a low degree of reliability. In this representation,

Figure 11-2

Relationship among reliability, relevance, and validity.

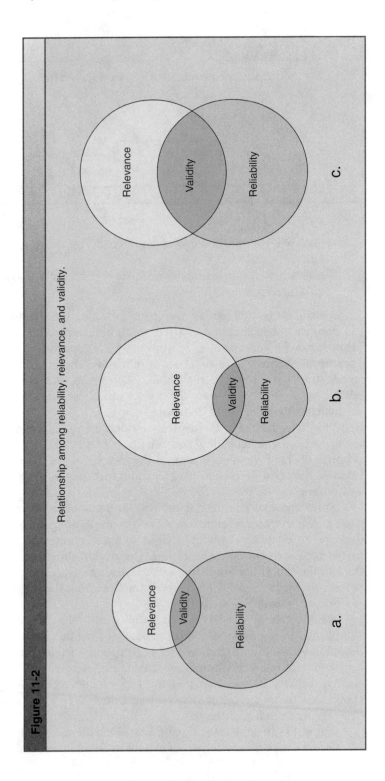

even when relevance is high, validity is low owing to the lack of reliability. Even when a nurse uses what might be considered the most relevant test for the situation, if the instrument has a low degree of reliability, it will also have a low degree of validity.

Figure 11-2c shows the desired capacity for an instrument—to have both a high degree of reliability and a high degree of relevance, thereby creating a high degree of validity. Whereas the other examples show that a test can be reliable but not relevant, or relevant but not reliable, a valid test will always have some degree of reliability and relevance. When validity is absent, the results of the testing are not truthful and making an informed or evidence-based decision is impossible. However, when validity is present, a nurse can be assured that the decision is based on truthful evidence.

Reliability as a Concept

As previously described, reliability focuses on the repeatability or consistency of data. To understand the theoretic constructs of reliability, one must understand the concept of the observed score. By definition, the observed score is the score that is seen; stated in other terms, the observed score is the actual score printed on the readout of an instrument.

An example of an observed score is the measurement of a patient's blood pressure. The systolic and diastolic pressures are determined based on the aneroid dial or digital liquid crystal display (LCD) readings associated with the first sound (systolic) and the last sound (diastolic) heard in the brachial artery. If the first sound occurs at a reading of 130 mm Hg, then this is the systolic observed score. If the last sound occurs at 85 mm Hg, then this is the diastolic observed score. These observed scores for blood pressure are not the true blood pressure scores for the patient, as those scores ultimately depend on factors such as the amount of error incorporated in the type of sphygmomanometer, the quality of the stethoscope, the quality of hearing of the person taking the blood pressure, the experience of the person taking the measurements, and placement of the cuff over the artery. Each of these nuances can add or subtract error within the readings, which increases the variability between the observed score and the true score. This variability can be described as the error score, thereby defining the observed score as the sum of the true score and the error score. As shown in **Figure 11-3**, any error within the measurement decreases the degree to which the observed score reflects the true score.

The true score exists only in theory, because all data collected are observed score data. A nurse can think of the true score as the

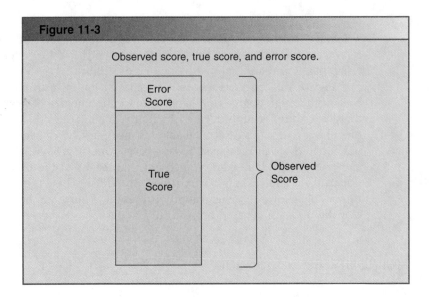

Figure 11-3

Observed score, true score, and error score.

perfect score of a test—that is, a score without any error and void of any misrepresentation. Of course, the world is not perfect and, therefore, neither are any data that might be collected. Thus a true score exists and never changes for a given period of time; changes occur only in the error score, which then determines the observed score.

? Think Outside the Box

Discuss the elements of trustworthiness as related to making decisions about the data found within a research study.

Reliability is the degree to which the observed score of a measure reflects the true score of that measure. Therefore, reliability could theoretically be calculated as the proportion of observed score variance that consists of true score variance (**Figure 11-4**).

In this equation, if no error exists, then the observed score variance and the true score variance are equal, and the reliability is 1.0. Conversely, when the observed score variance and the error score variance are equal, the reliability is 0. Therefore, reliability always falls within the range of 0–1.0, with a perfect reliability equaling 1.0 and no reliability equaling 0. For research purposes, high reliability measures are desired if at all possible. The general rule is that reliability coefficients greater than 0.80 are considered to be high. Note that if the reliability coefficient is calculated as 1.15, a calculation

---

Figure 11-4

Theoretical calculation of reliability.

$$\text{Reliability} = \frac{S^2 \text{ true}}{S^2 \text{ observed}} = \frac{S^2 \text{ observed} - S^2 \text{ error}}{S^2 \text{ observed}}$$

---

error has been made, because the range of reliability is between 0 and 1.0.

Forms of Reliability

Although the purpose of the theoretic concept of reliability is to determine the relationship between the true and observed scores of a measure, practical use of this concept allows a nurse to determine the relationship only between two or more observed scores. The relationship between these observed scores allows an individual to estimate reliability and to determine a range for the true score. The outcome of the calculation of the relationship between two or more observed scores is known as the correlation coefficient. The correlation coefficient is the practical calculation of the theoretic expression of the proportion of observed score variance that consists of true score variance, as described previously.

Given this basic understanding of reliability as a concept, it is now time to learn about the forms of reliability. Globally, reliability can be described as either interclass reliability or intraclass reliability. The most basic description of interclass reliability is the reliability between two and only two variables or trials, whereas intraclass reliability is the reliability between more than two variables or trials. The limiting factor that separates the two forms of reliability is the number of variables or trials that can be used in the calculation of the correlation coefficient. The number of variables also determines which statistic or equation is used to develop the correlation coefficient. Each of these considerations has its place in EBP depending on the number of variables a nurse uses to calculate the reliability coefficient.

Interclass Reliability

Interclass reliability is the reliability between two measures that are presented in the data as either variables or trials. Four types of interclass reliability are distinguished:

■ Consistency
■ Stability
■ Equivalency
■ Internal consistency

Each of these reliability coefficients is developed using a Pearson Product Moment (PPM) correlation. Most statistical packages or spreadsheet software can calculate PPM correlations; therefore, the actual equation is not included in this text. Although each interclass reliability coefficient uses the same formula, the calculated reliability coefficient is defined by the type of variables to be compared and the methods used for interpretation of the results. The previous statement becomes more evident as the types of interclass reliability are further defined.

Consistency

One type of interclass reliability to report is the consistency of a measure. Consistency simply describes the degree to which you can expect to get the same results when measuring a variable more than once on a single day. Consistency reliability is sometimes described as test–retest reliability, because it compares two trials of a single measure. An example of testing for consistency would be running two tests on a single blood sample from each subject to measure hemoglobin using a single hemoglobin analyzer. The question is whether the results from the hemoglobin analyzer are consistent within a single day. In **Table 11-1**, the subjects' hemoglobin from a single sample of blood was measured twice, and the reliability coefficient was calculated to be 0.996.

This coefficient simply means that 99.6% of the observed score variance is true score variance. Because the reliability coefficient is close to 1.0, the reliability of the instrument is high. The initial question with this data was whether or not the machine was consistent. The results demonstrate that it was consistent, with a consistency reliability coefficient of $r_{xx'} = 0.996$.

Stability

When results of trials or tests are collected over two or more days, consistency becomes stability. Suppose we take the same data from Table 11-1, this time imagining that the samples were tested over a two-day period. The question now becomes whether a blood sample is stable over a two-day period. Notice that the results remain constant, because nothing has changed except the theoretical timing of the tests. The reliability coefficient is still 0.996, but this time a nurse would interpret the results as the samples being stable over a two-day period, with a stability reliability coefficient of $r_{xx'} = 0.996$.

Table 11-1

Consistency and Stability of the ACTdif Analyzer

Subject Number	Test 1 (g/dL)	Test 2 (g/dL)
1	14.10	14.00
2	12.20	12.10
3	11.90	11.90
4	14.50	14.40
5	13.80	13.90
6	13.20	13.10
7	13.50	13.60
8	14.00	14.10
9	11.10	11.00
10	9.60	9.90
		$r = 0.996$

Both consistency and stability have their place in EBP. In the current example of hemoglobin testing, the consistency of the measures is described by determining that, for any time during a single day, the data would be repeatable. A nurse can expect the same results as long as no other factors have occurred in the interim, such as acute onset of anemia. In other words, the nurse is sure that the hemoglobin analyzer will give the same measure of hemoglobin for the same sample within the same day. Notice that nowhere in this example of consistency do we assume that the measurement gives the *correct* amount of hemoglobin, only that it indicates the presence of the *same* amount of hemoglobin. To determine if this is the correct amount of hemoglobin, the relevance and the validity of the instrument would have to be known.

When discussing this example in terms of stability, the key determination relates to the length of time that the blood samples remain stable. Hemoglobin analyzers usually have instructions that indicate the time frame for running samples before differing results would be seen. In most instances, the time frame is usually 24 hours. A question might arise concerning how the manufacturer determined this time frame. The answer simply is that the manufacturer developed a stability coefficient using the same techniques described previously.

Again, notice that nowhere in the example of stability is there any mention of the correctness of the amount of hemoglobin over a 24-hour period; the only consideration is that it is the same amount of hemoglobin measured for a 24-hour period. To determine whether this is the correct amount of hemoglobin over the 24-hour period, the relevance and the validity of the instrument and the measures would need to be determined.

Equivalency

Another type of interclass reliability to report is equivalency. This kind of reliability allows a person to report whether one type of test is equivalent to another. Equivalency reliability is calculated in the same manner as the consistency and stability coefficients described previously, except that a PPM correlation between two forms of a single test is calculated, rather than a single variable over two trials.

An example of testing for equivalency reliability would be comparing two methods of blood pressure measurement to determine if they are equivalent. In this case, the question is whether the systolic blood pressure results determined by an automatic blood pressure cuff are equivalent to those recorded from manual blood pressure measures using a stethoscope and sphygmomanometer. As shown in **Table 11-2**, subjects' systolic pressure was measured once with an automatic cuff and once using manual methods. The reliability coefficient was calculated to be 0.959.

This coefficient simply means that 95.9% of the observed score variance consists of true score variance. Because the reliability coefficient is close to 1.0, the reliability between the instruments is high. The initial question with these data was whether automatic cuff readings are equivalent to manual readings of systolic blood pressure. A person can now report that the two methods are equivalent, with an equivalency reliability coefficient of $r_{xx'} = 0.959$. These results indicate that either an automatic cuff or manual methods are acceptable for measuring systolic blood pressure, because they are equivalent. No matter which method is used, a nurse can expect to get similar measures from a single individual. Notice again that there is no mention

Table 11-2		
Equivalency of Automatic versus Manual Systolic Pressure Readings		
Subject	Automatic Cuff Systolic (mm Hg)	Manual Method Number Systolic (mm Hg)
1	150.00	155.00
2	130.00	128.00
3	125.00	129.00
4	124.00	120.00
5	122.00	125.00
6	148.00	144.00
7	133.00	135.00
8	146.00	143.00
9	117.00	120.00
10	121.00	120.00
		$r = 0.959$

of the correctness of the data, only the similarity of the data. To determine if the blood pressure measures are correct, the relevance and the validity of the measures would need to be determined.

Internal Consistency

The final type of interclass reliability discussed here is the internal consistency of written tests. Internal consistency reliability is sometimes described as split-halves reliability, because it entails comparing two halves of a written test. To calculate the internal consistency of a written instrument, the instrument responses are divided into two equal halves. The sum of each half is calculated to make the comparison.

The simplest means for dividing a test in half is to compare the sum of the odd-numbered question responses with the sum of the even-numbered question responses. If possible, the questions should be matched between each half based on their content and difficulty. Another possible method is to make the a priori assumption that both halves are equal because the questions were randomly placed in order during the development of the written test. As with the other types of interclass reliability, the PPM correlation is used to develop the reliability coefficient.

Data for a ten-item pain questionnaire are presented in **Table 11-3** to demonstrate the principle of internal consistency. Each item of the pain questionnaire is scored from 0 (strongly disagree) to 5 (strongly agree). The questionnaire is then divided into odd and even scores, with the sum of the scores for the odd-numbered items and the sum of the scores for the even-numbered items presented in the table. The question under consideration is whether this questionnaire has internal consistency. As with the previous types of reliability, the reliability coefficient is reported; here, it is 0.761. This coefficient simply means that 76.1% of the observed score variance consists of true score variance. Notice that the internal consistency is lower than in previous examples. The fact that the reliability coefficient is lower does not mean that the questionnaire is not reliable—just that it is less reliable than it could be.

? **Think Outside the Box**

Look around your clinical setting. Which tools or instruments are present, and how are they typically used for data collection? Do they include surveys of employees, patients, or consumers? Are the tools or instruments used appropriately?

Table 11-3		
Internal Consistency of a Ten-Item Pain Questionnaire		
Subject	Odd-Numbered Item Scores	Even-Numbered Item Scores
1	25.00	21.00
2	18.00	14.00
3	16.00	18.00
4	12.00	14.00
5	10.00	10.00
6	18.00	19.00
7	15.00	18.00
8	12.00	9.00
9	14.00	15.00
10	17.00	13.00
		$r = 0.761$

Figure 11-5
Spearman–Brown prophecy.
$$r_{xx'} = \frac{k \times r_{xx'}}{1 + r_{xx'}(k-1)}$$

The initial question for these data was whether the pain questionnaire was internally consistent. We can now report that it has some internal consistency, with a reliability coefficient of $r_{xx'} = 0.761$, but there is at least some error present in the questionnaire. In other words, the questionnaire is not perfectly consistent internally, so the results from using the questionnaire will not be an accurate reflection of the true score. This does not mean that this questionnaire should not be used, but rather that a person needs to be careful in the interpretation and use of the results of the questionnaire. When using written item tests, individuals can actually estimate how reliability will change as a result of adding items to the questionnaire. To estimate a new reliability for a written questionnaire with added items, the Spearman–Brown prophecy formula (**Figure 11-5**) could be used.

Where $r_{kk'}$ is the new reliability coefficient, $r_{xx'}$ is the original reliability coefficient, and k is the total items on the new questionnaire divided by the number of items on the original questionnaire, the Spearman–Brown prophecy can be determined. In the example given

---

Figure 11-6

Spearman–Brown prophecy example.

$$r_{xx'} = \frac{2 \times 0.761}{1 + 0.0761(2 - 1)}$$

---

in Table 11-3, the reliability coefficient was 0.761. To calculate the reliability of the questionnaire if 10 questions were added, a person would solve for $r_{kk'}$ using the following information shown in **Figure 11-6**.

The original reliability coefficient is 0.760 and the number of total items on the new questionnaire divided by the total items on the original test is 2. Notice that by increasing the number of items on the questionnaire to 20, the new reliability coefficient for the questionnaire becomes 0.864. This coefficient is higher than the original value. Thus adding items to the questionnaire improves this tool's internal consistency and strengthens the interpretation of its results. As discussed earlier, as reliability and relevance increase, so does validity. Thus, if the questionnaire being used has a high degree of relevance, the addition of more questions to the questionnaire (assuming they are relevant) would increase the reliability of the questionnaire, thereby improving the validity of its results.

Intraclass Reliability

Now that we have an understanding of interclass reliability, it is time to move on to intraclass reliability. As discussed earlier, the basic difference between interclass reliability and intraclass reliability is the number of variables that can be analyzed. Interclass reliability testing allows for the reliability analysis of only two variables, whereas intraclass reliability testing allows a researcher to develop a reliability coefficient for more than two variables.

Suppose we wanted to measure the reliability among three different pain scales. One of the scales requires only 2 minutes for completion, the second scale requires 10 minutes for completion, and the third scale requires 30 minutes for completion. The nurse would prefer to use either the 2-minute or 10-minute scale for efficiency, but the 30-minute scale is currently being used. Although the data could be analyzed using three PPM correlations to determine the equivalency reliability coefficients for these tools, this kind of analysis would miss a very important portion of the error: In the PPM interclass analysis, the statistic estimates only the error between the items,

---

Figure 11-7

Intraclass reliability coefficient using ANOVA.

$$r_{xx'} = \frac{MS_{between} - MS_{within}}{MS_{between}}$$

---

but it ignores the error within the item that reflects the differences in individuals taking the test.

In contrast, the intraclass reliability coefficient uses analysis of variance (ANOVA) to determine not only the error *between* the tests, but also the error *within* the tests. Using ANOVA allows for construction of a better estimate of the overall reliability of the scales and the errors that reduce the observed score variance, which is the true score variance. Thus, whereas PPM analysis allows for only a two-dimensional view of reliability, ANOVA supports a three-dimensional view of reliability. Notice that the basic terms of reliability remain the same. In the current example, a nurse is still estimating the equivalency of the scales, but now an error that might exist within each individual scale is included.

Figure 11-7 shows the equation used in determining a reliability coefficient using ANOVA. In this equation, a reliability coefficient is developed using the mean square between scales and the mean square within scale data from the ANOVA table.

Table 11-4 presents data for the example of the three pain scales. These ANOVA data include the between-cells mean square of 2908.233 and the within-cells mean square of 35.100. As shown in **Figure 11-8**, the reliability coefficient is determined by substituting the numbers represented in the table into the ANOVA equation for reliability (Figure 11-7).

In this example, the equivalency reliability is 0.988 for the three scales. We can now state that the 2-minute pain scale is equivalent to the 10-minute pain scale and the 30-minute pain scale. The evidence for replacing the longer 30-minute test with the more efficient 2-minute test is now documented, because the tests are equivalent. The same ANOVA reliability equation can be used to determine consistency, stability, and equivalency, depending on the intended use of the data.

Objectivity

An area of intraclass reliability that many times is overlooked is the measure of objectivity. Objectivity is the reliability of scores assigned

Table 11-4

Intraclass Reliability Using ANOVA

Subject Number	Scale		
	2-Minute Scale	10-Minute Scale	30-Minute Scale
1	15.00	35.00	60.00
2	12.00	30.00	51.00
3	9.00	22.00	40.00
4	10.00	25.00	42.00
5	11.00	19.00	43.00
6	14.00	31.00	45.00
7	6.00	20.00	38.00
8	3.00	15.00	33.00
9	12.00	22.00	45.00
10	11.00	21.00	45.00

Source of Variation	SSq	DF	MSq	F
Between cells	5816.467	2	2908.233	82.86
Within cells	947.700	27	35.100	
Total	6764.167	29		

Figure 11-8

Intraclass reliability coefficient using ANOVA.

$$r_{xx'} = \frac{2908.233 - 35.10}{2908.233} = 0.988$$

by judges or reviewers. In theory, if three individuals see the same performance, they should score the performance based on the merits of the performance, such that their scores are not affected by internal biases that each may possess. When no bias is evident, the scores should be similar among the judges.

A good example of objectivity (or lack of objectivity) comes from the 2002 Winter Olympics figure skating competition, in which three judges rated the performance of the Canadian skating pair. Two of the judges assigned scores of 9.9 and 9.8 for the pair's performance, but a third judge scored the pair at 7.8. If no biases were associated with the scoring method, then the third judge should have been expected to score the performance in the 9.7–9.9 range.

Objectivity also has relevance for EBP. The Apgar score—a tool for assessing the health of newborn infants—offers an example of objectivity in healthcare practice. If three medical professionals are in the delivery room, the Apgar scores each assigns to the newborn should be equivalent. This factor can be tested using the same ANOVA techniques described in the previously given pain scale example, albeit with scores for each observer, rather than each scale, being used. A researcher could determine if the Apgar scores are objective. If they are not, the researcher could meet with the observers to determine where differences occurred.

By now, it should be clear that the same formula (either PPM or ANOVA, depending on the number of trials) is used to determine the reliability of any measure. The only difference in the results relates to the interpretation based on the intended use of the data.

Accuracy

Another item that is important when determining the intraclass reliability of a test is the test's accuracy. The measure of the accuracy of a test is known as the standard error of measurement (SEM). The SEM reflects the fluctuation of the observed score attributable to the error score. Computing the SEM allows a researcher to determine confidence intervals for the observed score based on the standard deviation of the test and its reliability. The relationship between the true score and the observed score was discussed earlier in this chapter. The SEM allows a researcher to provide a range for which the true score is present.

The equation shown in **Figure 11-9** is used to calculate the SEM. Notice that in this equation, the reliability coefficient of the test and the standard deviation of the sample are used.

? Think Outside the Box

On most clinical units, many different tools are regularly used, such as thermometers, glucometers, sphygmomanometers, and weight scales. Are these tools accurate? How can you be sure that they are reliable and valid for what they are being used to evaluate? *Are* they valid and reliable tools?

Figure 11-9

Standard error of measurement.

$$SEM = s \sqrt{1 - r_{xx'}}$$

Figure 11-10

SEM for consistency of a hemoglobin analyzer.

$$SEM = 1.496 \sqrt{1 - 0.996}$$
$$= \pm 0.0946 \text{ mg/dl}$$

The SEM can be determined for any of the prior examples. For Table 11-1, the standard deviation of the sample is 1.496, and the reliability coefficient is 0.996. Using the equation in Figure 11-9, we can compute the SEM as ±0.0946 mg/dL (**Figure 11-10**).

In a normal distribution, 68% of the sample scores fall between ±1 standard deviation of the mean. Thus, for this example, we have 68% confidence that the hemoglobin scores will fall between ±0.0946 mg/dL of the measured score. If a ±2 standard deviation from the mean is used, a 95% confidence interval for the scores is expected. To find the SEM for ±2 standard deviations from the mean, we multiply the SEM by 2 (the number of standard deviation units). In our example, we have 95% confidence that the true hemoglobin score will fall between ±0.1892 mg/dL of the measured score. If a blood sample is run in the analyzer and the hemoglobin level is found to be 14.0 mg/dL, we would therefore have 95% confidence that the true score is between 13.1080 mg/dL and 14.1892 mg/dL. Notice that as the standard deviation increases for a set of scores, the SEM increases. Also, as the reliability of a set of scores decreases, the SEM increases. To proclaim a tool as giving an accurate measure, test scores need a relatively low standard deviation and a high reliability coefficient.

Up to this point, we have examined accuracy as it relates to continuous data. But what happens when a test uses nominal data—how do we determine its accuracy? In the case of nominal data, we use the χ^2 (chi-square) statistic and its corresponding phi coefficient as a measure of accuracy. Think of the phi coefficient as a correlation or reliability coefficient for nominal data. A χ^2 statistic and its corresponding phi coefficient would most likely be used when you are trying to determine whether a new test is equivalent to a "gold standard" test. All of the same rules apply just as they have in the previous discussion of reliability for continuous data; however, now you are simply determining the accuracy of the new test based on its "pass or fail" performance compared to the "gold standard" test.

Be aware that reliability and accuracy can be sensitive to situational changes. Just because a test is reliable in one situation or within one group, it may not always be reliable when the situation or group changes. This consideration is especially important concerning written items. Factors that can affect reliability and accuracy include the following issues:

- *Fatigue.* Fatigue of the person taking the test or collecting the data can decrease reliability.
- *Practice.* The more practiced a person becomes at taking a test or in collecting data, the more reliability is improved.
- *Timing.* The more time that passes between test administrations, the more the reliability of the test is decreased.
- *Homogeneity of the testing conditions.* The more homogeneous the testing conditions (e.g., same room, same time taken to collect data, same time of day), the better the reliability.
- *Level of difficulty.* The more difficult a test or data collection procedure, the lower the reliability.
- *Precision.* The more precise the measurement (1/100 or 1/1000 decimal), the better the accuracy.
- *Environment.* Environmental changes such as ambient pressure or temperature variations can decrease reliability.

The more control maintained over these factors, the better the reliability and accuracy of the resulting data. Accuracy and reliability improve the decision-making process in EBP.

Validity

To this point in the chapter, the knowledge necessary to understand the reliability and accuracy of the data collected has been provided. The fact that a test has accuracy and reliability does not mean that the test is valid, however. A valid test is defined as a test that truthfully measures what it purports to measure. Validity can be classified as either logical or statistical in nature. Logical validity requires inference and understanding of the subject being measured. Statistical validity uses statistical formulae to compare the test in question with a specific criterion or known valid measure. In EBP, validity is further delineated into three types: content-related validity, criterion-related validity, and construct-related validity. Depending on the measure, either one type or several types of validity can be used to determine if a measure is a valid one.

Content-Related Validity

Content-related validity is based on the logical thought process and interpretation of the measure. Many people refer to this quality as face or logical validity. The American Psychological Association (APA,

1985) defines content-related validity as "demonstrating the degree to which the sample of items, tasks, or questions on a test is representative of some defined content" (p. 10). A humorous restating of this concept is the cliché, "If it looks like a duck and quacks like a duck, then it must be a duck." A valid test using content-related validity should logically measure the content being reported.

Consider the pain scale example introduced earlier in this chapter. Content-related validity would assume that if it logically asks questions concerning the specific nature and degree of pain for a patient, then it must be measuring the pain of the individual. Another example arises with the stadiometer: If the stadiometer is a ruler, and a ruler measures distance, then it must logically be able to measure height. Both of these examples show the use of a logical thought process to validate the measure as a truthful representation of what the instrument reports to measure.

The fact that a test has content validity does not always mean that the test is valid. Other nuances may add error to the test and negate the test's content validity. Consider the practice of measuring of blood pressure at the arm, which is an accepted, valid method for measuring blood pressure. But what happens when the person obtaining the measurement is inexperienced or does not place the cuff in the proper position? The result will be an invalid measurement owing to the use of an improper measurement procedure. Any deviations in measurement procedures decrease the reliability of the test, thereby invalidating the data collected with the instrument.

The criteria for content-related validity can be traced back to the process used in developing the test, the interpretation of the results, and a well-defined protocol for collection of the data. In developing content-related validity, the researcher needs to be aware of extraneous factors that can affect the outcome of the test and render the test invalid. Whenever content-related validity for an instrument is relied upon, a set of strict guidelines concerning the use and collection methods of the instrument need to be in place to ensure that the validity of the instrument is not rendered useless by these factors.

Criterion-Related Validity

Criterion-related validity is based on a comparison between the test being used and some known criterion. According to the APA (1985), criterion-related validity involves "demonstrating test scores are systematically related to one or more known criteria" (p. 11). Criterion-related validity is the statistical validity identified earlier in this section. (Terms such as "statistical validity" and "correlational validity" are sometimes used as synonyms for "criterion-related validity.") The same statistical technique used to determine reliability (i.e., PPM) is used to develop a validity coefficient.

Consider the following example: measurement of oxygen saturation of arterial blood in patients. The criterion for arterial saturation would be blood gas analysis from an arterial line; however, this type of measurement brings the risk of complications and should not be used during a routine office visit. An alternative method for measuring oxygen saturation is via an infrared monitoring device that attaches to the fingertip. The infrared monitor is minimally invasive, can be used with the general population without risk, and is supposedly valid for estimating arterial oxygen saturation. To verify that the alternative method of infrared monitoring is valid, a researcher would identify a small sample of patients, subject those patients to both tests, and compare their actual blood gas results with the infrared monitoring scores. The PPM would be calculated to quantify the comparison, which would be between the alternative test to be used and the known criterion. The results would have a validity coefficient associated with the infrared monitoring model instead of a reliability coefficient. Interpretation would be done in the same manner used to interpret the reliability coefficient.

Criterion-related validity can be subdivided into concurrent validity and predictive validity, based on the time between the collection of data using the alternative method test to be validated and the criterion measurement. Concurrent validity can use the PPM statistic for validity coefficient development. With predictive validity, however, the researcher is not limited to using the PPM correlation; a linear or logistic regression can be used to develop a validity coefficient. Concurrent validity coefficients are developed simultaneously for the criterion and the alternative method test, whereas predictive validity is not limited by time.

The arterial blood oxygen saturation testing described previously is an example of concurrent validity. In this example, both criterion and alternative method measures are collected at the same time to develop the validity coefficient.

The criterion in predictive validity can be measured years after the collection of alternative method test data. Testing for the occurrence of heart disease is an example of predictive validity. A patient's total cholesterol, high-density lipoprotein (HDL) cholesterol, and low-density lipoprotein (LDL) cholesterol levels, along with other measures, are used to predict the future occurrence of atherosclerosis. Atherosclerosis—the criterion in this example—does not occur until later in life, whereas the lipid profiles, which are the alternative method test, are collected years earlier. In the predictive validity example, if a PPM correlation is used, the validity coefficient might be low because the criterion measure is a nominal value. In this case, a researcher might use logistic regression techniques to predict the probability of occurrence and develop the validity coefficient from the probability of occurrence rather than simply from the dichotomous variable (i.e., either a person does or does not have heart disease). A good point to remember is that whenever the criterion is a continuous variable, there is a better chance of having a high validity coefficient due to the possibility of improved true score variance and lower error score variance.

? Think Outside the Box

Discuss how you could make sure that each person who collects data as part of a research project does the collection in the same manner to ensure reliability of the study results.

When a dichotomous or nominal variable is used as the criterion, a researcher should expect to have a lower validity coefficient due to a decline in true score variance and an increase in error score variance. An example of this mystery is presented in **Table 11-5**.

In this example, the criterion measure of atherosclerosis is presented both as a dichotomous variable and as a probability of occurrence based on a logistic regression formula. The alternative test for the validity coefficient is the total cholesterol levels of the subjects collected when they were 40 years of age. Notice that when a continuous variable is used as the criterion in this example, the validity coefficient is 10% higher compared with use of a dichotomous

Table 11-5			
Effects of Variable Scale on Validity Coefficient			
Subject Number	Heart Disease (Yes or No)	Probability of Heart Disease	Total Cholesterol Level
1	0	40%	145
2	1	75%	200
3	1	89%	225
4	0	45%	170
5	0	30%	160
6	1	65%	195
7	0	40%	165
8	1	85%	250
9	1	88%	300
10	0	50%	180

Heart disease and total cholesterol $r = 0.777$

Probability of heart disease and total cholesterol $r = 0.879$

criterion. When using dichotomous variables as measures of validity, a researcher can expect to have lower validity coefficients than when using continuous variables. This decline in the validity coefficient reflects the lack of variability within the dichotomous measure—the lack of variability decreases the effectiveness of determining the true score of the measure. If the true score measure is decreased, then the error score measure is increased, which also affects reliability.

Many times, cross-validation techniques are used to develop a validity coefficient from a predictive validity criterion. Cross-validation simply implies that the researcher uses one group of subjects to develop the regression equation to predict the criterion and then gathers data from a second separate, but similar, group to develop the actual validity coefficient. Cross-validation techniques are generally used in developing new prediction models for a criterion.

Construct Validity

The most abstract of validity procedures is construct validity. Construct validity refers to the concept of "focusing on test scores that are associated with a psychological characteristic" (APA, 1985, p. 9). In practice, construct validity attempts to develop validity for measures that exist in theory but are unobservable.

The best example of this type of validity in EBP is the measure of pain perceived by a patient. Although we know pain exists, direct measurement of pain is somewhat convoluted and is affected by the psychological traits, tolerance levels, and perceptions of the patient. The tool most commonly used to measure pain today is the analog pain scale, which measures pain on a one-dimensional scale of 1 to 10. To develop a more precise pain scale that measures several dimensions of pain and has a high validity coefficient, constructs must be developed that can measure these traits associated with pain. Thus we can think of construct validity as the combination of content validity and statistical validity to develop a validity coefficient for an abstract variable such as pain.

To develop construct validity of a variable, the variable must first be defined as specifically as possible. The researcher would then need to identify all of the constructs associated with the variable and to define them as specifically as possible. These definitions would prove helpful in developing the measurement scales and tools to quantify the variable. In the case of the pain example, pain might be defined as the degree to which a physical symptom causes discomfort at greater than normal levels for a patient. In using this definition, the constructs associated with this variable need to be identified and defined. Notice in the definition of pain that the term "degree" is used, which assumes that some type of quantifiable scale with specific unit differences is available to quantify the intensity and severity of the variable. Also, the term "discomfort" is used in the definition, which assumes that some type of non-well-being exists. In this case, intensity is one construct, severity is another construct, and discomfort is the final construct that needs to be defined and measured.

To start the process of developing a pain scale, think about the physical pain that you have experienced previously in relation to the constructs of intensity, severity, and discomfort. If your experience with pain is limited, you might seek the help of others who have more experience with pain or investigate current publications in pain research to help you with the definition and development of these constructs. For the current example, assume the definitions for your constructs are as follows:

- Intensity is the degree of pain.
- Severity is the degree of debilitation associated with pain.
- Discomfort is the degree of the measure associated with the patient's pain tolerance.

In this example, it is assumed that these three constructs are measurable and part of the content that defines the overall construct of pain.

Once you have defined the constructs, you need to determine the type of scale that can be used to measure each one. For intensity, you might decide to use a scale of 0 to 10, where 0 is defined as the absence of pain and 10 is defined as the most excruciating pain imaginable. For severity, you might have to develop a scale using terms that reflect a decline in functional capacity associated with debilitation. For discomfort, you might use a scale that reflects the type of pain, such as sharp, dull, or throbbing.

After developing the scales for the constructs that are included in the measurement of pain, you must determine how each scale should be weighted to reflect the absolute construct of pain. Again, you might want to rely on personal experience when developing your construct weights; alternatively, you might wish to seek expert opinions or explore previous research to help in developing your weighting system.

When you have accomplished this last step, you have a measure that logically measures pain (content validity). You are ready to test the merits of the measure by applying it to comparable groups to determine the statistical validity of the measure. In using statistical validation measures, you are attempting to prove the following hypothesis: Those individuals with diseases that are not associated with pain should score low on the pain scale, and those individuals with diseases or disorders associated with a high level of pain should score high on the new pain scale. By combining the logical validation of the pain scale with the statistical interpretation of the pain scale, you have developed construct validity for a measure of pain. As you become more comfortable with the process of developing construct validity for abstract or unobservable measures, you will find that the greater the number of definable constructs, the greater the validity gained by the measure.

Conclusion

This chapter focused on two key principles of research: reliability and validity. Whereas reliability and relevance can exist independently of each other, validity cannot exist without the presence of both reliability and relevance.

The two basic statistical techniques used to determine reliability and validity are the PPM correlation and the ANOVA test. As with most techniques, the selection of which to use is based on the number of variables being compared. When there are only two variables, a researcher would use PPM; when more than two variables are being compared, the ANOVA technique would be used. Both techniques generate a coefficient between an absolute value of 0 and 1.0, and the presence of a coefficient greater than 1.0 signifies an error in the calculations.

The interpretation of the coefficient is the only change that should occur regardless of the technique used. In the case of reliability, the coefficient can be used to interpret the consistency, stability, equivalency, or objectivity of the measure depending on which aspects were used to determine the estimate. A researcher can also use the reliability coefficient in conjunction with the standard deviation of the sample to determine the accuracy of the measure using the SEM equation. With reliability and accuracy determined, a nurse can be sure that comparable measures are similar and can be interpreted as consistent, stable, equivalent, or objective within a defined range of error. In the case of validity, these techniques can be used to develop a validity coefficient for concurrent validity or predictive validity based on the time between the collection using the alternative method test, or a validity coefficient for construct validity to improve the interpretation of the measure beyond simple content validation.

Summary Points

1. Trustworthiness of study data is only as good as the instruments or tests used to collect the data.
2. Reliability and validity are the most important concepts in the decision-making process when designing research studies.

3. Reliability is the determination that an instrument consistently measures the same thing.
4. Validity is the determination that an instrument measures what it is supposed to measure.
5. Validity cannot exist without reliability and relevance.
6. Reliability and relevance can exist independently of validity.
7. The correlation coefficient is the degree (positive or negative) of the relationship between the variables.
8. Interclass reliability is the consistency between two measures that are presented in the data as either variables or trials.
9. The three types of interclass reliability are consistency, equivalency, and internal consistency.
10. Intraclass reliability allows for the development of a reliability coefficient for more than two variables.
11. Within intraclass reliability, objectivity and accuracy need to be considered.
12. The three types of validity are content-related validity, criterion-related validity, and construct-related validity.
13. Content-related validity is the level at which a sample of items, tasks, or questions represent the defined content.
14. Criterion-related validity reflects the demonstration that test scores are systematically related to one or more identified measures.
15. Criterion-related validity is subdivided into concurrent validity and predictive validity.
16. Construct-related validity concentrates on the test scores that are associated with a psychological characteristic.

RED FLAGS

- If reliability and validity are missing from the data, an informed decision concerning the trustworthiness of the results of a research study cannot be made.
- If validity is documented in a study without any indication of reliability and relevance, concerns about the trustworthiness of the results should be raised.
- If a tool is documented as being used within a study, the report should provide information concerning the validity and reliability indices for the tool.

Multiple Choice Questions

1. When making good decisions in evidence-based practice, _____ of the data is necessary.

   A. confirmability
   B. trustworthiness
   C. independence
   D. timing

2. Reliability is defined as the case in which an instrument

   A. Consistently measures the same thing.
   B. Measures what it is supposed to measure.
   C. Measures demographic data.
   D. Consistently measures the same sample.

3. Reliability and relevance may exist

   A. With dependence on validity.
   B. With only independence of validity.
   C. Independently of validity.
   D. None of the above.

4. A valid test will _____ have some degree of reliability and relevance.

   A. never
   B. sometimes
   C. frequently
   D. always

5. When measuring blood pressure, the actual score is the

   A. Observed score on the instrument.
   B. Estimated score determined by the nurse.
   C. Perfect score without error.
   D. First sound heard by the nurse.

6. Reliability coefficients greater than _____ are considered to be high.

   A. 0.50
   B. 0.60
   C. 0.70
   D. 0.80

7. As an example of consistency and stability in EBP, when a urinalysis is done four times in a 24-hour period, the urine sample needs to be the _____ amount.

   A. correct
   B. same
   C. smallest
   D. largest

8. Dividing scores on a pain questionnaire (with 0–5 items) into odd-numbered and even-numbered scores is a mechanism that can be used to determine

   A. External consistency.
   B. Relevance.
   C. Internal consistency.
   D. Validity.

9. A research study was developed to consider the assessment of skin color. Nurses on a medical–surgical unit were asked to record their judgments of the skin color from four pictures of individuals with differing skin tones. This process is an example of which area of reliability measurement?

   A. Accuracy
   B. Objectivity
   C. Feasibility
   D. Equivalency

10. Which test is used to establish the measurement of the accuracy related to reliability?

    A. ANOVA
    B. Standard error of measure (SEM)
    C. Pearson Product Moment (PPM) correlation
    D. Reliability coefficient

11. To establish a test as an accurate measurement of reliability, the test scores need a relatively _____ standard deviation and a _____ reliability coefficient.

    A. high; high
    B. low; low
    C. low; high
    D. high; low

12. Factors that can affect the reliability, objectivity, and accuracy of a tool or test include

    A. Practice, timing, and environment.
    B. Fatigue, subjects, and environment.
    C. Precision, homogeneity of the test conditions, and the researcher.
    D. Sequencing, practice, and level of ease.

13. Validity can be classified as

    A. Universal.
    B. Concise.
    C. General.
    D. Logical.

14. A criterion for content-related validity determination is

    A. The inclusion of extraneous variables.

    B. Establishment of brief guidelines for using the tool.

    C. A well-defined protocol for data collection.

    D. The clarification of nuances that might add errors.

15. A researcher was comparing alternative methods for establishing a child's core body temperature for a study. The testing included the measurement of anal, oral, and aural temperatures. This example reflects which type of validity determination?

    A. Construct-related validity

    B. Criterion-related validity

    C. Content-related validity

    D. Predictive validity

16. A study presented the results from the development of a new tool. This tool was established to measure the level of anxiety perceived by children. Which type of validity would this study need to document for the tool?

    A. Content-related validity

    B. Criterion-related validity

    C. Construct-related validity

    D. Concurrent validity

Discussion Questions

Use the following data to answer questions 1–4.

Patient #	Oral Temperature (°F)	Temperature (°F)
1	98.6	98.7
2	99.4	99.3
3	101.2	101.3
4	98.6	98.6
5	100.5	100.7
6	99.7	99.4
7	101.0	101.1
8	98.4	98.6
9	102.9	102.5
10	103.1	102.9

Patient #	Oral Temperature (°F)	Tympanic Temperature (°F)
1	98.6	98.7
2	99.4	99.3
3	101.2	101.3
4	98.6	98.6
5	100.5	100.7
6	99.7	99.4
7	101.0	101.1
8	98.4	98.6
9	102.9	102.5
10	103.1	102.9

1. Is tympanic temperature a similar measure of temperature?

2. Which type of reliability coefficient have you developed with these data?

3. What is the accuracy of tympanic temperature?

4. Is tympanic temperature a valid measure of patient temperature based on the information provided in the second table?

5. Using the example of the pain scale provided on page 284, define and develop five additional constructs that might be used to measure pain.

Suggested Readings

Baumgartner, T., & Jackson, A. J. (1999). *Measurement for evaluation in physical education and exercise science* (6th ed.). Dubuque, IA: McGraw-Hill.

Cunningham, G. K. (1986). *Educational and psychological measurement.* New York: Macmillan.

Glass, G. V., & Hopkins, K. D. (1996). *Statistical methods in education and psychology* (3rd ed.). Englewood Cliffs, NJ: Prentice Hall.

Golafshani, N. (2003). Understanding reliability and validity in qualitative research. *Qualitative Report, 8*(4), 597–607.

Morrow, J. R., Jackson, A. W., Disch, J. G., & Mood, D. P. (2000). *Measurement and evaluation in human performance* (2nd ed.). Champaign, IL: Human Kinetics.

Thomas, J., & Nelson, J. (2005). *Research methods in physical activity* (5th ed.). Champaign, IL: Human Kinetics.

Reference

American Psychological Association (APA). (1985). *Standards for educational and psychological testing.* Washington, DC: Author.

Chapter 12

Data Analysis

James Eldridge

Chapter Objectives

At the conclusion of this chapter, the learner will be able to

1. Identify the types of statistics available for analyses in evidence-based practice
2. Define quantitative analysis and qualitative analysis
3. Discuss how research questions define the type of statistics to be used in evidence-based practice research
4. Choose a data analysis plan and the proper statistics for different research questions raised in evidence-based practice
5. Interpret data analyses and conclusions from the data analyses

Key Terms

- ➤ Analysis of variance (ANOVA)
- ➤ Central tendency
- ➤ Chi-square
- ➤ Interval scale
- ➤ Mean
- ➤ Median
- ➤ Mode
- ➤ Nominal scale

➤ Ordinal scale

➤ Pearson chi-square

➤ Qualitative analysis

➤ Quantitative analysis

➤ Ratio scale

➤ Statistical Package for the Social Sciences (SPSS)

➤ *t*-test

Introduction

So far in this text, the authors have methodically explained how to move from the formulation of the hypothesis to the data collection stage of a research project. Data collection in evidence-based practice (EBP) might be considered the easiest part of the whole research experience. The researcher has already formed the hypothesis, developed the data collection methods and instruments, and determined the subject pool characteristics.

Once the EBP researcher has completed data collection, it is time for the researcher to compile and interpret the data so as to explain them in a meaningful context. This compilation and interpretation phase is completed using either quantitative data analysis or qualitative data analysis techniques. Quantitative analysis is defined as the numeric representation and manipulation of observations using statistical techniques for the express purpose of describing and explaining the outcomes of research as they pertain to the hypothesis. In other words, quantitative analysis uses numerical values to explain the outcomes of a research project. In contrast, qualitative analysis techniques use logical deductions to decipher gathered data dealing with the human element and do not rely on numerical values or mathematical models to explain the results. In other words, qualitative analysis uses words and phrases to explain the outcomes of a research project.

An example of the contrast between these two types of analyses would be a research project involving the study of a specific treatment for the reduction of back pain. To determine if the treatment was effective, data would be collected so as to compare two groups of individuals with back pain: One group would receive the treatment, while the other group would not receive the treatment. Using an analog pain scale, the researcher would collect numerical data to determine if differences were apparent between the treatment group and the no-treatment group. This would be a form of quantitative analysis. Using the same group of subjects, the researcher could also observe the patients' movement characteristics, attitude, and facial expressions during both pre-treatment and post-treatment phases and have the patients chronicle their improvement through the use of a written journal. This process would be a form of qualitative analysis.

In the example using quantitative analysis techniques, the researcher could report significant differences between the end treatment values of the treatment and no-treatment groups—for example, there was a significant difference between the mean post-treatment pain indices values of the treatment group and those of the no-treatment group. In the qualitative analysis example, the researcher would state the results in a different way—for example, the treatment group exhibited a greater range of motion while walking and sitting, with an observed decline in facial wincing; furthermore, the patients had a better attitude and were less likely to snipe at the nurse while undergoing the post-test procedures.

Notice that in the qualitative analysis example, no mention of statistical differences is made; only a description of the observed differences and changes is included. The only time a researcher can report a significant difference is when he or she has used quantitative analysis techniques to interpret the data. In this chapter, the learner will discover when and how to use these two techniques in the reporting and explanation of a project's results.

Quantitative Analysis

Measurement Scales

As described previously, quantitative analysis requires the use of numeric data to describe and interpret the results. It is often referred to as statistical analysis; in reality, however, statistical analysis is a subunit of quantitative analyses. Before a researcher can understand the nuances of quantitative analysis, he or she must first understand the types of numeric data that are available for analysis. Numeric data are classified into four measurement scales: (1) nominal, (2) ordinal, (3) interval, and (4) ratio. These four scales are listed here in hierarchical order, with the nominal scale being the least precise measurement scale and the ratio scale being the most precise measurement scale in describing results.

The nominal scale is the simplest of the measurement scales, because it is used for identification or categorization purposes only. This level of measurement lacks numeric order, magnitude, or size. Examples of nominal scales include race, gender, and patient identification number. A scale for race might collect data in the following way: Anglo equals 1, African American equals 2, Hispanic equals 3, and other race equals 4. In this scale, the number assigned to each race is indicative of group identification only, with no other assumption of magnitude, order, or size. The reason that we use the numerical scale rather than the word terms for race is because most statistical analysis packages have a difficult time interpreting word terms, especially when capitalization and misspellings occur.

The second measurement scale in the hierarchy is the ordinal scale. This scale is more precise in measuring items as compared to the nominal scale. It incorporates order or ranking, yet lacks magnitude and size. A researcher using an ordinal scale is unable to make direct comparisons between ranks, because he or she does not know whether the difference between a ranking of 1 and 2 is very small or very large. The only known aspect is that a ranking of 1 is greater or better than a ranking of 2. A medical example of an ordinal scale is the transplant recipient list for a donor heart. A transplant recipient is given a number that identifies his or her order on the list based on symptoms, severity, cross-matching/typing, and time of request. When a donor heart becomes available, the person ranked highest on the list who meets the criteria of proper cross-matching/typing, being symptomatic, with the highest level of illness severity, and the longest time on the donor list receives the heart. Potentially, two patients with the same symptoms, severity, and cross-matching/typing might be separated in the order only by the time (sometimes a few seconds) at which they were placed on the list. Thus the different aspects have no magnitude or set units of measure between each numeric value. This example illustrates how an ordinal scale represents order but lacks magnitude and size. For both nominal and ordinal scales, mathematical calculations have no meaning, because the scales are unable to represent the magnitude and size of the variable.

The final two scales of measurement in the hierarchy are considered continuous scales, because each incorporates both order and magnitude within its description. Continuous scales allow for mathematical calculations so as to give the results meaning. Researchers can truly describe significant differences because each number in the scale represents a unique place of order within the scale, and there is equal distance between it and the number directly above and below it in the order.

? Think Outside the Box

Compare and contrast quantitative versus qualitative research techniques for analyses.

The third scale of measurement is the interval scale. This scale is more precise than the nominal and ordinal scales because it incorporates both order and magnitude within the description; at the same time, it lacks a defined size or, for want of a better term, an "absolute" zero point. An example of the interval scale is the Fahrenheit temperature scale. The degrees in the Fahrenheit scale are ordered from high to low. Each degree within the scale has an equal distance from the next degree; however, the point taken as zero in the scale is arbitrary. Using the term "arbitrary zero" in a scale means that the zero point is not defining a complete lack of quantity, but rather just serves as a starting point for the measurement. In the Fahrenheit scale, the point chosen as zero is arbitrary, because you can actually have a score that is below zero. This same consideration also applies when using the Celsius scale for temperature.

The final and most precise scale in the hierarchy is the ratio scale. This scale combines the attributes of the interval scale with the addition of an absolute zero point. The best example of a ratio scale is weight, whether measured in pounds or kilograms. The weight scale has order: 1 pound weighs less than 2 pounds. It has magnitude, and the difference between 1 pound and 2 pounds is the same as the difference between 2 pounds and 3 pounds. Finally, it has an absolute zero point, in that 0 pounds means there is a complete absence of weight.

This section of the chapter has opened with the description of the measurement scales because the measurement scale used determines the type of statistic analysis performed. It is important to understand that the more precise a scale, the more stable the statistic used to calculate the outcome implies. Consider the measure of pain discussed earlier in this chapter. When determining pain, a physician might use a nominal pain scale that implies only the absence or presence of pain (1 = pain, 0 = no pain), or a physician could use the ratio analog pain scale that implies degrees of pain. If the physician used a nominal scale, no differences between the groups (treatment versus no treatment) could be identified, because all of the patients in both groups still exhibited pain at the end of the study. In the analog pain example, however, the physician used a ratio scale so that the degree of pain could be measured. Although none of the patients completely lacked pain, it is clear that the group receiving the treatment had a lower degree of pain at the end of the study when compared with the no-treatment group. Remember, precision not only adds reliability and validity to the study, but it also enhances the statistical power and enthusiasm of the results.

Descriptive Statistics: Nominal and Ordinal Data

The first step and lowest order of any quantitative analysis is the description of the data in numeric terms. As described earlier, the measurement scale used for each item on an instrument determines

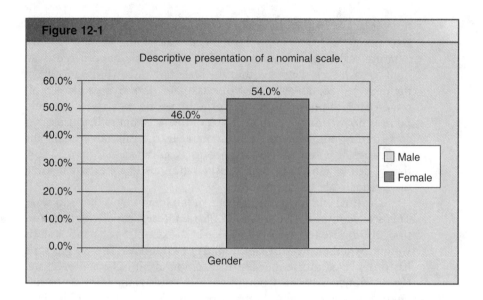

Figure 12-1

Descriptive presentation of a nominal scale.

how the data are presented in a descriptive form. Reporting of data for instrument items that use a nominal or ordinal scale usually takes the form of frequencies or percentages of the response for the item. For example, demographic data for a sample might be reported using variables such as gender, race, marital status, or educational status. Data of this type are presented in the form of percentages, such as the percentage of males and females in the sample (**Figure 12-1**).

Novice researchers often make the mistake of reporting nominal or ordinal data in the form of means; this is absolutely incorrect. Because nominal and ordinal data have no magnitude or size, measures of central tendency such as a mean and standard deviation are meaningless with these data.

Interval and Ratio Data

Central Tendency
What is central tendency? Central tendency is a way to allow the researcher to show the audience how the scores are distributed around a central point. Central tendencies are described in three ways: the mean, the median, and the mode.

The mean, or average, of a set of scores is determined by the sum of the scores divided by the total number of scores. Consider the example of taking a patient's systolic blood pressure five times. The systolic scores are 125, 130, 122, 128, and 130 mm Hg. Notice that these scores are ratio scale data, because there is an absolute zero point (meaning no pressure or the absence of any pressure might be

---

Figure 12-2

Mathematical representation of the mean.

$$\text{Mean} = \frac{\sum x}{n}: \text{where } X \text{ is the observed score and } n \text{ is the number of scores}$$

$$= \frac{\sum 125, 130, 122, 128, \text{ and } 130}{5}$$

$$= \frac{635}{5}$$

$$= 127$$

---

measured). The calculation of the mean of these scores is shown in **Figure 12-2**.

The average (mean) for the systolic pressure scores is 127 mm Hg. Notice that 127 mm Hg does not appear in the set of original scores. Rarely does the mean actually equal one of the scores in the observed list; rather, it represents a best estimate of the central point of all the measured scores. As discussed in Chapter 11, measurement error is inherent in all instruments. The mean allows a researcher to develop a central point within the data, incorporating the error within the measure. The process and rationale for doing so are explained in more detail in the discussion of the standard deviation that appears later in this chapter.

The median is the second measure of central tendency. The median is the middle score of a set of data. It represents the 50th percentile; thus it allows the researcher to show the exact point at which half of the scores fall above the median and half of the scores fall below the median. In the previous systolic pressure example, the median of the scores 125, 130, 122, 128, and 130 is 128 mm Hg. Notice that in these readings, the score of 128 is the second to the last score. If the median is the middle number, then how can 128 be the median score? A specific point needs to be made when determining the median. The data should always be ordered from lowest to highest when determining the median. In this case, the data for systolic pressure should be ordered as follows: 122, 125, 128, 130, and 130.

The final measure of central tendency is the mode. The mode is the most frequently observed score within a variable's data. In the previous example, the systolic pressure of 130 mm Hg is the mode of the data because it occurs twice, while all other scores appear only once. Whereas the mean is the most stable measure of central tendency (meaning it represents the absolute possible middle score), the mode is the least stable measure of central tendency (meaning it represents only the most frequently occurring score). As a researcher increases the number of observations within a variable, the chances are that the mean, median, and mode will be more representative or equal to each other.

Variability

A second issue when describing interval and ratio data is the variability of the data. Variability describes how the data vary between each score and also from the mean. There are two types of variability that the EBP research might report: the range of the data and the variance or standard deviation of the data.

The range of the data is calculated by subtracting the lowest score for the variable from the highest score for the variable. In the previous example involving systolic blood pressures, the range of the data is 130–122 mm Hg, or 8 mm Hg. This calculation simply means that the highest score and lowest score vary by only 8 mm Hg. When reporting this range, the reader can infer that because the mean of the data was 127 mm Hg and the range was 8 mm Hg, then the scores ranged from 123 to 131. In such a case, the reader of the report must assume that the variability was uniform. This rating reflects that the scores varied from the mean evenly: In other words, the upper scores varied 4 mm Hg from the mean, and the lower scores varied 4 mm Hg from the mean. With the aforementioned assumption, the reader infers some error, because the actual scores ranged from 122 to 130 mm Hg. When reporting the range of 8 mm Hg and the mean of 127 mm Hg, however, the range was 123 to 131 mm Hg.

One other point to remember is that the range is unstable if the data being used include numerous outliers, either above the mean or below the mean. For example, in the systolic pressure example, assume that the data were 125, 130, 122, 128, and 160 mm Hg. The mean for these data is 133 mm Hg (approximately 6 mm Hg higher than the mean found in the first example), and the range is 38 mm Hg. Notice that the inclusion of a single high value increased the range by 30 mm Hg. Also notice that when interpreting the data, the reader would assume falsely that with a mean of 133 mm Hg, the data would range from 114 to 152 mm Hg. In this case, the description of the data is lacking, because the outlier of 160 mm Hg negatively affects the description.

The second measure of variability in describing data is the standard deviation, which is the square root of variance. Variance is the measure of the spread of scores around the mean based on the squared deviations of the observed scores from the mean of the data. The concept of a standard deviation allows a researcher to develop a description of the scores' variability from the mean based on a normal distribution. The standard deviation, which can be determined using

---

Figure 12-3

Mathematical representation of standard deviation.

$$\sqrt{\frac{\sum x^2 - \frac{(\sum x)^2}{n}}{n-1}}$$ where X is the observed score and n is the number of scores

---

the formula in **Figure 12-3**, provides the ability to describe the data based on a normal distribution and the percentage of the normal distribution expected to occur between each standard deviation unit.

As shown in **Figure 12-4**, the researcher can more fully describe the pattern of the data by using both the mean and the standard deviation. The standard deviation can be interpreted as meaning that the reader of the data can expect 68.26% of the observed scores to fall plus or minus one standard deviation from the mean. Conversely, the reader can expect less than two-tenths of 1% of the scores to fall plus or minus one standard deviation from the mean. In presenting both the mean and the standard deviation, a researcher describes the data in terms of a normal distribution, allowing the reader of the results to get a mental picture of how the scores compare to the normal distribution.

Consider the systolic pressure example once again. With scores of 122, 125, 128, 130, and 130 mm Hg, the mean is 127 mm Hg, with a standard deviation of 3.46 mm Hg. When data are presented in this form, the reader can visualize that 68.26% of the scores fell between 123.54 and 130.46 mm Hg. The reader can also determine from the mean and the standard deviation that less than 0.26% of the scores were less than 116.62 mm Hg or greater than 137.38 mm Hg. In looking at the data described in this manner, the reader begins to understand that most of the scores from this sample were within the normal range for systolic blood pressure.

❓ Think Outside the Box

Discuss how statistics can be used in your evidence-based practice.

This type of analytical presentation emphasizes the verbal descriptions that are made when describing the sample demographics ("The sample when beginning the study had normal systolic blood pressures"). Some people might shy away from reporting the mean and the standard deviation in their research reports because of math phobia. This fear is unwarranted, because most statistical software

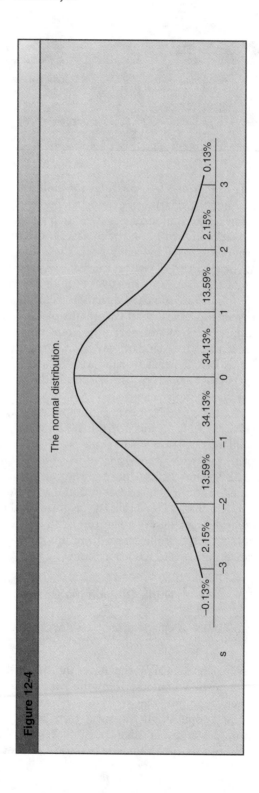

Figure 12-4

The normal distribution.

Table 12-1	
Hemoglobin Scores	
Patient ID	**Hemoglobin**
1	14.10
2	12.20
3	11.90
4	14.50
5	13.80
6	13.20
7	13.50
8	14.00
9	11.10
10	9.60

packages make the process of computing these values very simple. In the current world of research, most researchers utilize a statistic software package, such as the Statistical Package for the Social Sciences (SPSS), to complete all of the calculations for the data collected.

From this point forward in this text, all data analysis is described to the student. To finish the lesson on the mean and standard deviation, the student is asked to determine the mean and standard deviation of a set of scores for hemoglobin content (**Table 12-1**). In this example, all of the scores would need to be totaled and divided by 10.

Inferential Statistics

Once a researcher has described the study subjects through descriptive analysis, it is time to quantitatively analyze and present the data for the results. To accomplish this task, a researcher must understand not only the scales of measurement, but also the type of variable. Research design typically includes two types of variables—the dependent variable and the independent variable. The dependent variable is the criterion that determines the entire purpose of the research. The independent variable is the variable that affects the change in, or is related to, the dependent variable. A dependent variable can be categorized as the outcome variable or the effect variable, while the independent variable is categorized as the manipulated variable or the cause variable. **Table 12-2** lists other differences between the dependent and independent variable.

An example of a statement using an independent variable and a dependent variable would involve a researcher attempting to determine if there is a difference between use of a statin drug and use of

---

Table 12-2

Differences Between Dependent and Independent Variables

Independent Variable	Dependent Variable
Cause	Effect
Manipulated	The consequence
Measured	Outcome
Predicted to	Predicted from
Predictor	Criterion
x	y

Table 12-3

Statistical Choice for Measurement Scales of Dependent and Independent Variables

Independent Variable	Dependent Variable	Statistical Test
1 nominal	1 nominal	Chi-square
1 nominal (2 groups)	1 continuous	t-test
1 nominal (2 groups)	1 continuous	One-way ANOVA
2 nominal	1 continuous	Two-way ANOVA

ANOVA = analysis of variance.

---

niacin alone in reducing cholesterol level. The dependent variable in this case is cholesterol level (the outcome measured in mg/dL); the independent variable is the type of treatment (statin or niacin). Determining which variable is the dependent variable and which is the independent variable is only the first step in identifying the statistic to use for data analysis, however. The second step is to determine the scale of measurement for both the dependent variable and the independent variable. The scale of measurement for each of these variables then determines the proper statistic for analysis of the data. General guidelines for choosing the proper statistic based on the measurement scale of the dependent and independent variables are presented in **Table 12-3**.

Chi-Square

Whenever the dependent variable is scaled nominally, the chi-square statistic is typically used for its analysis. The chi-square (χ^2) value suggests whether an association exists between nominally scaled variables.

An example of a research design that warrants a chi-square analysis would be the case in which a researcher wants to know if there are differences between men and women in undergoing annual checkups (yes or no). The dependent variable for these data is whether the person underwent an annual checkup, while the independent variable is gender. With the use of a statistical software package, the chi-square value could be calculated quite easily. Once the calculation is completed, the determination of any difference between men and women in terms of whether they underwent an annual checkup could be made by reviewing the Pearson chi-square statistic and the significance of the test. Generally, most research studies seek to find statistical differences at the $p < 0.05$ level. Anything greater than 0.05 is considered not significant.

This is an appropriate time to point out that in data analysis, the results are either significant or not significant. The p value does not impose magnitude. Therefore, even if the results have a significance of 0.0001, this finding does not mean that the results are "extremely" significant—just that they are significant.

t-Test

Now that we have described the analysis of a nominally scaled dependent variable, it is time to learn how to determine which test to use for a continuous scaled dependent variable. Review Figure 12-3 to refresh your memory. The number of nominal variables and levels within the nominal variables for the independent variable determines which statistic (t-test or analysis of variance [ANOVA]) should be used. If the independent variable has one nominal variable with two groups (e.g., gender), the researcher would use a t-test to determine statistical differences between the groups.

Two types of t-tests can be calculated—the independent t-test and the dependent t-test. An independent t-test is used when a single continuous dependent variable is being compared, while a dependent t-test allows a researcher to compare two continuous variables as long as the variables are related.

An example of a dependent t-test would be a comparison of the pre-treatment and post-treatment cholesterol levels of a group of individuals receiving a statin drug as single-agent therapy. Interpretation of the t-test statistic is the same for both variables; the nuance relates to the number of dependent variables and whether they are related.

The independent t-test statistic determines if a difference is present in a single dependent variable between the two groups. An example of a research design that warrants a t-test analysis would be a researcher who wants to know if there are differences between men and women in terms of their hemoglobin content. The dependent

Table 12-4		
Quantitative Analysis: Data for *t*-Test Analysis		
Patient ID	**Gender**	**Hemoglobin**
1	Male	14.10
2	Female	12.20
3	Male	11.90
4	Female	14.50
5	Female	13.80
6	Female	13.20
7	Male	13.50
8	Male	14.00
9	Male	11.10
10	Female	9.60

variable for these data is hemoglobin content, which is a ratio-scaled continuous variable; the independent variable is gender. Data are provided in **Table 12-4** to assist in determining the answer to this question.

Once the results are input and statistics are calculated using a statistical software package, the determination of the difference between men and women in hemoglobin levels could be identified by assessing the significance of the test. Again, remember that most research studies seek to find statistical differences at the $p > 0.05$ level.

? Think Outside the Box

Describe the different numerical values used in the clinical setting. Discuss which level of measurements each of those types of values represent (i.e., blood pressure readings, fasting blood sugars, weights). Differentiate among the different measurement scales that you use on a daily basis. Does this understanding change the way you think about the values that you use when delivering care?

ANOVA

The final statistical analysis to be discussed for interpreting data is the analysis of variance (ANOVA). As described previously in the t-test section, the number of nominal variables and levels within the nominal variables for the independent variable determine which statistic (t-test or ANOVA) should be used. If the independent variable has one nominal variable with more than two groups (e.g., race), an ANOVA test would be used to determine statistical differences.

Two types of ANOVA can be calculated—the one-way ANOVA and the two-way ANOVA. The one-way ANOVA is used when a research study is comparing a single nominal independent variable. The two-way ANOVA allows the researcher to compare two nominal independent variables. An example of a two-way ANOVA would involve comparing men and women (one independent variable) by trial (pre-treatment versus post-treatment; the second independent variable) in terms of their cholesterol levels. This example would be considered a 2 × 2 design, which is used in many clinical trials.

Interpretation of the ANOVA statistic is the same for both variables; the nuance relates to the number of independent variables. The one-way ANOVA statistic determines whether a difference is present in a single dependent variable among the several groups within a single independent variable.

An example of a research design that warrants an ANOVA analysis would be a researcher who wants to know if there are differences among people of various ethnicities in terms of their hemoglobin content. The dependent variable for these data is hemoglobin content, which is a ratio-scaled continuous variable, while the independent variable is race (White, African American, or Hispanic). Data are provided in **Table 12-5** to assist in answering this question. Notice that in the data entry for race, the variables are dummy coded (1 = White, 2 = Hispanic, and 3 = African American). These are treated as nominal scale variables.

To determine if there is a difference among people of these races in terms of their hemoglobin levels, the significance of the test would need to be calculated using a statistical software package. Again, remember that most research studies seek to find statistical differences at the $p > 0.05$ level.

A final note about ANOVA techniques: When completing either a one-way ANOVA or a two-way ANOVA, the statistical program will require the ANOVA to be defined as a one-tailed or two-tailed test. This simply means that the researcher must determine whether the differences among the data are expected to occur in a single direction on the normal curve or in both directions on the normal curve. A single-tailed test suggests that the expected differences for all groups will occur in a single direction, either above the mean (an increase) or below the mean (decrease). A two-tailed test assumes that group differences are expected to change in a bidirectional manner, where one group may have a decrease from the mean while another group may have an increase from the mean. An example of a single-tailed test would be the measurement of body temperature with the onset of a disease. The researcher might expect that body temperature will increase from the normal temperature of 98.6°F only with the onset of a disease, so the ANOVA in this study will be a single-tailed test.

Table 12-5		
ANOVA Model		
Patient ID	Race	Hemoglobin
212	1	8.119
172	2	16.029
183	2	14.569
152	2	17.624
153	2	15.242
154	2	19.942
182	2	16.111
186	2	14.230
213	3	16.951
237	1	12.400
105	1	12.350
106	1	12.106
107	1	11.811
149	1	12.972
150	1	13.930
151	1	12.038
181	2	13.703
227	2	16.433
228	2	13.446
128	2	14.953
129	2	12.624
130	2	13.169
142	2	14.987
159	2	12.596
170	3	15.996
171	3	11.476
179	1	11.233
187	1	12.253
222	1	14.090
173	1	14.060

An example of a two-tailed test would be the measurement of body weight among a dieting group and a control group. The researcher might expect that body weight will decrease in the dieting group, whereas it will increase with the control group, so the ANOVA will be a two-tailed test.

Reporting the Results of Quantitative Analysis

The final step in the quantitative analysis of data is disseminating the results in an intelligible form. Put simply, a researcher must thoroughly describe the sample using the descriptive analysis techniques. Once the sample is described, each inferential statistic needs to be described within the results. The a priori probability value (usually

$p > 0.05$) must be stated. Finally, the statistical tests need to be reported, including what their probability is and whether these results are significant. These analyses allow a researcher to develop the discussion by comparing the results of the study with the findings from other research and inferring whether these results have substantial implications for practice.

Qualitative Analysis

The second major form of analysis that an EBP researcher may perform is a qualitative analysis. As described previously, qualitative analysis incorporates observation and language to develop an in-depth description of the results. Where quantitative analysis describes results and outcomes based on numeric data, inferential statistics, and sample size, qualitative analysis relies on the observational method of the researchers and their ability to describe the in-depth intricacies of the observations to explain outcomes and develop theories for the research. The final outcome of most qualitative analyses is not based on significant differences from the numeric data, but rather consists of a refined conceptual framework of the research that is improved through logical reasoning.

Another way to think about the difference between quantitative and qualitative analysis is to frame it in the terms of the reasoning process. Quantitative analysis uses the deductive reasoning process— that is, a top-down method of analysis. With this approach, the researcher begins with a theory on a topic, then narrows the scope to one or more hypotheses, and finally hones in on conformational results collected from a specific sample. In contrast, qualitative analysis most times uses the inductive reasoning process—a bottom-up analysis that goes in the opposite direction of the deductive process. With this approach, the researcher starts with observations of a specific pattern and, from those observations, develops hypotheses and theories. Once these theories are developed, then the quantitative method can be used to test those theories and generalize the results to a population. Many times, the final outcome of a qualitative analysis is not a set of specific results, but rather a set of specific questions or hypotheses in need of quantitative analysis.

Two types of qualitative analysis apply to the EBP practitioner— the case study and the program evaluation. Each of these types of analysis occurs at some time during a nurse's professional practice. Each has both commonalities and distinct characteristics that are based in the foundation of observation. The major skills that all EBP researchers must possess to ensure well-derived products from qualitative analyses are good language skills and keen observational techniques.

Notice that observation is the key element in all qualitative analyses. As a result, most qualitative research plans focus on small groups of individuals to develop the conceptual framework that encompasses the final deductions, unlike quantitative analyses that use large samples to derive the results. Also, comparison data are minimal, because qualitative analysis, although not restrained by the assessment of significant differences, lacks the distinct comparable traits that are inherent in the use of quantitative analysis.

The Case Study

The case study is the most commonly practiced type of qualitative analysis occurring in EBP research. Case studies are individualized and personal. Many of the case studies gleaned from EBP eventually lead to larger quantitative analysis trials. In developing a case study, the researcher's initial response is to assume that all aspects of the case are important and to take a broad overview of the topic in an attempt to explain the outcomes.

In any qualitative analysis, focus on the conceptual framework determines the success or failure of the end product. The conceptual framework explains the dimensions of the study, the key factors, the variables, and the relationship among different variables. The EBP researcher must focus on and define the conceptual framework prior to implementing a case study. Effective preparation and focus can help eliminate unnecessary observations and shorten the time for completion of the study.

To develop a conceptual framework for a case study, or any other qualitative analysis, the EBP nurse must be well versed in the area of study and thoroughly familiar with research previously conducted on the topic (i.e., the literature). The conceptual framework many times starts as a new observation that piques the curiosity of a researcher. In the process of becoming interested, the researcher begins to focus his or her observations, collecting data through a written journal or diary of the observations, and then attempts to develop a coherent framework that explains the novel observations. In nursing practice, patient files may be reviewed and described to develop the conceptual framework for the analysis.

Once a conceptual framework sets the boundaries of the analysis, the research questions must be developed. This is done in the same manner as in any research—through review of the literature and comparison of the case with the previous findings of other research. Case studies, like program evaluations, must be described in depth to improve the impact of their findings. A lack of depth in such descriptions may lead subsequent reviewers of the research to discard it as being poorly substantiated.

Once the conceptual framework is completed and the research questions are defined, it is time to develop the means to explain the observations in the context of the questions. A researcher should focus and include only those material observations that are relevant. Inclusion of minutiae and irrelevant observations in the report of a study tend to detract from the impact of the overall analysis. The relevant findings should be described in detail and previous research should be used, when available, to help derive the conclusions. The end product of the effective completion of this process is often the identification of questions needing further study.

The Program Evaluation

The program evaluation is another method of qualitative analysis that the EBP researcher may use to evaluate a specific program rather than an individual case. Program evaluation allows the EBP researcher to observe the workings of a specific program, rather than a single case, and develop explanations for the success or failure of the program.

Like the case study, the program evaluation needs a well-defined conceptual framework through which to judge success or failure. Many times the program evaluator will ask the program participants to complete a self-study exercise listing the items that each participant perceives as important to the successful implementation of the program. The evaluator will then review the self-study and compare it with previously successful programs that incorporated the same conceptual framework. The researcher may also review characteristics of the site where the program implementation occurs to determine if site-specific barriers are present that might potentially hamper the successful implementation of the program.

The end product of a program evaluation should include well-defined areas of success within the program and identification of all observed barriers in the program that might increase the likelihood of failure. The final product of a program evaluation should include well-founded conclusions that will improve the likelihood of successful implementation of the program. Many times the end product will either help strengthen the implementation of the program or determine that, in the present state and site reference, the program needs to be reconceptualized.

Conclusion

Data analysis is one of the most stressful aspects of the research process because of the complexity of the endeavor. Table 12-3 is designed to help address some of the confusion related to which tests to use. Care must be taken to select the appropriate data analysis test, thereby ensuring the broad applicability of the study's findings. For quantitative data, focus on the level of measurements for the different variables is of paramount importance. Consideration of the appropriate central tendency measurement has application when determining which statistical test to use. For most researchers, the statistical tests are calculated using statistical software. The researcher must then make sense of the results that are provided.

Summary Points

1. Quantitative analysis uses numeric values to explain the outcome of a research project.
2. Qualitative analysis uses words or phrases to explain the outcomes of a research project.
3. Nominal scales use only group identification or categories to organize data.
4. Ordinal scales use ranking to organize data.
5. Interval scales have an arbitrary zero point.
6. Ratio scales have an absolute zero point.
7. Measures of central tendency include the mean, median, and mode.
8. Variability of the data describes how data vary between each score and from the mean.
9. The standard deviation statistic provides the ability to describe data based on a normal distribution and the percentage of the normal distribution expected to occur between each standard deviation unit.
10. A chi-square test is used to analyze data when the dependent variable is scaled nominally, to determine if an association exists between the variables.
11. A t-test is used to analyze data that include one nominal variable with two groups.
12. ANOVA is used to analyze data that include one nominal variable with more than two groups.
13. Case studies often lead to larger quantitative analysis trials.

RED FLAGS

- Means are not calculated for nominal data.
- Large standard deviations imply a wide range within the individual scores. This result suggests there is greater variability and less consistency within the resulting data.
- Outliers within the data set can skew the results of analysis of those data.
- If the data consist of a nominal level of measurement for the variable, the chi-square (χ^2) statistic would be the statistical test of choice.
- Chi-square (χ^2) tests reflect association between variables.

Multiple Choice Questions

1. Which statistic is often used for nominally scaled variables?

   A.   t-test
   B.   ANOVA
   C.   Chi-square
   D.   Pearson product moment

2. What level of measurement is most often associated with categorical data such as gender?

   A.   Nominal
   B.   Ordinal
   C.   Interval
   D.   Ratio

3. Which inferential procedure is appropriate when there is one nominal-scale dependent variable and one nominal-scale independent variable?

   A.   Chi-square
   B.   t-test
   C.   One-way ANOVA
   D.   Factor analysis

4. Inferential statistics are used to decide if differences among treatment groups are due to the

   A.   Significance.
   B.   Dependent variable.
   C.   Confounding variable.
   D.   Independent variable.

5. Selection of the appropriate statistical technique is based on

   A.   The research question.
   B.   The level of measurement of the independent variable or variables.
   C.   The level of measurement of the dependent variable or variables.
   D.   All of the above.

6. What do statistically significant findings imply?

   A.   The results are very important.
   B.   The results are not very important.
   C.   The results are likely due to chance differences among groups.
   D.   The results are likely due to real differences among groups.

7. A researcher investigated the relationship between vitamin C (none, 500 mg, 1,000 mg) and workers (office, outdoors) in terms of the frequency of colds. Which of the following is (are) the dependent variable(s)?

    A.   Colds

    B.   Vitamin C

    C.   Colds and workers

    D.   Vitamin C and workers

8. Which of the following is an inferential statistic?

    A.   Mode

    B.   t-test

    C.   Standard deviation

    D.   Range

9. Which statistical test has a dependent variable that is nominal in nature?

    A.   Chi-square

    B.   t-test

    C.   ANOVA

    D.   Two-way ANOVA

10. The standard deviation is

    A.   The square of the mean deviation.

    B.   The square of the variance.

    C.   The square root of the variance.

    D.   The square root of the sum of squares.

11. The t-test is used to

    A.   Adjust for initial differences within the groups.

    B.   Estimate the error of prediction.

    C.   Test whether two groups differ significantly.

    D.   Test whether more than two groups differ significantly.

12. Use of a one-tailed versus a two-tailed test of significance of the difference between two samples is determined by

    A.   Whether there is expected overlap between the error curves of the two sample distributions.

    B.   Whether the difference is expected to be in one direction only.

    C.   The size of the samples relative to population size.

    D.   Whether the subjects were matched or chosen randomly.

Discussion Questions

1. A nurse has decided to research the following PICOT question: "Adult clients who are admitted to the cardiac unit with congestive heart failure are more likely to develop nosocomial infections than other cardiac clients admitted to the cardiac unit." A quantitative research design is planned for this project. From the PICOT question, determine the variables, the levels of measurement of each variable, and the statistical test to be used.

2. A research study assessing vital signs for 15 clients resulted in the following results.

Client Number	Oral Temperature (°F)	Pulse Beats per Minute	Respirations Breaths per Minute	Blood Pressure
1	97.6	80	12	160/80
2	98.6	60	20	154/90
3	98.6	54	32	132/60
4	99.0	92	16	90/62
5	98.0	86	18	200/140
6	98.4	84	22	116/76
7	99.2	74	28	132/80
8	100.0	72	18	124/78
9	98.6	90	20	140/90
10	98.6	88	32	160/90
11	98.6	64	30	100/50
12	98.8	68	20	118/84
13	98.4	74	18	120/88
14	98.2	50	14	132/74
15	97.6	100	32	190/110

Calculate the mean, median, mode, range limits, range, and presence of outliers for each of the vital sign indices.

3. A research project is envisioned to analyze preintervention and postintervention cholesterol levels for a group of high school students participating in an after-school athletic program. Which type of statistical test could be used for this study and why?

Suggested Readings

American Psychological Association (APA). (2001). *Standards for educational and psychological testing.* (5th ed., pp. 8–9). Washington, DC: Author.

Baumgartner, T., & Jackson, A. J. (1999). *Measurement for evaluation in physical education and exercise science* (6th ed., pp. 57–109). Dubuque, IA: McGraw-Hill.

Colling, J. (2004, June). Coding, analysis, and dissemination of study results. *Urology Nursing, 24*(3), 215–216.

Cunningham, G. K. (1986). *Educational and psychological measurement.* New York: Macmillan.

Glass, G. V., & Hopkins, K. D. (1996). *Statistical methods in education and psychology* (3rd ed., pp. 31–77). Englewood Cliffs, NJ: Prentice Hall.

Happ, M. B., Dabbs, A. D., Tate, J., Hricik, A., & Erlen, J. (2006, March/April). Exemplars of mixed methods data combination and analysis. *Nursing Research, 55*(2), S43–S49.

Magee, T., Lee, S., Giuliano, K., & Munro, B. (2006). Generating new knowledge from existing data: The use of large data sets for nursing research. *Nursing Research, 55*(2S), S50–S56.

Morrow, J. R., Jackson, A. W., Disch, J. G., & Mood, D. P. (2000). *Measurement and evaluation in human performance* (2nd ed., pp. 65–70). Champaign, IL: Human Kinetics.

Owen, S., & Froman, R. (2005). Focus on research methods. Why carve up your continuous data? *Research in Nursing & Health, 28*(6), 496–503.

Priest, H., Roberts, P., & Woods, L. (2002). An overview of three different approaches to the interpretation of qualitative data. Part 1: Theoretical issues. *Nurse Researcher, 10*(1), 30–42.

Seibers, R. (2002). Data in abstracts of research articles: Are they consistent with those reported in the article? *British Journal of Biomedical Science, 59*(2), 67–68.

Thomas, J., & Nelson J. (2005). *Research methods in physical activity* (5th ed., pp. 110–212). Champaign, IL: Human Kinetics.

Chapter 13

The Research Critique Process

Carol Boswell and Sharon Cannon

Chapter Objectives

At the conclusion of this chapter, the learner will be able to

1. Provide a rationale for completing a research critique
2. List the necessary elements in a research critique
3. Evaluate evidence needed for clinical decision making
4. Use evidence-based practice guidelines to manage holistic nursing practice

Key Terms

➤ Critique

➤ Hypothesis

➤ Qualitative research

➤ Quantitative research

Rationale for Doing a Research Critique

When a critical question in nursing practice has been posed, the immediate reaction is often itself a question: What's in the literature? A common assumption made by most people is that the printed words are absolute or true. This assumption is even more commonplace when the literature is a researched study. Unfortunately, not all published research is scientifically sound. As a result, it is imperative that a nurse be able to critically assess a report.

According to Burns and Grove (2009), in the 1940s and 1950s nursing research generated critiques that were less than pleasant. Consequently, little nursing research was undertaken until the 1980s and 1990s. No studies are without some imperfections, but that is not a valid excuse for failure to conduct research. The basic concept of research management is that the researcher makes decisions about the research plan and justifies those decisions. If the researcher has done a good job with the justifications, then the strength of the results is supported. When poor justifications for the research decisions are evident, the strength of the results must be questioned. As a result of this realization, scrutiny focusing on the limitations and strengths of studies are now commonplace. This shift from criticism to analysis provides a more positive approach to examining the usefulness of the scientific data generated. Fain (2009) has suggested that nurses must critically assess research studies to determine the appropriate application to practice. Melnyk and Fineout-Overholt (2005) support this sentiment in relation to research and evidence-based practice (EBP). In EBP, research provides the evidence that guides clinical practice in making decisions about the care nurses provide.

? Think Outside the Box

Why would you want to do a critique? Is one enough? What are some of the reasons for doing research critiques?

According to Polit and Beck (2008), a research critique is a mechanism to provide feedback for improvement. They suggest that nurses who can critically review a study make valuable contributions to the body of nursing knowledge.

Finally, considering a rationale for a research critique can be found in the definition of the word "critique" as offered by *Webster's II College Dictionary* (1999): a "critical review or commentary, especially one dealing with a literary or artistic work" (p. 268). If one thinks of nursing as both an art and a science, then a critical review of nursing research can be seen as a work of art. Studies withstanding the test of time through careful exploration of findings and implementation in nursing EBP allow nurses to practice the art and science of the profession.

Elements of a Research Critique

Perhaps, before considering the elements of a research critique, we should discuss the types of critiques. Burns and Grove (2009) have identified nine types of critiques, ranging from a student critique to the critique of research proposals:

- Students learn to critique in their nursing education programs.
- Practicing nurses analyze studies for evidence on which to base the care provided.
- Educators approach critiques from the aspect of improving instruction.
- Nurse researchers focus on building a program of research emphasizing the review of studies in one specific area.
- Abstracts are frequently reviewed for use in presenting research findings.
- Presenting research at meetings, conferences, and workshops allows participants to verbally critique studies.
- Several nursing journals publish critiques of published articles, with the authors of the original article subsequently responding to concerns raised with the critique. These types of critiques often take the form of letters to the editor.
- An article submitted for publication undergoes a review by peers (peer-reviewed journals) who assess the quality of the study.
- Requests for funding for research studies from agencies such as the National Institute of Nursing Research (NINR) are subjected to scrutiny.

Critiques are essential to EBP and are expressed in the various forms just discussed.

Regardless of the type of critique, each critique includes certain elements. Brink and Wood (2001) have suggested that "the purpose of a research critique is to determine whether the findings are usable for you" (p. 57). Some general questions can be associated with the elements of a critique.

Study Purpose

The first element of a research critique generally involves determining the purpose of a study. Questions to be asked about this element include the following:

- Is the purpose clear?
- Is it relevant to your practice?
- Is there a need for the study?
- Will the study improve nursing practice and add to the body of nursing knowledge?

Answers to these questions guide the critique. If the responses are negative, then the notion of EBP flowing from the study is questionable.

Research Design

A second element involves the design of the research. Questions to ask about this element include the following:

- Is there a framework/theory to guide the study?
- If there is no framework/theory, are you able to identify how data will be collected?
- Who will be studied?
- What is the plan for conducting the study?
- Are the research plan decisions justified adequately?

"Designing and producing research is a complex activity" (Brockopp & Hastings-Tolsma, 2003, p. 59). Adequate planning is important to allow the use of the best evidence for incorporation in nursing practice. A well-thought-out design allows for assurance that the evidence has practicality. The research design can be likened to a set of instructions allowing the builder to put together the pieces of a puzzle resulting in a usable product.

? Think Outside the Box

Which aspects of a research article do you perceive as important, and why?

Literature Review

Another element to consider is the literature review focusing on the problem presented. Questions to ask about this element include the following:

- Is the literature review comprehensive?
- Is the literature review current—that is, has the literature been published within the last 5 years?
- Are there benchmark publications?
- Are the majority of sources primary or secondary?

- Is the literature review well organized, including an introduction and a summary?
- Does the literature review include a section for a model/theory?

A thorough literature review allows for assessment of the credibility of the present study. Of major importance in beginning a research study is the need to ask, "What has been written about the problem?" The literature review provides the foundation for the study's significance and relationship to practice.

Research Question/Hypothesis

The next element of a research critique is the research question(s) or hypothesis(es). This element of the critique is of extreme importance, as it should reflect the purpose of the study. Research questions in EBP are the "who, what, when, where, why, and how" guiding the nursing care provided to patients. Thus it is essential to assess the following issues:

- Is the research question clearly stated?
- Does it match the purpose of the study?
- Are the research question decisions justified adequately?
- Is there a theory/framework/model that establishes a relationship with the question?

A study sometimes contains a hypothesis rather than a research question. Polit and Beck (2008) define a hypothesis as "a prediction about the relationship between two or more variables" (p. 755). Simply put, a hypothesis may predict, propose, suppose, explain, or test a quality, property, or characteristic of people, things, or settings. We have all talked about or discussed "hypothetical situations." A hypothesis proposes a solution. Questions to ask about a hypothesis include the following:

- Are all variables described?
- Is the hypothesis clearly stated?
- Does the hypothesis reflect the purpose of the study?
- Are the hypothesis decisions justified adequately?
- Is there a theory/framework/model that establishes a relationship with the hypothesis?

The establishment of the research question or hypothesis is paramount to the focusing of the study. Each aspect of the wording within the questions or hypotheses needs to be clear and concise to allow for the effective concentration of the research endeavor. The PICOT statement can facilitate the development of the research question or hypothesis. The PICOT process drives the literature review and can evolve into the research question or hypothesis based on the outcomes of the literature review.

Study Sample

Another element of the research critique focuses on the sample. Questions regarding the sample should include the following:

- Who is identified as the target population?
- How were the subjects chosen (e.g., randomly, conveniently)?
- Who is included (e.g., males, females, children, adults)?
- Who is excluded (e.g., elderly, pregnant women, minorities)?
- How large is the sample?
- Are the sampling plan decisions justified adequately?
- Were ethical considerations clearly addressed within the sampling process?

Answers to these questions can help the nurse decide if decisions about patients and clinical problems are relevant. Clarification of the sample population must be denoted. Each aspect of the sampling process should be carefully and thoroughly described within the discussion of the project.

Data Collection

Essential to the critique is a description of how the data were collected. Questions about this element include the following:

- What steps were taken to collect the data?
- How often were data collected and for how long?
- Which instruments or tools were used?
- Who designed the tools?
- Are the tools valid and reliable?
- Are the tools adequately described so that readers can understand what the score means?
- Were data analysis procedures appropriate?
- Are the plans for data collection and analysis decisions justified adequately?
- Were ethical considerations adequately addressed within the data collection process?

Data collection gives information about the research question or hypothesis. Quantitative data, for example, are often collected by a survey mechanism that provides a score for analysis. In such a case, a clear understanding of how and where the data were collected, the description of the instrument (tool) that was used, and how the results were analyzed statistically is essential. In contrast, the data collected for a qualitative study are presented in narrative format.

? Think Outside the Box

Debate the importance of including the theoretical foundation for a study in the report of its findings. Frequently, this aspect seems to be omitted in research articles owing to the page restrictions imposed by the journal.

Study Results

A critique should provide the results of the study. Questions about results include the following:

- Is the research question answered or the hypothesis proved?
- Were there limitations?
- Can generalizations be made?
- Did the results support what was reported in the literature?
- Were there any unexpected findings?
- Did the outcomes affirm the theory used as the basis of the study?

The elements of the critique summarize the study, including what was found and how the findings might be applied to similar situations. The summary of the findings needs to be carefully presented to allow for generalization to other settings and populations.

Study Recommendations

The final element of the research critique is the section presenting the author's recommendations. Questions for this element include the following:

- Are suggestions for further use in practice included?
- Is there an identified need for further research?
- Could you make a change in your practice based on the results of this study?
- What are the benefits to using the information learned?

The necessary elements in a research critique can be organized as answers to a series of questions. Those questions then form the basis for the process of conducting a research critique. As an individual attempts to investigate the quality of a study, these questions can provide a beginning place for the critique.

Process for Conducting a Research Critique

The word "critique" can also be defined as "a critical review or commentary, especially one dealing with works of art or literature; a critical discussion of a specific topic; the art of criticism" (Editors of the American Heritage Dictionaries, 2005, p. 1). Although "research critique" is the term frequently used, several other terms—such as "critical analysis," "review," "evaluation," and "appraisal"—can also be associated with the process (CyberNurse, 2005). Any of these terms could be, and are, used as the modus operandi for assessing a published research article.

To gain a true understanding and appreciation of the process of a research critique, one must recognize the expectations for conducting the process. As the definition implies, it is undertaken to allow individuals to carefully and thoroughly examine a research endeavor. The outcome is not anticipated to be a negative grilling of the project to identify all of its shortcomings. Wood and Ross-Kerr (2006) affirm this point: "In your best judgment, you decide if what you have read will serve your purpose" (p. 65). The materials need to be practical and applicable to your individual practice setting and the patient situation.

According to guidelines developed at San Jose State University (2005), studies should be scrutinized for their merits, limitations, implications, and consequences. Each and every report needs to be assessed with a critical eye toward each unique setting. As Rodger (1997) notes, the resulting critique should be "balanced, including strengths and weaknesses, and constructive, providing suggestions for how the study might be improved" (p. 1). It is envisioned as a review or analysis of the research undertaking. Both the strengths and limitations within the process of the research study are judiciously examined to verify that the ending results can truly be generalized to the target population.

? Think Outside the Box

If nurses do not value research, their engagement with the critique process and their participation in research studies are decreased. Identify steps and incentives that might be used to get you and your peers involved in doing research critiques or research projects.

By completing an effective research critique, a reviewer becomes aware of both the strengths and the shortcomings of the research project. As a consequence of identifying these concerns, the assessor can efficiently incorporate the results into practice based on this in-depth knowledge of the study findings. Thus the incorporation of the results into nursing practice is based on an understanding of the comprehensiveness of the study.

Every study has limitations, because researchers must inevitably make multiple methodological judgments that influence the significance, integrity, and value of the resulting research outcomes (San Jose State University, 2005). No study is ever perfectly conducted unless it is not done on humans, but even nonhuman studies frequently have limitations and weaknesses. It is true that research conducted on laboratory animals can be controlled with greater domination than projects in which humans are the subjects. Put simply, when working with laboratory animals, the variables can be manipulated. If the same project were envisioned using human subjects, however, the ethical ramifications could be increased, because manipulation of the variables for human subjects might result in damages. Human research always has nuances that must be considered when the results are proposed to be incorporated into practice.

As nurses are asked to become involved with the critiquing of research articles for EBP, several formidable factors emerge and must be dealt with. Several Internet sites are available to use as resources for exploring the development of research critiques geared toward EBP (**Table 13-1**).

? Think Outside the Box

Look at some research articles. Can you identify within them any discussion related to patient preferences that is part of evidence-based practice? Discuss your thoughts about your findings.

Table 13-1

Suggested Resources for Research Critique Formats

http://www.sonoma.edu/users/n/nolan/n400/critique.htm

http://www.camden.rutgers.edu/dept-pages/nursing_ugrad/Fall2004/Research/Research_Written_Critique_Format_F04.pdf

http://www.uwm.edu/~brodg/Handout/critique.htm

http://www.fadavis.com/kearney/StudentWebAncillary/ch06_ex01.cfm

http://www.umsl.edu/~lindquists/critique.html

Note: Access to these Web sites was verified on March 15, 2009.

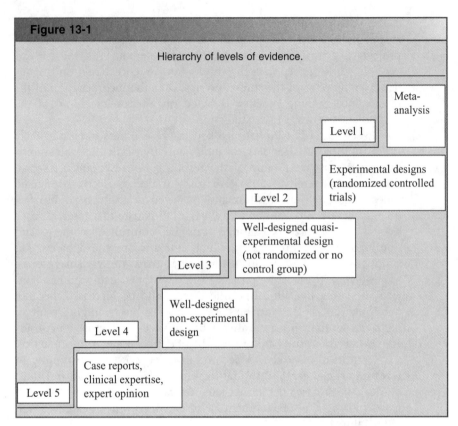

Figure 13-1

Hierarchy of levels of evidence.

Level 1 — Meta-analysis

Level 2 — Experimental designs (randomized controlled trials)

Level 3 — Well-designed quasi-experimental design (not randomized or no control group)

Level 4 — Well-designed non-experimental design

Level 5 — Case reports, clinical expertise, expert opinion

Source: Adapted from United States Prevention Service Task Force (USPSTF). (2007). *Grade definitions after May 2007.* Retrieved February 24, 2009, from http://www.ahrq.gov/clinic/uspstf/gradespost.htm.

One topic drawing an increasing amount of attention as part of the movement toward incorporation of research critiques into EBP is the grading of the evidence. Numerous organizations, including the Agency for Healthcare Research and Quality (AHRQ), Joanna Briggs Institute, and Cochrane Collaboration, among others, have developed "levels of evidence" hierarchies in an effort to help reviewers categorize the strengths and weaknesses of various studies (see **Figure 13-1**). Quantitative and qualitative types of research design are designated as a specific level within the hierarchy of research study designs. One drawback at this time with the levels of evidence is the management or classification of mixed method studies. Reviewers must make their own decisions about classifying such studies as quantitative or qualitative, because no level for mixed method studies has been established. A quick Internet search can provide multiple levels for consideration. After the critique of the article is completed, the information assessed is awarded a specific grade based on the strength of the evidence presented in the publication. For the most part, the "levels of evidence" categories developed by the various organizations are compatible, with only minor differences based on the agency being apparent.

The Agency for Healthcare Research and Quality (AHRQ) has also developed a "tool for evaluating the strength of the evidence" (United States Prevention Services Task Force, 2007); see **Figure 13-2**. With this tool, the evidence is assigned a level of strength based on the anticipated harm to the patient. With the integration of EBP into the research critique process, the classification of research projects in terms of the "level of evidence" and the strength of the evidence using instruments such as the AHRQ tool seeks to improve the clarity of the information available for making clinical decisions about the modification of policies, procedures, and clinical guidelines.

Another factor—the austere style of journal articles—also triggers some concerns. The amount of space allocated to articles within journals is prescribed by the companies that publish those journals. As a result of these restrictions regarding page length and word count limits, key elements within the research process must be succinctly presented within the published research article. Depth of discussion about the basic research principles must, therefore, be limited or even omitted. Unfortunately, discussions of the operational definitions for key variables; models, plans, and systems; and conceptual or theoretical frameworks are often omitted due to space restrictions. Classic research studies include a description of the theory/framework and concepts underlying the study, but many other studies use a model, plan, or system for the research.

Another aspect of the process that deters nurses from participating in research critiques is the unfamiliar jargon. Statistical aspects are quite intimidating to many practicing nurses. The definitions used within research to discuss sampling, variables, hypotheses, and quantitative and qualitative methods are typically foreign to the practicing nurse. Although many of these are common terms, such as "independent," "dependent," "convenience," and "variable," they often take on new meanings within a research project. This specificity of the terms within research leads to conflict and misunderstanding for novice evaluators of research. In the future, nurses will be increasingly confronted with the expectation that they will center their practice on evidence. Because nurses must become proficient at reading and understanding research reports to incorporate their findings into EBP, they need to take a deep breath now and plunge into the critiquing process.

The ability to accomplish critical appraisals is a skill that must be developed through repeated practice. The University of Saskatchewan College of Nursing (2005) has acknowledged that completing research critiques "will become a rewarding intellectual challenge that keeps

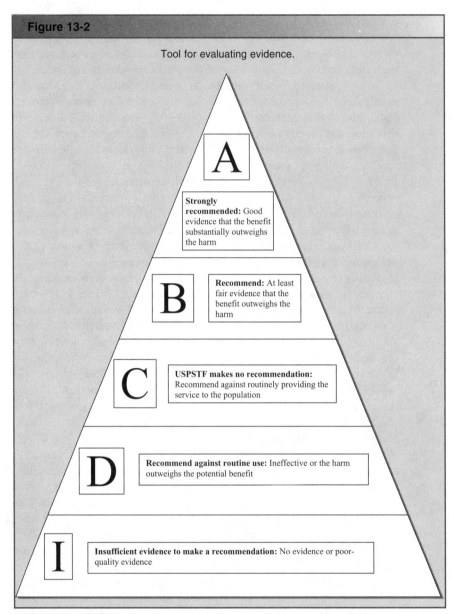

Figure 13-2

Tool for evaluating evidence.

A

Strongly recommended: Good evidence that the benefit substantially outweighs the harm

B

Recommend: At least fair evidence that the benefit outweighs the harm

C

USPSTF makes no recommendation: Recommend against routinely providing the service to the population

D

Recommend against routine use: Ineffective or the harm outweighs the potential benefit

I

Insufficient evidence to make a recommendation: No evidence or poor-quality evidence

Source: Adapted from United States Prevention Service Task Force (USPSTF). (2007). *Grade definitions after May 2007.* Retrieved February 24, 2009, from http://www.ahrq.gov/ clinic/uspstf/gradespost.htm.

getting easier and more interesting with experience" (p. 3). The most valuable advice for developing expertise in this process is to continue doing research critiques, because practice does diminish the confusion and overwhelming nature of the process. By reading research articles, nurses become increasingly accustomed to the format and terminology. Evidence-based nursing practice mandates that nurses begin to build a knowledge base by the "steady diet" approach—specifically, by digesting at least one research report each week. By accepting the challenge to become comfortable with research reports, nurses will find that the different aspects of the report become more familiar, even commonplace—and, therefore, less threatening. Not all nurses will strive to carry out research activities, but it is imperative that all nurses become comfortable with the use of research results to advance the discipline of nursing and ultimately improve nursing care.

Initially, some general areas of the research study must be considered. The author(s) of the study needs to be evaluated. Precisely who is completing the research, including those persons' job titles and qualifications to conduct the project, needs to be carefully contemplated. After the author information is pondered, an assessment of the study title provides valuable information. The title of the project should provide a clear, concise description of the project. It should stimulate a prompt perception of the fundamental nature of the paper (Cyber-Nurse, 2005). At this point, the abstract is examined to further clarify the focus for the research endeavor. The abstract should condense the main points from the research project. A quick read of the abstract and discussion sections should provide valuable insight into the complexity and applicability of the study to a unique practice setting.

Holder (2003) has identified four key aspects to carefully address when initiating a research critique:

- Understanding the purpose and problem, while determining if the design and methodology are consistent with the study purpose
- Determining if the methodology is applied properly
- Assessing if the outcomes and conclusions are believable and supported by the findings
- Reflecting on the report's overall quality, strengths, and limitations, and whether they contribute to knowledge and suggestions for improvement in the study

According to the guidelines developed by San Jose State University (2005), the research critique process involves the following steps (**Table 13-2**):

1. Read the entire study carefully.
2. Examine the organization and presentation.
3. Identify terms you don't understand.
4. Highlight each step of the research process.
5. Identify the strengths and weaknesses objectively.
6. Suggest modifications for future studies.
7. Determine how well the study followed the rules for ideal study.

Table 13-2	
Critique Worksheet	
Topic	**Discussion**
Title of the study	
Author credentials	
Purpose of the study (in your own words)	
Literature written about the problem	
Theory/framework, concepts, and the relationship to nursing	
Research question or hypothesis	
Dependent and independent variables	
Definitions given	
Tools and their reliability and validity information	
Sample description	
Study ethics description (i.e., institutional review board [IRB] information)	
Data collection procedures	
Data analysis	
Results, recommendations, and implications for practice	

These guidelines are fairly general, but they do provide a place to start. A careful, general reading of the entire study must be the beginning point for any critique. According to Holder (2003), the examiner should "read the research report in its entirety to get a sense of the study and its contribution to knowledge development, then read again paying attention to the questions appropriate to each stage of the critiquing process" (p. 2). The use of a photocopy of the article may facilitate the research critique process, because areas can be highlighted, questions can be added to the margin, and key points can be circled.

As the reader begins this initial review of the research project, he or she will develop a feel for the organization of the article, along with the manner of presentation for the entire research process. At this point, the examiner will become aware of the complexity of the identified material. To become somewhat relaxed with the content, he or she should expect to read the article several times. Each time the article is read, the examiner comes to terms with a different aspect of the article. Frequently, an initial question relates to the researcher's ability to verbalize the process in a manner that nurses can understand and be able to utilize in practice. The reader may also find that some of the initial questions raised in the introductory section are answered in other sections within the article. After this general overview of the article, a more critical examination of the documentation can then be completed.

Table 13-3	
Rules for an Ideal Study	
Research problem	• Significance of problem noted • Clarification of aim of study • Practicality of study • Clarity, significance, and documentation
Review of literature	• Organization of literature • Progression toward study question through previous research reports • Rationale and direction for the study presented
Study conceptual framework/theory	• Clear link between conceptual framework/theory and research question/purpose • Any maps/models logically presented
Research questions or hypotheses	• Expressed appropriately and clearly • Logically related to the research purpose/aim and framework/theory
Variables	• Concepts identified within the framework/theory used • Variables operationally defined • Conceptual definition consistent with operational definition of each variable
Research design	• Design appears appropriate • Clearly defined protocol for conducting research project • Any treatment closely scrutinized to guarantee consistency • Threats to internal validity minimized • Logically connected to the sampling method and statistics used
Sampling method	• Method appropriate to result in representative sample • Biases identified • Human rights protected • Setting described and appropriate for target population
Measurements	• Instruments sufficient for measuring the study variables • Instrument validity and reliability levels • Instrument scoring techniques clearly described
Data collection	• Techniques for using observation clearly described • Methods for recording measures clearly described • Inter-rater reliability described when appropriate • Process clearly, consistently, and ethically described
Data analysis	• Procedures suitable for the type of data collected • Analysis procedures clearly portrayed • Outcomes offered in a comprehensible way

Source: Modified from San Jose State University. (2005). *Reading and critiquing research.* Retrieved December 26, 2006, from http://www.sjsu.edu/upload/course/course_969/Reading_and_CritiquingResearch.ppt.

Each aspect within a research article is examined to identify areas of concerns and assets (**Table 13-3**). The evaluator will benefit from taking the time to highlight each of the steps of the research process, spotlighting the hypothesis(es), literature review, sample, ethical considerations, and research design. During this focused examination, any limitations identified by the researchers should be noted. Another area to recognize explicitly is the operational definitions, which reflect the standards used within the research project to clarify the specific variables. After noting the operational definition for each variable, a reviewer should not have many additional terms that require explanation. The evaluator should define any term that continues to be unfamiliar to enable him or her to better understand the entire process.

Every reader should develop a habit of looking up unfamiliar terms instead of skipping over them, which simply causes those terms to remain unfamiliar. The objective of critiquing any research report is to become familiar with the language and procedures used regularly within the scheme.

At this point in the research critique, the reviewer attempts to identify the strengths and limitations of the research process described in the report. The reviewer should be aware that the limitations so identified might actually be a consequence of the lack of space allowed within the documentation of the research endeavor rather than representing the intended omission of the aspect. All journal articles have space limitations, which can result in some items being cut because of space considerations rather than because they were lacking in the study.

One major challenge for novice research readers is the evaluation of statistics. In considering this aspect of any research process, the key point is to ask for help. The guidelines developed by the University of Saskatchewan College of Nursing (2005) strongly suggest that reviewers either find someone to provide help in this area or obtain a book similar to *Statistics for Dummies* to aid in the assessment of the statistical data. Nurses who practice evidence-based nursing are not expected to become statisticians. Nurses are, however, expected to acknowledge their limitations and seek help from statisticians and others as needed to improve their evaluation of research results for incorporation into everyday nursing practice.

Critically Assessing Knowledge for Clinical Decision Making

The various aspects of EBP are of fundamental importance in considering the assessment of knowledge related to clinical decision making. According to guidelines provided by the University of Saskatchewan College of Nursing (2005), "The evidence you will require to guide your practice in a matter of clinical importance will not come from reviewing a single independent study" (PowerPoint® slide 8). The practicing nurse comes to the research critique process with a foundation of clinical experience. Thus the critique of the research endeavor is tempered by this clinical expertise. Yoder (2005) suggests that "clinical decisions require that one use a problem-solving approach to clinical practice that integrates a systematic search for and critical appraisal of the relevant evidence to answer the clinical questions" (p. 91). Every nurse has been taught a problem-solving methodology. During the review of research, it becomes essential for nurses to utilize this critical thinking framework, which has already been incorporated into practice, to validate and conceptualize the research critique process. The idea behind a research critique is to provide a systematic process for critically appraising research projects. Within this process, nurses must become comfortable with looking at all aspects of the various studies to assess any strengths and limitations that might be apparent. Carefully considering these different aspects of the report facilitates critical thinking concerning the results reported and the applicability of those results to the workplace.

One aspect of paramount importance to be considered within any research critique is the determination of the sampling process. According to Pajares (2005), "The key word in sampling is representative" (Section VI.E.4). Determining the appropriateness of the sampling method is critical in any study appraisal. When a convenient sampling method is used, the rationale and limitations related to this methodology must be meticulously discussed.

Decisively Evaluating Quantitative Research Evidence

Quantitative research reports tend to be slightly easier to critique because of the concreteness of the quantitative research design. The various aspects of quantitative research reports document the expectations for all of the various elements of the article—that is, the introduction, literature review, hypothesis(es), sampling, research design, statistical testing, and discussion. Although each of these areas includes considerable levels and components, the clarity of the descriptions of these aspects is more distinct than in qualitative methodologies.

According to Carter (2006), the critiquing of quantitative research reports should address four basic areas: comprehension, comparison, analysis, and evaluation. Each of these four levels of review adds a different dimension to the resulting scrutiny. Comprehension and comparison provide the overall appraisal of the report. Analysis then takes the investigation of the report to the level of reflecting on the continuity among the different parts (Carter, 2006). At this point of assessing the report, the principal concern is whether the hypothesis flows into decisions made about the sample, and whether that sample is appropriately managed by the research design. The final aspect of the review carefully considers the meaning and significance of the study process for implementation into nursing practice. The focus here is to determine whether the findings, implications, and recommendations presented in the study report are truly supported and presented.

A key aspect of this review process that is unique to the quantitative research appraisal is the use of a conceptual or theoretical framework (Pajares, 2005). Although it can be provided in any of the research methodologies, this framework is essential in all quantitative research endeavors. Having said this, within printed articles documenting quantitative research, the discussion of the conceptual/theoretical framework is frequently omitted to satisfy the journal's page length requirements. Of course, the omission could also reflect the researcher's failure to include a conceptual/theoretical framework as part of the study design. The total omission of this framework would be a marked limitation within a quantitative research methodology. When a lack of theoretical foundation for a study is determined (yet the study outcomes appear to be applicable to your setting), sending a query to the authors about the issue may be helpful to determine the status of the theoretical foundation.

Decisively Evaluating Qualitative Research Evidence

When evaluating qualitative research endeavors, the examination of the entire process assumes a slightly different perspective from that employed with a quantitative research endeavor. Assessment of the clarity of the purpose and statement of the phenomenon remains consistent with that of any other methodology critique. These components must be presented upfront. From that point onward, the specificity of the qualitative design must be considered. Broad research questions, instead of hypotheses, are frequently employed within this type of research design. The literature review may follow the data collection process rather than driving the research endeavor from its inception. A framework may or may not be clearly presented as part of the study report. Qualitative research reviews must carefully discuss the researcher–participant relationship, because this aspect is a critical component of the data collection process. Ethical considerations also play significant roles in determining the appropriateness of this methodology.

Carter (2006) has elucidated five standards to keep in mind when conducting a qualitative research critique. First, the research report must present a comprehensible depiction of the research environment, data collection process, sampling process, and the researcher's thought process. A second standard relates to the importance of congruence among the methodological aspects. According to Carter (2006), this section should indicate "rigor in documentation, procedural rigor, ethical rigor, and auditability" (Critique of qualitative research, 2). The third standard is the analytical preciseness: The researcher's thoughts and decisions related to the data should be evident in the report. The fourth standard stresses the importance of addressing the theoretical connectedness presented within the report. The fifth standard identified suggests that the relevance (value of the study) needs to be apparent within the documentation of the research project. Appropriate examination of each of these facets within a research report should yield a strong, valid depiction of the research project.

The data collection aspect of the study is a crucial component of the presentation of qualitative research projects. The reader must be walked through the entire process, from identification of the participants to the management of the data collected from them. The congruence of these data with the research purpose, question, and tradition needs to be assessed. The researcher is obliged to discuss how the field engagements and observations ought to build trust and ensure validity of the data collected. Another aspect that should be identifiable within the report is the ongoing and concurrent nature of data collection and analysis. Because data collection and analysis occur in tandem in qualitative research, the codes used as categories and the process utilized to determine data saturation must be explicitly discussed in the report. The research report should also address triangulation, peer review of the research process, articulation of researcher biases, member checking, and external audit by expert consultants.

A final aspect that must be noted within qualitative research reports is the sampling data. Because the sample population in such studies is usually small and focused, a description of this population is critical to allowing the reader to determine if the study findings are generalizable to other populations.

Qualitative research often employs additional terminology that must be defined and clarified, which can cause further confusion and frustration. As a result, the critique of qualitative research tends to be an area that is best entered into after learning how to conduct critiques of quantitative research endeavors. Put simply, qualitative research tends to be less structured than quantitative research.

Decisively Evaluating Mixed Method Evidence

Mixed method research embraces both quantitative and qualitative design aspects. According to Creswell (2003), the mixed method approach takes advantage of the strengths of both quantitative and qualitative research by employing sequential, concurrent, and transformative strategies of inquiry. As a critique of a mixed method research study is undertaken, the reader must, therefore, consider the presentation of both methodologies within the discussion. A unique aspect of a mixed method research critique is the expectation of a stated rationale for the use of this method.

The quantitative and qualitative data in a mixed method research report are frequently presented separately, which allows the reader to concentrate on one type of data prior to considering the other type. Quantitative data are customarily presented initially and followed by the qualitative data. The discussion section should integrate the two types of data, thereby strengthening the study's findings. When a transformative study design is employed, this section should address the advancement of the agenda for change or reform that has developed as a result of the research.

Employing EBP Guidelines: Instruments for Holistic Practice

EBP requires that multiple related articles be correlated to provide a sum of evidence rather than a single data set. Contradictory evidence must be reconciled through the evaluation and association of data from multiple quality research projects. Of course, this process of reconciling contradictory evidence and multiple research discussions generates additional questions that need to be investigated at some point in time.

According to the Oncology Nursing Society (2005), the EBP process comprises six steps:

1. Identify the problem.
2. Find the evidence.
3. Critique the merit, feasibility, and utility of the evidence.
4. Summarize the evidence.
5. Apply the ideas to practice.
6. Evaluate the results.

Each of these steps, with the exception of the application to practice (Step 5), can be visualized within the research critique process. Research critiques require the identification of the problem; an examination of the literature review; a critique of the merits, feasibility, and use of the research process; summarization of the research process; consideration of the applicability of the research results to practice; and evaluation of the results.

Summary Points

1. Critiques of research are essential to EBP and allow nurses to practice the art and science of the profession.
2. There are nine types of critiques.
3. The necessary elements in a research critique can be compiled in a series of questions for the process of critiquing research.
4. Critiques should be balanced, identifying both strengths and limitations in the study report examined.

5. Journal articles have restrictions on page limits and word limits, which sometimes results in information being omitted.
6. Jargon in research reports often deters nurses from doing research critiques.
7. The critical appraisal of research is a skill to be developed through repeated practice.
8. General areas of the research study include author qualifications, study purpose, study design, the sample, the research methodology, the outcomes, limitations, and strengths of the research, and recommendations.
9. Nurses in EBP do not need to be statisticians, but they do need to be comfortable asking for help when evaluating the statistical analysis portion of a research report.
10. Quantitative research studies are concrete in nature and should include a theoretical framework.
11. Qualitative research studies contain broad research questions, are unstructured, and must consider ethics.
12. Mixed method research embraces both quantitative and qualitative aspects of study design.
13. Research critiques should consider the applicability of the research results to practice.

RED FLAGS

- A critique is not a negative process, but rather should entail a careful examination of all aspects of the research process.
- A research critique should identify gaps within the study's research process.
- Future research possibilities should be identified as part of the original study and the critique of that study.
- Recommendations for advancement of the nursing profession should be documented in transformative research.
- For EBP, multiple related articles need to provide a sum of evidence rather than a single data set.

Multiple Choice Questions

1. Nurses must critically assess research studies to
   A. Understand that all research is scientifically sound.
   B. Determine the applicability of their findings to practice.
   C. Know that all studies are perfect.
   D. Identify a negative approach to research utilization.

2. Of the nine types of critiques, which of the following are considered essential to EBP?
   A. Student, practicing nurse, and peer review critiques
   B. Abstracts, presentations, and e-mail critiques
   C. Program of research, letters to the editors, and lay-journal critiques
   D. National Institute of Nursing Research, educator groups, and newspaper critiques

3. The purpose of a study applies to EBP when it
   A. Adds to the body of nursing knowledge.
   B. Is complete and requires multiple readings.
   C. Is relevant to the authors.
   D. Is hard to find in the literature.

4. A hypothesis may be described by which of the following terms?
   A. Results, introduces, criticizes, reviews
   B. Findings, improvements, collections, sets
   C. Studies, plans, appreciates, concerns
   D. Proposes, predicts, supposes, tests

5. An essential component of a critique is a description of how the data were collected. Which of the following statements provides the best data collection description?
   A. Data collection was timely and used a tool developed by the researcher.
   B. Multiple tools were used to collect the data.
   C. The data was collected at 2-week intervals using a pre-test/post-test procedure.
   D. The score for the tool is easily understood and needs little description.

6. Results of the study should include
   A. Unexpected findings.
   B. Unanswered questions.
   C. Pictures of subjects.
   D. Endorsements of peers.

7. A research study recommendation should include
   A. No further need for research.
   B. No benefits for use in practice.
   C. Ways to change practice based on results.
   D. Ways to avoid using the results in other studies.

8. The definition of a research critique is understood to imply
   A. Analytical examination or commentary of a research report.
   B. A negative assessment related to the weaknesses of a research report.
   C. An analytical evaluation of the literature review.
   D. A positive assessment of the research design.

9. Although many aspects are discussed within a research critique, the basic aspects that the critique is attempting to identify are
   A. Hypothesis(es) and literature review.
   B. Strengths and limitations.
   C. Research design and sampling methodology.
   D. Shortcomings and critical problems.

10. Evidence-based nursing practice requires that nurses initiate a pattern to facilitate effective utilization of research results. The best method for improving a nurse's ability to incorporate research results into practice is
    A. Planning a monthly session to complete a literature review.
    B. Completing a critique of a single research project.
    C. Assessing at least one research report on a weekly basis.
    D. Reviewing abstracts from selected research projects.

11. Several basic guidelines can be used to make the research critiquing procedure less threatening. Which of the following reflects the utilization of these guidelines?
    A. The nurse reads the entire discussion section carefully to gain an overview of the research report.
    B. The nurse identifies shortcomings that are unfamiliar, to clarify the limitations within the study.
    C. The nurse reads the entire study meticulously to acquire a general understanding of the research report.
    D. The nurse identifies modifications for the selected research report.

12. Quantitative research design tends to be easier to critique due to the
    A. Length of the research reports.
    B. Incorporation of triangulation into the process.
    C. Use of convenient sampling methodology.
    D. Concreteness of the research design.

13. When attempting to critique a qualitative research endeavor, individuals must be able to

    A.   Easily identify the hypothesis(es).

    B.   Carefully assess the data collection and management processes.

    C.   Quickly determine the conceptual framework utilized.

    D.   Effectively understand the statistical results.

14. One unique aspect present in reports of mixed method research projects is a(an)

    A.   Rationale for the utilization of the method.

    B.   Clear delineation of the sampling method.

    C.   In-depth discussion of the methodology.

    D.   Listing of the strengths and limitations.

Discussion Questions

1. You and your peers, as staff nurses, have found a research article that has the potential to change the way you practice. List questions about the report elements that could guide your critique of the study.

2. Select an article on a research project for your practice area and complete the critique worksheet in Table 13-2. After completing the critique of the article, give the article a "level of evidence" rating and a "strength of evidence" score. Would you change your practice based on the information in this article?

3. You are a manager on a medical–surgical acute care unit. Your facility is moving toward an EBP format. Each unit has been charged with establishing a process for involving the staff nurses in this transformation. You have decided to implement a journal club for staff nurses to review and critique research articles for potential inclusion in evidence-based policies. What would you set as the ground rules for the implementation of this journal club activity?

Suggested Readings

Daggett, L., Harbaugh, B. L., & Collum, L. A. (2005). A worksheet for critiquing quantitative nursing research. *Nurse Educator, 30*(6), 255–258.

Pellechia, G. L. (1999). Dissemination of research findings: Conference presentations and journal publications. *Topics in Geriatric Rehabilitation, 14*(3), 67–79.

Riley, J. (2002). Understanding research articles. *Tar Heel Nurse, 64*(3), 15.

Valente, S. (2003). Critical analysis of research papers. *Journal for Nurses in Staff Development, 196*(3), 130–142.

References

Brink, P. J., & Wood, M. J. (2001). *Basic steps in planning nursing research from question to proposal* (5th ed.). Sudbury, MA: Jones and Bartlett.

Brockopp, D. Y., & Hastings-Tolsma, M. T. (2003). *Fundamentals of nursing research* (3rd ed.). Sudbury, MA: Jones and Bartlett.

Burns, N., & Grove, S. K. (2009). *The practice of nursing research: Appraisal, synthesis, and generation of evidence* (8th ed.). St. Louis, MO: Saunders Elsevier.

Carter, K. (2006). *How to critique research.* Retrieved February 19, 2009, from http://www.runet.edu/~kcarter/Course_Info/nurs442/chapter12.htm

Creswell, J. W. (2003). *Research design: Qualitative, quantitative, and mixed methods approaches* (2nd ed.). Thousand Oaks, CA: Sage.

CyberNurse. (2005). *Reading and critiquing research.* Retrieved December 1, 2005, from http://www.cybernurse.org.uk/research/Reading_and_Critiquing_Research.htm

Editors of the American Heritage Dictionaries. (2005). Dictionary definition: critique. In *The American heritage dictionary of the English language* (4th ed.). Retrieved March 8, 2009, from http://education.yahoo.com/reference/dictionary/entry/critique

Editors of Webster's II College Dictionaries. (1999). *Webster's II new college dictionary.* Boston: Houghton Mifflin.

Fain, J. A. (2009). *Reading, understanding, and applying nursing research: A text and workbook* (3rd ed.). Philadelphia: F. A. Davis.

Holder, B. (2003). *The research critique.* Retrieved December 26, 2005, from http://virtual.clemson.edu/group/odce/summer1_03/nursT807/pdf

Melnyk, B. M., & Fineout-Overholt, E. (2005). *Evidence-based practice in nursing and healthcare: A guide to best practice.* Philadelphia: Lippincott Williams & Wilkins.

Oncology Nursing Society. (2005). *Evidence-based process.* Retrieved March 8, 2009, from http://onsopcontent.ons.org/toolkits/evidence/Process/index.shtml

Pajares, F. (2005). *The elements of a proposal.* Retrieved February 19, 2009, from http://www.des.emory.edu/mfp/proposal.html

Polit, D. F., & Beck, C. T. (2008). *Nursing research: Generating and assessing evidence for nursing practice* (8th ed.). Philadelphia: Lippincott Williams & Wilkins.

Rodger, B. L. (1997). *Guidelines for critique of research reports.* Retrieved February 19, 2009, from http://www.uwm.edu/~brodg/Handout/critique.htm

San Jose State University. (2005, March 1). *Reading and critiquing research.* Retrieved December 26, 2005, from http://www.sjsu.edu/upload/course/course_969/Reading_ and_Critiquing Research.ppt

United States Prevention Services Task Force (USPSTF). (2007). PowerPoint presentation entitled "Using evidence to inform and improve clinical prevention, 2007 AHRQ Annual Conference." Bethesda, MD: Author.

University of Saskatchewan College of Nursing. (2005). *Reading, summarizing, and critiquing research reports.* Retrieved December 26, 2005, from http://usask.ca/nursing/classes/323/notes/Lec5.pdf

Wood, M. J., & Ross-Kerr, J. C. (2006). *Basic steps in planning nursing research: From question to proposal.* Sudbury, MA: Jones and Bartlett.

Yoder, L. H. (2005). Evidence-based practice: The time is now! *Medsurg Nursing,* 14(2), 91–92.

Chapter 14

Application of Evidence-Based Nursing Practice with Research

Sharon Cannon and Carol Boswell

Chapter Objectives

At the conclusion of this chapter, the learner will be able to

1. Synthesize key components from evidence-based nursing practice and research utilization to drive the provision of quality nursing care
2. Demonstrate proficiency in one component of evidence-based practice using the principles of the research process

Key Terms

➤ Evidence-based practice

➤ Integrative reviews

➤ Meta-analysis

➤ Research use

➤ Systematic reviews

Introduction

In Chapter 1, evidence-based practice (EBP) was defined as a process of utilizing confirmed evidence (research and quality improvement), decision making, and nursing expertise to guide the delivery of holistic patient care. The recent need for and acceptance of EBP is apparent in the literature. In a 2006 survey conducted by Sigma Theta Tau International (STTI, 2006), results suggested that a majority of the nurses needed evidence on a weekly basis to guide practice. Approximately 90% of the participants indicated a moderate to high level of confidence in EBP. The results of this survey again support the premise that EBP is a driving force for the use of scientific data in the decision-making process in the provision of nursing care. In addition, as Finkelman and Kenner (2007) state, "Nurses need to be involved in safety and quality research and to participate in evaluating how nursing care is connected to safety and quality" (p. 4). Their statement is a direct result of the Institute of Medicine's imperative to ensure patient safety. Nurses' involvement in gathering evidence to support safe, quality nursing care is essential for the future growth of the profession and most important to the patients receiving the care.

Understanding the research process is the first step in using evidence in everyday nursing practice. Following the initial historical background provided about research in nursing in Chapter 1, the chapters of this book have focused on the research process. Examples of evidence-based practice have been given to demonstrate how EBP is applied in specific components of the research process.

Difficulty in analyzing the evidence has been identified as a major obstacle to research use. The preceding chapters of this book have provided information that is intended to assist the modern-day nurse in the analysis of research findings, with their subsequent application to nursing care. This chapter is designed to "pull the pieces together" by suggesting a practical approach for research utilization in evidence-based nursing practice.

To get a clear understanding of the interconnectedness of EBP and research, a flowchart is provided here to conceptualize the relationship (see **Figure 14-1**). As a problem is identified, a PICOT statement is formed. This PICOT statement drives the review of the literature, with each part of the PICOT statement providing key words to narrow the search for relevant articles during the literature review. Once the literature has been collected and reviewed, gaps and consistencies within the literature can be determined. Based on these gaps or consistencies, the next step toward establishing a thorough foundation constructed on the evidence can be embraced. These gaps and consistencies can either lead to a research study or a quality improve-

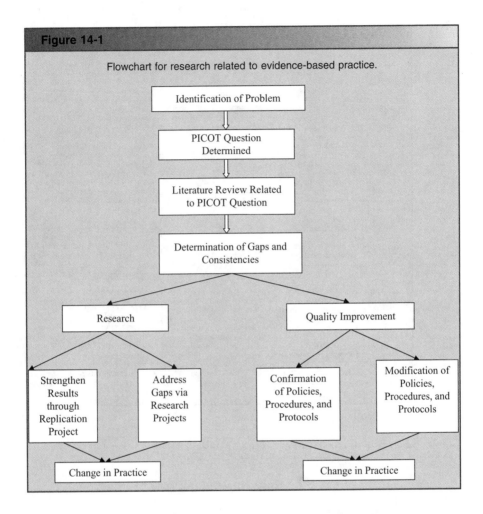

Figure 14-1

Flowchart for research related to evidence-based practice.

ment project. If the evidence indicates that a policy, procedure, or protocol needs to be investigated, then a quality improvement process is instituted for that purpose. If the gaps and consistencies suggest that further research is required to arrive at an answer for the identified problem, then a full research project would need to be planned and implemented.

If research is the direction in which the nurse should proceed, the best process for arriving at a sound conclusion would need to be determined (see **Figure 14-2**). As a research endeavor is planned, the methodology for best addressing the problem must be selected. The flowchart in Figure 14-2 identifies the steps commonly followed when conducting quantitative or qualitative research. The steps are somewhat the same for both types of research, but they do reflect the uniqueness of the research approaches.

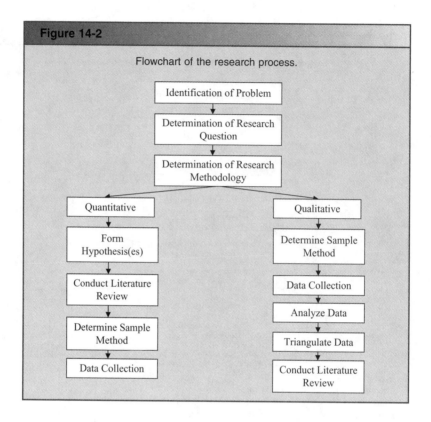

Figure 14-2

Flowchart of the research process.

Process for Evidence-Based Practice

? Think Outside the Box

Frequently, a laboring patient receives an epidural for pain management. A potential side effect of this procedure and the laboring process is difficulty with urination. To address this problem, the patient typically receives catheterization. Depending on several factors, either a straight (in-and-out) catheter or a retention Foley catheter is used. Both methods for managing urinary retention have both pros and cons.

- Based on the evidence, which option is the best choice to manage this health challenge for the laboring client?
- List PICOT questions that could be generated from this scenario.
- Which ethical considerations would need to be addressed prior to conducting a research study on this topic?
- How would you incorporate patient preferences into the evidence-based practice?

According to Myers and Meccariello (2006), "Outdated practices are barriers to decreased length of stay, favorable patient outcomes, and lowered costs" (p. 24). To move evidence-based nursing practice forward, a realistic approach for allowing bedside nurses to actively engage in the process must be determined and used. At each stage of providing holistic care, nurses have to be confident in asking the questions and seeking the best practices to advance the provision of effective nursing care. Omery and Williams (1999) set forth the initiative to ensure that careful and practical best evidence is used to propel healthcare decisions. Nurses must seek the best evidence to make sure that the care provided represents the optimal health care available for the specified treatment plan. By determining a functional method for documenting an EBP search, nurses can then gain confidence in the overall process of conducting and implementing EBP.

The process for EBP determination is different from the process for research utilization. Research utilization is covered in Chapter 13, which describes how to complete an assessment of a single research report (i.e., a research critique). The research utilization process carefully examines a distinct study to determine the strengths and limitations assumed within that one study and decide whether to apply its findings to nursing practice. Research utilization becomes a key aspect within the overall process of EBP, but it is only one piece of the EBP puzzle. For a nurse to be able to effectively utilize EBP, it is clear that he or she must be able to perform research critiques. Jolley (2002) supported this idea by emphasizing the need for all nurses to be able to use research, though not everyone has to necessarily be able to conduct research. To facilitate implementation of EBP, bedside nurses need to understand how to recognize those elements of a particular research process that either strengthen or limit the use of its results.

Armed with this understanding of the applicability of the research results to practice, a nurse can then determine which study results might be used to sustain best practices in EBP. Clearly, to make this determination, nurses do need to appreciate the intricacies of the research process. Bedside nurses should be able to identify the justifications that a researcher provides for selecting a specific method of sampling, data collection, research design, and data analysis. If a researcher has a valid explanation for the choices employed within a study, the results can be assigned a higher value and incorporated into practice. Having begun the work with research critiques discussed in Chapter 13, the nurse can then move to the next step of development to use those skills within the EBP process.

Melnyk and Fineout-Overholt (2005) suggest that the process of EBP involves five critical steps:

1. Raise the urgent clinical question using a format that includes the key aspects of the issue.
2. Assemble the most appropriate evidence that addresses the issue identified.
3. Evaluate the evidence critically to determine its validity, relevance, and applicability.
4. Assimilate the evidence into clinical practice.
5. Assess the changes resulting from the use of the best evidence.

Each of these steps must be carefully completed to come to a conclusion about the best practices for a nursing setting. If an EBP process does not include all of the five steps, the result does not take into consideration all of the available evidence related to the clinical question.

? Think Outside the Box

In recent years, more parents have begun seeking alternative birthing options. Some individuals elect to deliver at home due to the burden placed on them by rising healthcare costs. Others make this decision based on a desire to have a more natural birthing process. When complications occur during the birthing process, however, the baby may have to be admitted to an acute care setting. For newborn infants, the standard initial treatment process includes erythromycin eye ointment, injection of triple dye into the umbilical cord, and a vitamin K injection. If the parents voice concerns about these procedures, which steps would a nurse need to take to provide evidence-based information to alleviate their fears?

- List PICOT questions that could be generated from this scenario.
- Which ethical considerations would need to be addressed prior to conducting a research study on this topic?
- Which key words would be used in a literature search to locate evidence related to this EBP question?
- Which type of research project could be developed to further study this concern?
- How would you incorporate patient preferences into the evidence-based practice?

Although many models for EBP are currently being evaluated and modified, **Table 14-1** summarizes the key points in a quick and easy organizational design for evidence consideration. Within this format, the initial step is to refine the question confronting the nurse. Careful time and attention should be given to clarifying the five aspects

Table 14-1

Format for Documenting Aspects of Evidence-Based Practice

Question to Considered Within the Evidence-Based Practice Process

P (population of interest): _____

I (intervention of interest): _____

C (comparison of interest): _____

O (outcome of interest): _____

T (time): _____

Articles (Level of Evidence/ Evaluation of Strength of the Evidence)	Who Is Involved (Sample Size, Sampling Method, Population)	What Occurred (Qualitative, Quantitative)	Where Completed (Type of Agency, State, Country)	When (Year Research Done)	Why Research (Question)	How (Data Collection, Tool Used with Validity and Reliability, Statistical Tests, Qualitative Control)	Consistencies (How It Addresses the PICOT Question, How Alike with Other Studies Reviewed)	Gaps (How It Does Not Address the PICOT Question, What Did the Researchers State Still Needed to Be Studied)

Summary of Findings

Application of Findings to Evidence-Based Practice that Validates or Changes Policies and Procedures

driving the EBP question. As discussed previously, the question should consider the following aspects of the research issue (PICOT):

P: Population of interest (required aspect)
I: Intervention of interest (required aspect)
C: Condition of interest (recommended aspect)
O: Outcome of interest (required aspect)
T: Time (recommended aspect)

Each of these characteristics for the clinical questions was discussed in Chapters 1 and 4. The development of a clear and concise clinical question is of paramount importance, because the question directs the entire research process. Once the question is determined, the nurse needs to work with the librarian to determine key words and expressions to use in conducting the literature review. Having appropriate terms to use within the various search engines helps to ensure that the search results provide the structure for the subsequent analysis of the best practices. As Melynk (2003) has stated, "Evidence-based practice is a problem-solving approach to clinical decision making that incorporates a search for the best and latest evidence, clinical expertise, and assessment, and patient preference and values within a context of caring" (p. 149).

Malloch and Porter-O'Grady (2006) have classified investigations of best practices as meta-analyses, systematic reviews, or integrative reviews. The combining of these different study types identified through the literature review and search engine inquiry process provides the foundation for determining whether there is a need to change practice patterns. Meta-analysis incorporates a statistical technique to determine the rigorousness of the findings from multiple studies dealing with a focused question. A systematic review summarizes all quantitative evidence found through the literature search that is correlated to an identifiable research or clinical issue, employing a rigorous format to ensure completeness of the assessment. An integrative review also summarizes prior research studies on a selected topic but, in addition, draws conclusions from the summary concerning the studies examined.

To determine the level of evidence, Figure 13-1 on page 340 illustrates the ranking of the literature that is available. For example, Level 1 evidence (meta-analysis) is considered to be the highest-level, most important evidence that can be gathered. While Level 1 evidence is the most desirable, the researcher should not toss out evidence classified as being at the other levels. Sometimes the only evidence that is available is a case study (Level 5). A case study still can provide evidence for clinical decision-making purposes, though it is not the strongest form of support. The depth of the justification for using this

? Think Outside the Box

Evidence-based practice should cause members of the nursing profession to question most of their normal activities. A simple skill such as catheterizing an individual can result in an EBP question such as "How much urine should a nurse drain off the bladder at one time following a catheterization of a client?"

- List PICOT questions that could be generated from this scenario.
- Which ethical considerations would need to be addressed prior to conducting a research study on this topic?
- Which key words would be used in a literature search to locate evidence related to this EBP question?
- Which type of research project could be developed to further study this concern?
- How would you incorporate patient preferences into the evidence-based practice?

level of evidence provided by the researcher aids in the determination of the value of the results documented.

Once the level of evidence is established, the researcher needs to evaluate the strength of the evidence. A simple rating system for this aspect of evidence can be seen in Figure 13-2 on page 342. Depending on the study, the evidence may be very strong or insufficient. The rating tool provides the researcher with a means for further discriminating which studies have significance for the project being considered.

The form provided in Table 14-1 allows for either a systematic review or an integrative review. Once the PICOT question has been determined and the literature review completed, each of the identified articles/studies is carefully assessed. For each article (citation, level of evidence, and evaluation of strength of the evidence), who is involved (sample size, sampling method, population), what occurred (qualitative, quantitative, level of evidence), where completed (type of agency, state, country), when (year research was done), why (research question), and how (data collection, validity and reliability of any tool used, statistical tests, qualitative control [trustworthiness, confirmability, transferability]) are determined and documented. As these aspects of a research critique are completed on the different studies, consistencies (how the study addresses the PICOT question, how similar it is to other studies reviewed) and gaps (how the study does not address the PICOT question, what the researchers stated still needs to be studied) within the different studies begin to surface. The identification of consistencies within the various studies may either support the proposed changes in practice or confirm that best practices are currently being used. The detection of gaps within the studies suggests the need for further or more in-depth research into the topic under consideration. The idea of identifying consistencies and gaps within the different articles and research reports also incorporates the concept of similarities and omissions that may be present.

Figure 14-1 provides a schema for understanding the process underlying EBP. As a clinical problem is identified, individuals are directed to develop that problem concern into a PICOT format. The PICOT drives the literature search and the subsequent review of the literature discovered. From the literature review, the focus for the management of the problem is confirmed. When consistencies are identified in the literature, the nurse can elect to repeat the research concentration to strengthen the evidence related to the clinical challenge. Conversely, when gaps in the literature are recognized, additional research projects will be needed to address the gaps found. The third potential outcome is that the literature review might result in either a confirmation or a change in the agency's policies and procedures. In such a case, a quality initiative project may be needed to validate the practices, though further research might not be necessary.

Thus, within an EBP-focused endeavor, the outcomes could be either research projects (to replicate prior work or to address gaps) or quality initiatives (to validate clinical practice). Should the outcome lead to a research study, the research must be conducted in compliance with sound research design. By comparison, for quality initiative projects, any of the many quality initiative models—for example, Six Sigma, plan–do–check–act (PDCA), define–measure–analyze–improve control (DMAIC), Lean, and root cause analysis—can be utilized. The development of these models has been largely driven by manufacturing businesses, with the models subsequently being adapted to many quality improvement efforts and used in the healthcare arena to improve performance. Some methodologies, such as Six Sigma, rely heavily on statistics and research as their underpinnings. The Lean philosophy relies on standardization to improve both the process and the organization from a consumer approach.

Associations established from the results of the various studies need to be collected to add strength to the rationale for making any changes in policies and procedures related to the selected clinical question. If several studies produce equivalent results, then nursing practice should embrace the behavior as supported by evidence. Conversely, if multiple studies reflect a gap in knowledge related to the selected clinical question, then further research should be directed toward the identified segment of nursing practice. According to Pravikoff, Tanner, and Pierce (2005), "The finding that a lack of value for research in practice was the most frequently selected barrier to the use of research in practice is of greatest concern" (p. 48). When practicing nurses cannot or do not use research results to strengthen and sustain holistic nursing practice, the implementation of EBP at the bedside falls short of its potential.

After completing the grid portion of Table 14-1, time must be allocated to summarizing the findings. The nurse should pay careful attention to, and critically consider the meaning ensuing from, the consistencies and gaps identified. This painstaking contemplation of the discovered omissions and similarities serves to narrow the focus of the next steps within the process. By taking the time and energy to summarize and synthesize the information collected, the nurse becomes well versed in the current state of the clinical problem. Obtaining this clearer viewpoint related to the clinical problem allows the nurse to make an informed decision about what is needed next in dealing with this challenge.

The final section of Table 14-1 relates to the application aspect of EBP-related research. After completing each of these prior steps, the nurse has a basis for making recommendations for maintaining or changing a policy or procedure. The time taken to complete this exercise allows for any recommendations to be based on sound, factual data. The suggestions can then be effectively supported by a wealth of tested research endeavors. At this point, the nurse would take this review of the evidence and combine it with the decision-making method employed, personal expertise, and holistic client focus to drive quality, sound nursing care.

❓ Think Outside the Box

Frequently, an insulin drip protocol will seek to maintain a serum blood sugar level between 70 and 110 mg/dL. At one healthcare agency, a pilot research project revealed that the mean blood sugar for patients dismissed from a cardiac intensive care unit after three months was 148 mg/DL. The nurses questioned the protocol ranges as a result of this pilot study result.

- List PICOT questions that could be generated from this scenario.
- Which ethical considerations would need to be addressed prior to conducting a research study on this topic?
- Which key words would be used in a literature search to locate evidence related to this EBP question?
- Which type of research project could be developed to further study this concern?
- How would you incorporate patient preferences into the evidence-based practice?

Conclusion

According to Yoder (2005), "Both EBP and QI initiatives require ongoing evaluation of the practice environment, the appropriate use of data collection and evaluation, and the dissemination of the information learned through excellent communication process both from the top down and the bottom up" (p. 92). A variety of resources are available to help the nurse in strengthening the healthcare organization's EBP foundations and activities (**Table 14-2**). The current healthcare community requires nurses and other healthcare providers to be diligent in the determination and provision of holistic health care. The different treatments and plans of care put forth for clients must be based on factual, tested data. Each nurse must take responsibility for ensuring that the care provided is based on firm, accurate research data. These research data are then used to provide individualized health care to clients based on factual data, patient preferences, and nursing expertise.

? Think Outside the Box

Gather at least three of your peers and form a journal club. Select a topic of your choice and identify a PICOT question. Conduct an integrative review for the selected topic. What conclusions can you draw from the review? How will this new understanding change your practice?

Table 14-2

Suggested Resources to Support the Retrieval and Appraisal of Evidence

- Oncology Nursing Society (ONS) EBP Online Resource Center "Evidence Search" section (http://onsopcontent.ons.org/toolkits/ebp/process_model/evidence_search.htm)
- National Library of Medicine Web site, which allows free searches of MEDLINE through PubMed (www.ncbi.nlm.nih.gov/entrez/query.fcgi)
- National Guidelines Clearinghouse (www.guideline.gov)
- National Comprehensive Cancer Network (www.nccn.org)
- Agency for Healthcare Research and Quality (www.ahrq.gov)
- Cochrane Database of Systematic Reviews (www.update-software.com/publications/cochrane)
- University of Alberta: Evidence-Based Medicine Tool Kit (www.ualberta.ca/ebm/ebm.htm)
- Retired Nurses' Association of Ontario (RNAO): *Best Practice Guidelines* (www.rnao.org/Page .asp?PageID=861&SiteNodeID=133)
- Centre for Evidence-Based Nursing, York, United Kingdom (www.york.ac.uk/healthsciences/centres /evidence/cebn.htm)
- Joanna Briggs Institute (www.joannabriggs.edu.au)
- School of Health and Related Research (ScHARR), University of Sheffield: *Netting the Evidence* (www.shef.ac.uk/scharr/ir/netting)

Summary Points

1. Evidence-based practice (EBP) is the process of utilizing confirmed evidence (research and quality improvement), decision making, and nursing expertise to guide the delivery of holistic patient care.

2. Understanding the research process is the first step in using evidence in everyday nursing practice.

3. To move evidence-based nursing practice forward, a realistic approach for allowing bedside nurses to actively engage in the research process must be determined and used.

4. The process for research use carefully examines a distinct study to determine the strengths and limitations assumed within that one study.

5. Armed with an understanding of the applicability of the results to practice, a nurse can determine which studies can be used to sustain best practices in EBP.

6. The development of a clear and concise clinical question is of paramount importance, because this question directs the entire research process.

7. Meta-analysis uses a statistical technique to determine the rigorousness of the findings from multiple studies conducted to answer a focused question.

8. A systematic review summarizes all quantitative evidence found in a literature search that is correlated to an identifiable research or clinical issue, employing a rigorous format to ensure completeness of the assessment.

9. An integrative review summarizes prior research studies on a selected topic but, in addition, draws conclusions from the summary concerning the studies examined.

10. For each article (citation, level of evidence and evaluation of strength of the evidence), the who involved (sample size, sampling method, population), what occurred (qualitative, quantitative), where completed (type of agency, state, country), when (year research was done), why (research question), and how (data collection, validity and reliability of tools used, statistical analysis, qualitative control) are determined and documented as part of the evaluation process.

11. The identification of consistencies (how the research addresses the PICOT question, how similar the research is to other studies reviewed) within the various studies evaluated may either support potential changes in practice or confirm that best practices are currently being used.

12. The detection of gaps (how the research does not address the PICOT question, what the researchers stated still needed to be studied) within the studies evaluated suggests the need for further or more in-depth research endeavors on the topic under consideration.

13. Obtaining a clearer viewpoint related to the clinical problem allows the nurse to make an informed decision about what is needed next in this challenge.
14. Quality improvement activities are designed to incorporate research into the healthcare environment from a consumer approach.

RED FLAGS

- Research utilization and evidence-based practice are not the same thing.
- The recommendation for changing nursing practice must be based on sound evidence, not on the results from a single study.

Case Scenario

An Hispanic woman presents to the emergency room complaining of epigastric pain in atypical form, nausea, diaphoresis, and neck pain. The initial assessment reveals a 60-year-old, Hispanic female with a history of diabetes and hypertension. She has a granddaughter attending nursing school at the local community college. The client reports being a smoker with a family history of cardiac problems. She is 5 feet, 3 inches tall and weighs 185 pounds. She is a homemaker with no outside employment. For the most part, she reports a sedentary life style and denies alcohol consumption.

The ER physician orders an EKG and cardiac panel to rule out an acute myocardial infarction. Other tests ordered include a chest X-ray, urinalysis, and standard chemistry (CBC, troponins, creatinine protein). The tests reveal elevated troponin and EKG changes with an elevation in the ST segment. The client is diagnosed with a full-blown myocardial infarction. The ER physician mobilizes the cath lab team and orders a cardiology consultation. The client is transported to the cath lab for an angiogram, which reveals two blocked cardiac vessels.

After a double angioplasty is performed, the client is transferred to the cardiac care unit (CCU). After she arrives in the unit, the nursing staff assesses the client and determines that the angioplasty versus manual compression was completed with Perclose. The use of this closure for angioplasty has been a topic of debate in the CCU.

As a result of this case and others, the nursing staff elects to engage in an evidence-based practice activity to determine if the policies and procedures currently used on the unit reflect the best practices for this type of client and medical treatment plan. The PICOT question shown in **Table 14-3** was identified, and the EBP process was initiated.

As can be seen from the case study analysis in Table 14-3, there are gaps in the literature—specifically, a lack of actual research projects on the use of Perclose versus manual pressure. All of the literature reviewed consisted of case studies with reference to recommendations from the manufacturer of Perclose. If the nurses wished to continue further exploring the use of Perclose in this clinical scenario, they could use the gap table provided in Chapter 5 (Table 5-4 on page 130). However, the case study illustrates how EBP and research can lead to specific actions to improve nursing care, thereby improving patient outcomes.

Table 14-3

Documenting Aspects of Evidence-Based Practice

Question to Considered within the Evidence-Based Practice Process

P (population of interest): Hispanic adult 50 years or older
I (intervention of interest): Perclose usage for percutaneous arterial closure
C (comparison of interest): Manual pressure
O (outcome of interest): Decrease length of stay, decreased hematoma, decreased discomfort, decreased infection rate
T (time): Within 2 weeks from discharge from hospital

Articles (Level of Evidence/ Evaluation of Strength of the Evidence)	Who Is Involved (Sample Size, Sampling Method, Population)	What Occurred (Qualitative, Quantitative)	Where Completed (Type of Agency, State, Country)	When (Year Research Done)	Why (Research Question)	How (Data Collection, Tool Used with Validity and Reliability, Statistical Tests, Qualitative Control)	Consistencies (How It Addresses the PICOT Question, How Alike with Other Studies Reviewed)	Gaps (How It Does Not Address the PICOT Question, What Did the Researchers State Still Needed to Be Studied)
Geary, Landers, Fiore, & Riggs. (2002). Management of infected femoral closure devices. *Cardiovascular Surgery, 10*(2), 161–163. Level of evidence: 5. Strength of evidence: B.	4 males, 1 female, age range 63–73, purposive sampling	Qualitative, case study	New York, acute care unit, outpatient general hospital	2002	Examined Perclose	Case study; no indication of prophylactic antibiotic use, *Staphylococcus* infection	Population correct for age; all had infections, suture placement, antibiotics	Little research; recommendations came from manufacturer; no indication of ethnicity or manual pressure

(continues)

Table 14-3

Documenting Aspects of Evidence-Based Practice (continued)

Articles (Level of Evidence/ Evaluation of Strength of the Evidence)	Who Is Involved (Sample Size, Sampling Method, Population)	What Occurred (Qualitative, Quantitative)	Where Completed (Type of Agency, State, Country)	When (Year Research Done)	Why (Research Question)	How (Data Collection, Tool Used with Validity and Reliability, Statistical Tests, Qualitative Control)	Consistencies (How It Addresses the PICOT Question, How Alike with Other Studies Reviewed)	Gaps (How It Does Not Address the PICOT Question, What Did the Researchers State Still Needed to Be Studied)
Heck, Muldowney, & McPherson. (2002). Infectious complications of Perclose for closure of femoral artery puncture. *Journal of Vascular and Interventional Radiology, 13*(4), 427–431. Level of evidence: 5. Strength of evidence: B.	2 females, 1 male, age range 40–76, purposive sampling	Qualitative, case study	Three different institutions	2002	No specific question documented; report of cases, 3 days post-op	Case studies	Age range exceeds PICOT range; 2 cases had staphylococcal infection, one from bacterial source; concerns about suture placement	Neither manual pressure nor ethnicity noted in this study; refers to published trials
Tiesenhausen, Tomka, Allmayer, Baumann, Hessinger, Portugaller, & Mahler. (2004). Femoral artery infection associated with a percutaneous arterial suture device. *VASA: European journal for vascular medicine, 33*(2), 83–85. Level of evidence: 5. Strength of evidence: B.	77-year-old male, purposive sampling	Qualitative, case study	Austria	2004	No specific question documented; single case	Add to data; infection identified 4 weeks post hospitalization; seen in ER prior to final admission to hospital with sepsis; Perclose carries risk of femoral artery infections	Age complies with PICOT; sterile field must be maintained	Neither manual pressure nor ethnicity noted in this study; refers to research

Dumont. (2007). Blood pressure and risks of vascular complications after percutaneous coronary intervention. Dimensions of Critical Care Nursing, 26(3), 121–127. Level of evidence: 4. Strength of evidence: B.	Convenience sampling, 150 subjects, mean age 62.4, 45% women, 92% white	Case-matched control design	South Atlantic state, tertiary care teaching facility	2006	Determine which variables are significant individual predictors of vascular complications post-PCI—1); comorbidities: 2); physician-sensitive procedural factors (hemostatis method [Perclose compared with manual compression for hemostatis]), and 3)' nurse-sensitive procedural factors	Specific details not provided; data collected—body mass index, comorbidity, physician-sensitive procedurals, and nurse-sensitive procedural factors	Mean age within PICOT level; use of Perclose compared to manual pressure included; outcomes of interest addressed	Ethnicity not addressed
Lasic, Nikolsky, Kesanakurthy, & Dangas. (2005). Vascular closure devices: A review of their use after invasive procedures, American Journal of Cardiovascular Drugs, 5(3), 185–200. Level of evidence: 5. Strength of evidence: B.	Not a research article, so no sampling done	In-depth review of vascular closure devices	Not a research article	2005	Meta-analysis data related to complications and success rates; research reports discussed within the summary of the different closure devices	Not a research article	Outcomes related to Perclose usage provided	Not a research article, so no sampling done

Summary of Findings (Consistencies and Gaps from All Articles)

Perclose can reduce length of stay and improve outcomes. Proper use of Perclose and consideration of prophylactic antibiotic therapy should be implemented. All of the reviewed articles were case studies; no quantitative research was found, and no nurse-directed research was located. The length of time before infections were identified ranged from 3 days to 4 weeks. Use of sterile technique during the procedure is paramount.

Application of Findings to Evidence-Based Practice that Validates or Changes Policies and Procedures (Which policies and procedures does this information directly address and why?)

- All articles suggest prophylactic antibiotic use and strict adherence to the manufacturer's recommendations for ensuring a sterile surgical site.
- ER departments should review their policies concerning the assessment of post-angioplasty clients who present with vague symptoms, because the infection may be masked until it develops into a sepsis-type infection even as late as 4 weeks post procedure.
- Patient education should be addressed within policies to ensure that clients are taught to maintain a clean site at the incision area, to complete all antibiotic treatment ordered, and to report vague symptoms reflective of infections even up to 4 weeks post procedure.

Critical Thinking Exercise

Multiple ideas related to potential clinical questions are provided for your consideration here. Select one of these situations to use in working through the process outlined in Table 14-1. The situations are presented in a brief manner in the following list. Take the chosen idea and develop a PICOT question to best meet the needs at a selected healthcare agency of your choice.

1. One possible clinical question relates to whether a relationship between adequate pain control and length of stay in a community hospital setting could be determined.

2. Another clinical situation for investigation involves the determination of any relationship between glucose control during the operative period and length of stay in an acute care setting.

3. An alternative clinical circumstance relates to the effect of a one-on-one diabetic education course on the patient's HbA_{1c} level.

4. When a medication error occurs, the value of full disclosure to patients and/or family members in building trust and restoring confidence, as opposed to nondisclosure, with a look at the impact on perceived quality of care, could be investigated.

5. An additional idea involves determining whether the length of time and frequency of visits to patients' rooms by nursing staff affect the number of calls and the perception of quality of care by the patient and/or family members.

6. Maternal/child nurses understand that certain treatments (prophylactic eye treatments, vitamin K injections, PKU tests) are provided for all newborn children. What happens to children born outside of an acute care setting (e.g., home births)? What rationales do we have to support these treatments?

7. Childhood immunization is a state-directed process that applies to all school-age children. Certain immunizations (MMR, polio, DPT) are designated at key times prior to and during the school-age years. So what is happening with the growing number of home-schooled children? Are they receiving these immunizations? What happens when these children come into acute care settings without having received the expected childhood immunization series?

Suggested Readings

Coopey, M., & Clancy, C. M. (2006, July/September). Translating research into evidence-based nursing practice and evaluating effectiveness. *Journal of Nursing Care Quality, 21*(3), 195–202.

Marchiondo, K. (2006, January/February). Planning and implementing an evidence-based project. *Nurse Educator, 31*(1), 4–6.

Newhouse, R. P. (2006, July/August). Examining the support for evidence-based nursing practice. *Journal of Nursing Administration, 36*(7–8), 337–340.

References

Finkelman, A., & Kenner, C. (2007). *Teaching IOM: Implications of the IOM reports for nursing education.* Silver Spring, MD: American Nurses Association.

Jolley, S. (2002). Raising research awareness: A strategy for nurses. *Nursing Standard,* 16(33), 33–39.

Malloch, K., & Porter-O'Grady, T. (2006). *Introduction to evidence-based practice in nursing and health care.* Sudbury, MA: Jones and Bartlett.

Melnyk, B. M. (2003). Finding and appraising systematic reviews of clinical interventions: Critical skills for evidence-based practice. *Journal of Pediatric Nursing,* 29(2), 125, 147–149.

Melnyk, B. M., & Fineout-Overholt, E. (2005). *Evidence-based practice in nursing and healthcare: A guide to best practice.* Philadelphia: Lippincott Williams & Wilkins.

Myers, G., & Meccariello, M. (2006). From pet rock to rock-solid: Implementing unit-based research. *Nursing Management,* 37(1), 24–29.

Omery, A., & Williams, R. P. (1999). An appraisal of research utilization across the United States. *Journal of Nursing Administration,* 29(12), 50–56.

Pravikoff, D. S, Tanner, A. B., & Pierce, S. T. (2005). Readiness of U.S. nurses for evidence-based practice. *American Journal of Nursing,* 105(9), 40–51.

Sigma Theta Tau International. (2006). *Results of EBN survey.* Retrieved from an e-mail dated June 12, 2006, from Sigma Theta Tau International Honor Society of Nursing. NurseAdvance: Knowledge Solutions.

Yoder, L. (2005). Evidence-based practice: The time is now! *Medsurg Nursing,* 14(2), 91–92.

Glossary

Accessible data Data that can be linked into for use within a research study.

Accessible population Individuals and/or groups accessible for a specific participation study; frequently a nonrandom division of the target population.

Accuracy The correctness of the information used within the process.

Action research Applied research that is attentive to the resolution of nursing personnel's identified challenges.

Analysis A process of organizing and synthesizing data in such a way that research questions can be answered and hypotheses can be tested.

Anonymity A situation in which the identity and data provided by the research participant are shielded from everyone, including the researcher.

Applied research Research that concentrates on resolving functional questions to supply reasonably direct solutions.

Associative hypothesis A hypothesis stated in a way that indicates that the variables exist side by side and that a change in one variable is accomplished by a change in another variable.

Assumption A fundamental tenet that is recognized as truthful on the foundation of logic or reason but is devoid of evidence or confirmation.

Barrier An object, goal, or thing that obstructs or inhibits; a maximum value; a cut-off point.

Baseline The state or conduct of a participant preceding the initiation of a treatment regimen.

Basic research Research designed to generate elemental knowledge and theoretic agreement about crucial human and foundational innate processes.

Best practice Those nursing actions that produce the most desirable patient outcomes through scientific data.

Bias Any pressure that generates an alteration in the outcomes of an inquiry.

Biased sample A sample group that is analytically diverse from the target population.

Biophysiological Objective data that use a specialized piece of equipment to establish the physical and/or biologic condition of the subjects.

"Blind" review The appraisal of a document in which the identities of the author and the reviewer are concealed from the other party.

Bundling Multiple identified interventions that, taken together, enhance the clinical outcomes.

Case study A qualitative research method that concentrates on supplying a comprehensive description and scrutiny of an identified case situation.

Categorical variable A variable that diverges in type or kind but that has distinct values instead of values spaced along a continuum.

Causal–comparative research A type of nonexperimental research design in which the principal independent variable under investigation is a categorical variable.

Causal hypothesis A hypothesis stated in a way that indicates that one variable causes or brings about a change in another variable or variables.

Chi-square test for contingency tables Statistical test employed to establish if an association recognized in a contingency table is statistically significant.

Clinical pathway A document that has been prepared and validated to provide the acceptable management of a disease process; components of the pathway uphold the standards of practice.

Clinical relevance Degree to which a research inquiry addresses a problem of significance to the practice of nursing.

Clinical research Research calculated to produce knowledge to direct nursing practice.

Clinical trial A research process that assesses the efficacy of an aspect of clinical management, usually in a large and heterogeneous sample of participants.

Closed-ended question A question that is set up to force specific responses through the options provided within the question.

Cluster sampling A method of sampling in which a sizeable group is divided into consecutive subsampling of smaller units; a style of sampling in which groups are randomly selected.

Coding   Classifying portions of qualitative data with either symbols, explanatory words, or categorical narrative designations.

Code of ethics   Underlying ethical assumptions that are recognized by a discipline or organization to direct researchers; management of the research related to the safe handling of human subjects.

Coercion   Related to research endeavors, the specific and/or embedded use of threats and/or disproportionate rewards to get individuals to consent to take part in a proposed study.

Cohort   Several individuals presenting with a recognizable categorization or common attribute.

Comparative design   A design that does not entail any manipulation or control of the independent variable, such that the dependent variable is the only variable measured in two or more groups.

Comparison group   A company of participants whose results related to a dependent variable classification are used as a foundation for appraising the results of the grouping of designated significance; phrase employed in place of "control group" for studies not applying an exact experimental plan.

Complex hypothesis   A statement that specifies the relationship between and among more than two variables.

Concept   Theoretical foundation for inspection of specific activities or characteristics.

Conceptual definition   Characterization of the identified word, variable, or activity from the dictionary-specific explanation of the term.

Conceptual model   Systematic concepts or beliefs that are compiled in a logical representation based on their significance to a familiar premise; a conceptual framework.

Concurrently   Occurring at the same time (data or processes).

Concurrent validity   Validity verification that is based on the correlation between the calculated scores and criterion scores acquired at the same time.

Confidence interval   A range of numbers assessed from the sample that has a specific likelihood or probability of containing the population limitation.

Confidence limits   The final limits of a confidence interval.

Confidentiality   Protection of study participants that results in the individuals' identities not being linked to the information they provided, meaning that the information can be provided only in the aggregate; not revealing the data collected from study participants to any person except the researcher and designated staff.

Confounding variable   A type of extraneous variable that is not controlled for. A confounding variable regularly fluctuates with the independent variable and affects the dependent variable.

Constant   A single quantity or status of a variable.

Construct validity   The degree to which a higher-order concept is characterized in a specific inquiry.

Consumer A person who reads, evaluates, and appraises research conclusions while endeavoring to use and employ the results in practice.

Content analysis The practice of categorizing and combining qualitative results to establish the materializing premises and perceptions.

Content-related validity The extent to which the details in a tool effectively characterize the totality of the content that needs to be included.

Contingency table A table that places data in cells produced by the juncture of two or more categorical variables.

Continuous variable A term that can take on a wide range of values, such as from 0 to 100, or larger.

Control The procedure for managing the extraneous influences that could affect the dependent variable.

Control group Participants in an experiment who provide the baseline for the study, in contrast to the treatment group. Members of the control group they do not receive the experimental treatment.

Convenience sampling The process of selecting elements to be in the sample who are accessible and/or who volunteer; also called accidental sampling.

Convergent validity A type of construct validity.

Correlational coefficient The outcome of the calculation of the relationship between two or more observed scores.

Correlational design Any of a variety of nonexperimental research designs in which the primary independent variable of interest is a quantitative variable.

Corroboration The process of evaluating documents against other documents to establish the consistency within the conclusions provided.

Covert Covered up, hidden. Covert data are collected without the subject having knowledge of the collection of the information.

Criterion-related validity Based on the comparison of the tests being used with some known criterion.

Criterion The yardstick or benchmark used for predicting the accuracy of test scores.

Critique An impartial, analytic, and reasonable appraisal of a research report.

Cross-sectional study A study based on data collected at a solitary moment in time with the intent of concluding tendencies over time.

Cross-validation A method for triangulating qualitative data by confirming the results through some other process.

Database An organized body of related information arranged for speed of access and retrieval.

Data set The collection of information resulting from a research project.

Data triangulation The employment of multiple data sources and data management procedures to validate qualitative data.

Debriefing An interview conducted with the participants following the initial data analysis, during which aspects of the study are exposed, rationales for the employment of deception are explained, and questions that the participants may have about the results are resolved.

Deductive reasoning The practice of drawing explicit conclusions from broad tenets.

Demographic variable A term that refers to characteristics of the subjects in the study.

Dependent variable The outcome variable that is alleged to be influenced by one or more independent variables; the presumed outcome of the study.

Descriptive design A research study whose foremost intention is providing the truthful depiction of the distinctiveness of persons, situations, or groups and/or an accurate explanation or representation of the condition of a state of affairs or phenomenon.

Descriptive statistics Statistics that concentrate on recounting, summarizing, or explaining.

Dichotomous variable A characteristic that can be measured only in the sense that it is present or not present; often assigned a number for identification purposes, rather than to represent a quantity.

Directional hypothesis A statement that predicts the path or direction that the relationship between variables will take.

Discrete variable A variable that can take on only a finite number of values, usually restricted to whole numbers.

Effect size The expected strength of the relationship between the research variables; used in the calculation of desired sample size through power analysis.

Element The fundamental component that is chosen from the population.

Eligibility criteria The conditions employed by a researcher to indicate the detailed characteristics of the target population that are used to select participants for a study.

Emic term The point of view provided by the individuals directly involved in a situation.

Empiric Established by inspection, experiment, or practice (data and/or results).

Equivalence reliability A measure of reliability that is calculated in the same manner as the consistency and stability coefficients, except this time, instead of a single variable over two trials, the test is between two forms of a single test.

Error The difference between a factual score and an observed score.

Ethics The main beliefs, ideology, and guidelines that facilitate the maintenance of an issue that we appreciate and respect.

Ethnocentrism The practice of evaluating individuals from a diverse culture according to the principles of the evaluator's identifiable culture.

Ethnography A type of qualitative research that conscientiously illustrates the customs of a grouping of individuals.

Ethnohistory An investigation into the cultural history of a group of people.

Etic perspective An appreciation for the scientific consideration of reality from an external viewpoint.

Etic term An explanation of the social world under examination from an outsider's viewpoint.

Evaluation Identification of the significance, advantage, or worth of an object being examined.

Evidence-based practice A process of utilizing confirmed evidence (research and quality improvement), decision making, and nursing expertise to guide the delivery of holistic patient care.

Exclusion criteria Characteristics that, if present, would make persons ineligible for participation in a study, even if they meet all of the other inclusion criteria.

Expedited review A method by which a project is quickly appraised by selected members of the full institutional review board.

Experiment A setting in which a researcher impartially scrutinizes a situation that occurs in a rigorously restricted position, with one or more variables being manipulated while others are held steady.

Experimental control In research, the practice of eradicating the degrees of difference resulting from the extraneous variables.

Experimental design Research in which the independent variable is manipulated, a control group is established, and randomized selection of the participants is employed to select who does and does not receive the treatment or intervention.

Experimental group The participants who receive the experimental treatment or intervention.

External validity The degree to which the analysis outcomes can be generalized to a specific group of persons, settings, times, outcomes, and treatment variations.

Extraneous variable A variable that confuses the association between the independent and dependent variables; for this reason, it needs to be restricted either within the research design or through statistical procedures.

Face validity The degree to which a research tool correctly reflects what it is purposed to measure.

Field notes Annotations recorded by an observer during qualitative research endeavors.

Focus group A small group of people assembled to participate in a moderator-facilitated discussion geared toward the designated topic being researched.

Focus group interview A dialogue with a group of individuals assembled to respond and converse about a prearranged theme.

Formative evaluation An appraisal conducted to improve the evaluation process.

Framework The conceptual foundation of a study; sometimes classified as a theoretic framework, for projects centered on a theory, and as a conceptual framework, for projects with a connection to a definite conceptual model.

Generalizability The extent to which findings from a study can be extended from a sample of a population to the population at large.

Grounded theory A general methodology for developing new theory that is grounded in data that are systematically gathered and analyzed.

Hawthorne effect A change in a dependent variable that occurs as a result of the participants' recognition that they are engaged in a study.

Histogram A diagram that reveals the frequencies and profile resulting from a quantitative variable.

Historic research Research that uses a practice of methodically investigating past events or mixtures of events to explain what ensued in an earlier period.

Homogeneity The extent to which items are similar with regard to a select attribute.

Hypothesis A prediction or educated guess about the relationships among variables; the recognized proclamation of the researcher's prediction of the affiliation that exists among the variables under investigation.

Hypothesis testing The division of inferential statistics that focuses on how the sample data confirm or reject a null hypothesis.

Inclusion criteria Characteristics that must be met to be considered for participation in a study; also known as eligibility criteria.

Independent variable The variable in experimental research that is established as the cause or influence on the dependent variable; it may be identified as the manipulated (treatment) variable.

Inductive reasoning The practice of reasoning from detailed annotations to more common conceptualizations.

Inferential statistics The category of statistics focused on moving beyond the immediate data and conjecturing the distinctiveness of the populace established by the samples.

Informed consent The decision of an individual to participate in a research study based on an understanding of the project's purpose, procedures, risks, benefits, alternative procedures, and limits of confidentiality.

Interclass reliability The reliability between two measures that are presented in the data as either variables or trials.

Institutional review board (IRB) A council of individuals representing an institution who assemble to evaluate the ethical considerations related to proposed and ongoing research studies.

Instrument A tool that a researcher uses to accumulate information.

Internal validity The capacity to conclude that a contributory affiliation exists between two or more variables.

Inter-rater reliability The extent of agreement or consistency between two or more scorers, judges, or raters (operating independently) for attributes being measured or observed.

Intervention The experimental treatment or manipulation employed during a research endeavor.

Interview A data collection technique in which an interviewer poses questions to the interviewee.

Intraclass reliability A type of reliability that allows a person to develop a reliability coefficient for more than one variable.

In vitro Requiring the extraction of physiologic materials from a participant in a research study, frequently via a laboratory analysis.

In vivo Requiring the use of some apparatus to evaluate one or more elements of a participant in a research study.

Journal club A group that assembles on a regular basis to discuss and appraise research reports for the purpose of judging the possibility of implementing the findings.

k The magnitude of the sampling interval applied in systematic sampling.

Level of confidence The likelihood that a confidence interval to be used for a random sample will contain the population characteristics.

Likert scale A summated rating scale consisting of a series of items to which respondents are requested to indicate their level of agreement.

Literature review A rigorous examination of research related to a topic of interest that is documented to categorize a research problem or as the beginning of a research use project.

Longitudinal design A study design in which information is accumulated at various times for use in comparisons.

Manipulation An intervention or treatment initiated in an experimental or quasi-experimental study to assess the independent variable's impact on the dependent variable.

Margin of error One-half of the measurement of a confidence interval.

Maturation Any alteration that happens as a result of time that influences the participant's involvement related to the dependent variable.

Mean The mathematical average of a data set.

Measure of central tendency The distinct numeric value deemed generally predictable for the values of a quantitative variable.

Measure of variability A numeric indicator that exhibits information about the extent of variation present.

Median The 50th percentile.

Memoing Chronicling thoughtful observations about information learned from data collected in a research study.

Meta-analysis A process of quantitatively comparing the results from multiple research studies on a selected subject.

Mixed method research (multimethod research) A type of study in which a researcher uses qualitative research methodology for one phase of the study and quantitative research methodology for another phase of the study.

Mode   The most frequently occurring number in a data set.

n   Designation used to denote the total number of study participants; the sample size.

Naturalistic observation   Surveillance conducted in "real-world" surroundings.

NCNR   National Center for Nursing Research.

Network sampling   The inclusion of participants in a sample as a result of referrals from individuals already in the sample; also called snowball sampling.

NIH   National Institutes of Health.

NINR   National Institute for Nursing Research.

Nominal scale   A level of measurement that applies symbols, such as numbers, to describe, categorize, or recognize people or objects.

Nondirectional hypothesis   A statement that predicts a relationship between variables but not the path or direction of that relationship.

Nonexperimental design   A research study in which data are collected without introducing any treatment and no random assignment of participants to groups occurs.

Nonprobability sampling   A sampling strategy that does not include random selection of elements.

Nonsignificant results   The outcome of a statistical test demonstrating that the connection between variables could have transpired as a consequence of chance, at the designated level of significance.

Normal distribution   A unimodal, symmetric, bell-shaped distribution of the data analysis for a selected variable.

Norms   The written and unwritten regulations that denote acceptable behavior.

Novel data   New data collected as part of a research study.

Null hypothesis   A prediction or educated guess that no relationship exists between the designated variables.

Objectivity   The degree to which two researchers working independently would reach comparable findings or conclusions.

Observation   Inconspicuous surveillance of people as they engage in everyday activities.

Obstacle   Something that resists, hampers the forward progress, or reroutes movement in a certain way or path.

Open-ended question   A question that permits the respondent to answer without any restrictions or barriers.

Operational definition   The characterization of a concept or variable in terms of the operations or procedures by which it is to be measured for a specific research endeavor.

Ordinal scale   A rank-order level of measurement.

Outcome validity The capacity to generalize concerning assorted, but interrelated, dependent variables.

Overt Accomplished with full knowledge of the subjects under investigation (referring to data collection).

Phenomenology A type of qualitative research in which the researcher endeavors to comprehend how individuals experience a phenomenon.

PICOT The five components of an evidence-based question: patient population of interest, intervention of interest, comparison of interest, outcome of interest, and time.

Pilot study A miniature edition of a study, or trial run, completed prior to the implementation of the full study.

Population The complete group of individuals (or objects) possessing various characteristics to which a researcher wants to generalize the sample results; sometimes referred to as the universe population or target population.

Power A level at which the likelihood of rejecting the null hypothesis when it is false is set.

Power analysis A statistical calculation of the number of subjects needed to accurately reject a null hypothesis.

Predictive validity A characteristic based on the time between the collection of the alternative method tests to be validated and the criterion measured. It does not limit the researcher to using the Pearson Product Moment (PPM) to develop a validity coefficient, as a linear or logistic regression can also be used.

Primary sources First-hand testimony to facts, findings, or events; reporting of the research results structured by the individual who conducted the study.

Probability sampling Use of a specific sampling strategy using some form of random selection of elements.

Problem statement A declaration of the research problem, occasionally verbalized in the form of a research question.

Purposive sampling A nonprobability sampling process in which the researcher chooses study participants based on personal decisions about which individuals would be most representative of the general population; also identified as judgmental sampling.

Qualitative design The analysis of phenomena, characteristically in a comprehensively and holistic manner, through the compilation of abundant narrative notes based on an adaptable research model.

Qualitative researcher A researcher who concentrates on investigation or theory creation using qualitative information.

Qualitative research question An inquisitive sentence that poses a query about a selected practice, concern, or phenomenon to be investigated.

Quantitative analysis The numeric representation and manipulation of observations using statistical techniques for the express purpose of describing and explaining the outcomes of research as they pertain to the hypothesis.

Quantitative design The scrutinizing of a phenomenon that contributes to the collection of meticulous measurement and quantification, while using a painstaking and manipulative strategy.

Quantitative research question A question that asks about the affiliation that exists concerning two or more variables.

Quasi-experimental design An experimental research design in which individuals are not randomly assigned to groups, but rather the researcher manipulates the independent variable and implements specific controls to augment the internal validity of the outcome.

Questionnaire A self-report data collection tool completed by research participants.

Quota sampling A nonrandom selection of participants by which the researcher identifies specific properties and/or characteristics that are used to establish the sample and determines sample size for the groups to increase their representativeness.

Random assignment (randomization) A selection system that creates assignments in a manner that augments the probability that the comparison groups will be equivalent on all extraneous variables.

Random sampling Selection of a sample such that every member of a population has an equal possibility of being included in the sample.

Random selection Picking a group of individuals from a population where every member of the population has an equal chance of being included in the sample.

Range The variation between the uppermost and lowest numbers in a data set.

Ranking The arranging of responses into ascending or descending sequence.

Ratio scale A level of measurement that has a true zero position, while also having the characteristics of the nominal (labeling), ordinal (rank ordering), and interval (equal distance) scales.

Reliability The extent to which a tool measures the attribute it is intended to evaluate; a measure of consistency.

Replication The premeditated duplication of research procedures in a second examination with the intent of determining whether previous outcomes can be duplicated.

Representative sample A sample that bears a resemblance to the target population.

Research A methodical examination that uses regimented techniques to resolve questions or decipher dilemmas.

Research design The inclusive design for addressing a research question that incorporates the outline, plan, or strategy used to enhance the integrity of the study.

Research ethics A series of principles used to guide and aid researchers in determining the most important goals for reconciling contradictory principles.

Research hypothesis A testable statement that predicts the relationship between two or more variables in a population of interest.

Research problem An unfathomable, bewildering, or inconsistent state that can be explored through regimented investigation.

Research proposal A written text that recapitulates the preceding literature, distinguishes the research topic to be resolved, and stipulates the processes that will be followed to answer the research questions.

Research question A statement of the particular inquiry the researcher desires to resolve through a research endeavor.

Research utilization The application of selected facets of a scientific analysis through a process unconnected to the fundamental research.

Researcher bias An intentional or unintentional manipulation of a study so that it achieves results consistent with what the researcher intends to uncover.

Response rate The proportion of individuals in a sample who participate in a research project.

Retrospective research The analysis of existing data to address the question to be answered.

Retrospective question A question that asks individuals to remember something from a previous time.

Sample A division of a population chosen to participate in a study.

Sample size The number of individuals included in a sample.

Sampling The practice of extracting a designated group from a population.

Sampling bias Misrepresentations that occur when a sample is not representative of the target population from which the group was extracted.

Sampling error The variation between a sample statistic and a population parameter.

Sampling interval The total number within the target population divided by the preferred sample size; denoted by k.

Sampling plan The plan for selection of the study participants proposed prior to the beginning of the study; it specifies the eligibility criteria, the sample selection process, and, in the case of quantitative studies, the number of subjects to be used.

Saturation In qualitative research, the point at which sufficient data have been accumulated for all new data to produce redundant information.

Scientific merit The extent to which an inquiry is methodologically and theoretically complete.

Search engine A Web-based tool providing access to needed data. It takes a person to the information and helps to retrieve the information in a format that is accessible visually on screen at an onsite library or in downloadable written/readable format.

Secondary data (secondary analysis) Data initially accumulated by various persons for a purpose other than the present research.

Secondary source Second-hand explanation of proceedings or facts; explanation of a study or studies organized by someone other than the primary researcher.

Sequential The following of one item after another item.

Significance level The boundary used by the researcher to denote the point at which the null hypothesis will be rejected; also known as the alpha level.

Simple hypothesis A statement that specifies the relationship between two variables.

Simple random sampling A population group extracted by a formula in which each member of the population has an equivalent possibility of being chosen.

Snowball sampling A type of sampling in which every research contributor is asked to recommend additional prospective research participants; also referred to as network sampling.

Standard error of measure A statistic that reflects the fluctuation of the observed score due to the error score.

Statistical significance An idiom demonstrating that it is improbable that the results achieved in an examination of sample data would have been produced by luck at a particular level of probability.

Stratified sampling A random selection of study participants from two or more levels of the population.

Subject A person who supplies information in a study. This term is predominantly used in quantitative research studies.

Systematic sampling The selection of research study participants such that each kth individual (or facet) in a sampling frame is selected.

Table of random numbers An inventory of numbers that are generated in a random sequence.

Target population The total population to whom the research outcomes are to be generalized.

Test A device used to determine the selected intelligence, talents, behaviors, health status, or cognitive endeavor that is under investigation.

Test–retest reliability A calculation of the uniformity of scores over time.

Theoretical sampling The qualitative research process of selecting new study participants based on emerging findings from previous data collection and analysis; followed until the point of data saturation.

Theory A rationalization that challenges how a phenomenon functions and why it functions as it does; a generalization or series of generalizations employed methodically to clarify certain phenomena.

Triangulation The application of various methods to accumulate and decipher facts about a phenomenon, and then merge those data to create a precise portrayal of realism.

Trustworthiness An expression used in the appraisal of qualitative data; it is measured based on the decisive factors of credibility, transferability, dependability, and confirmability.

Type I error Discarding a true null hypothesis.

Type II error Failing to discard a false null hypothesis.

Validity The extent to which a research tool measures what it is proposed to measure.

Variable A characteristic of a person or entity that fluctuates.

Vulnerable human beings Distinct groups of individuals whose rights require particular protection because of their inability to grant informed consent or because their state of affairs consigns them to higher-than-average risk of adverse effects from a proposed treatment or intervention.

Index

Italicized page locators indicate a figure; tables are noted with a t.

O